SOUTHWEST
MEDICINAL
PLANTS

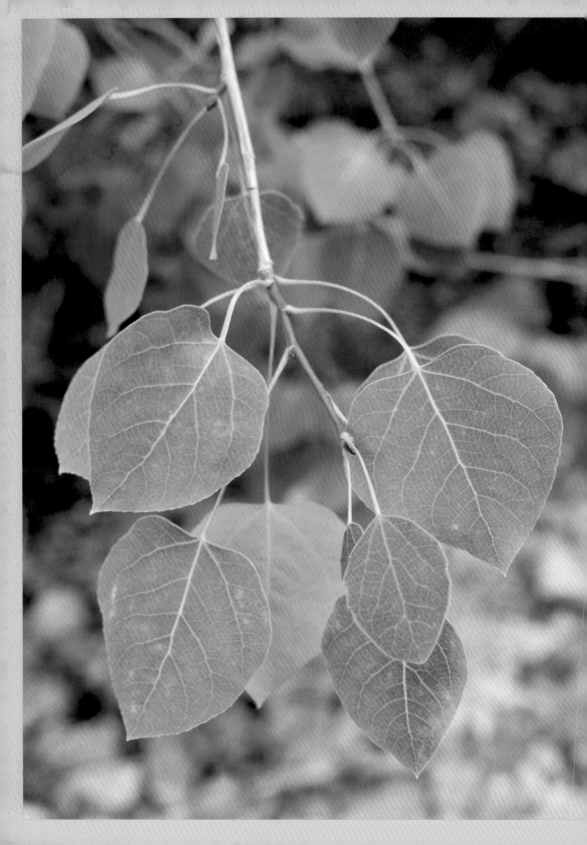

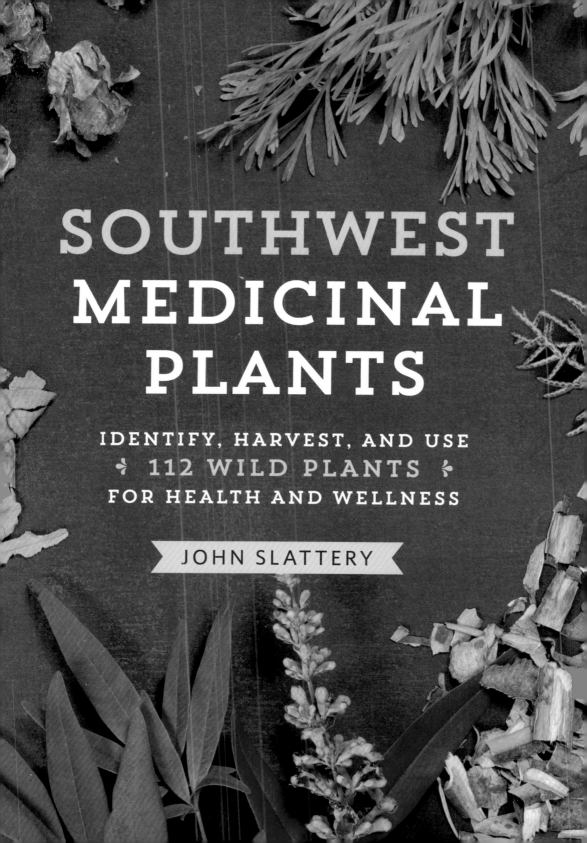

SOUTHWEST
MEDICINAL
PLANTS

IDENTIFY, HARVEST, AND USE
❧ 112 WILD PLANTS ❧
FOR HEALTH AND WELLNESS

JOHN SLATTERY

Frontispiece: The leaves of aspen, *Populus tremuloides*.
All photos are by the author, with the exception of those on
pages 159, 160, and 161, which are by Kelly Kindscher,
and the one on page 113, which is by Hugo.arg, Wikimedia.

Published in 2020 by Timber Press, Inc.,
a subsidiary of Workman Publishing Co., Inc.,
a subsidiary of Hachette Book Group, Inc.
1290 Avenue of the Americas
New York, NY 10104
timberpress.com

Printed in China on responsibly sourced paper
Third printing 2023
Text and cover design by Adrianna Sutton

The Hachette Speakers Bureau provides a wide range of authors for
speaking events. To find out more, go to hachettespeakersbureau.com or
email HachetteSpeakers@hbgusa.com.

ISBN 978-1-60469-911-1
A catalog record for this book is available from the Library of Congress.

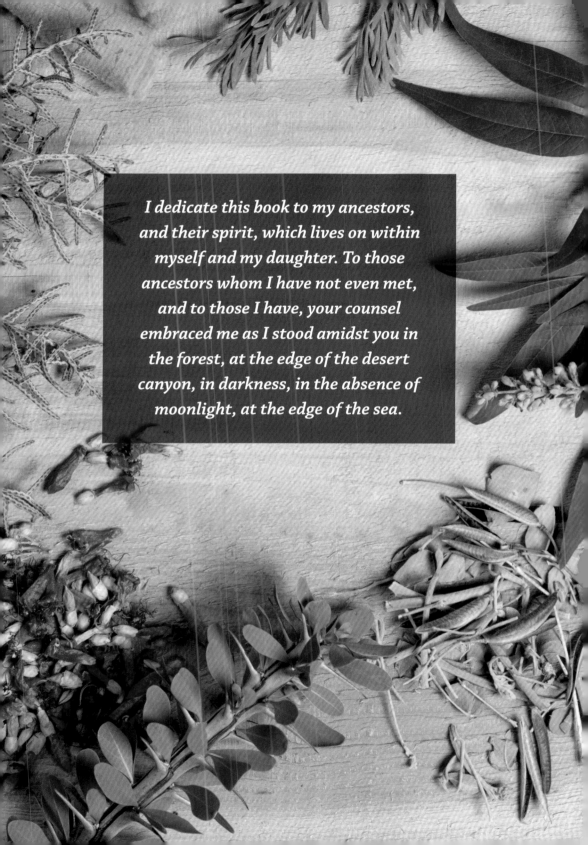

I dedicate this book to my ancestors, and their spirit, which lives on within myself and my daughter. To those ancestors whom I have not even met, and to those I have, your counsel embraced me as I stood amidst you in the forest, at the edge of the desert canyon, in darkness, in the absence of moonlight, at the edge of the sea.

CONTENTS

❖ PREFACE ❖

When I initially sought out books on herbalism, I didn't really know what I was looking for. I wanted to learn more about plants. I knew I wanted to become better educated about the world around me, in the spirit of seeking to understand the interconnectedness of life, and my place within it. But I didn't yet comprehend how vast and limitless the potential information gathering is (this was before Google). I sought to have a grasp on this knowledge, the knowledge of how to heal with plants, in such a way that I could call upon any of it, and within a moment have it at my fingertips. This was my discipline, my dream. I had no idea how far-fetched and impossibly grandiose it truly was.

Settling into a weekly walk through our desert home landscape with my then-2-year-old daughter, I stopped to feel the place I was in. To listen to it with the utmost openness and as much silent receptivity as I could muster. Her playfulness amid all Nature was a continual reminder of how little one truly needed to "know" to enjoy this world we live in. To enjoy it is to become part of it. To listen deeply. In a poignant moment, I began to hear the desert speak to me again. A voice that I had been missing. A reawakening to an old friendship, a deep knowledge waiting to unfold from within, and all around me. I allowed myself to journey with this voice as my daughter amused herself by the stream, declaring all the wonderful things she was noticing.

Messages come as if from the Earth herself, guiding me, teaching me, telling me where to go and what to look for. It's as if I'm on a treasure hunt and there is nothing more important than finding that which I don't even have a name for yet, but I'll know it when I see it. This is the healing, the reawakening, the coming back to life that occurs as I step out into the wild in the spirit of companionship with the plants, with no preconceived notions about how I should do it, or where I should go. I simply begin to move—and listen.

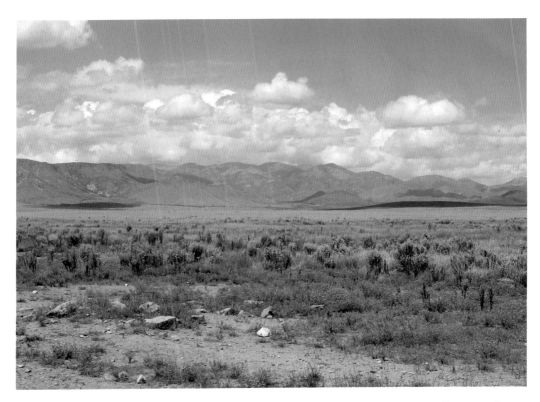

I hope that my daughter develops this type of relationship with Nature, on her own terms, in her own time. If there is one thing I feel we have done, that has injured us the most, it is to divorce ourselves from Nature's daily embrace by sequestering our senses to a place that is highly controlled and artificial. For all our modern advancements, we have left so much of great value behind.

The cold, damp air of early February penetrates my lungs, searing them, making them heavy. The chill up my spine provokes me to move across the desert floor toward the next rays of low-hanging early morning sunshine. We are exploring, my daughter and I, amused by this interplay between our imagination, the diversity of Nature around us, and our senses. We feel a sense of freedom, which for the moment we don't speak to but simply enjoy. Cold, sweet water comes out of the mountain spring, wetting the sand beneath our feet;

we savor it one taste at a time. For now, there will be no talk of scientific names, no plant quizzes, no studying of animal tracks and identifying the contents of their last meals. We are immersed, at one with our home place, seeding our consciousness back into the Earth, trusting in her ability to regenerate and renew us with no true loss of self. The truest healing is to let go of ourselves and our misconceived hold on the world around us, and to simply "be," in harmony with it all.

I invite you to entrain your heart to your landscape once again, as you did as a young child, finding your way with curiosity, awe, and wonder for all that you saw in Nature. Healing with plants is more than drinking a cup of tea, or making tinctures. Their spirits call us to return to a place of splendor and delight within ourselves, reigniting our creative spark, healing our bodies, minds, and spirits.

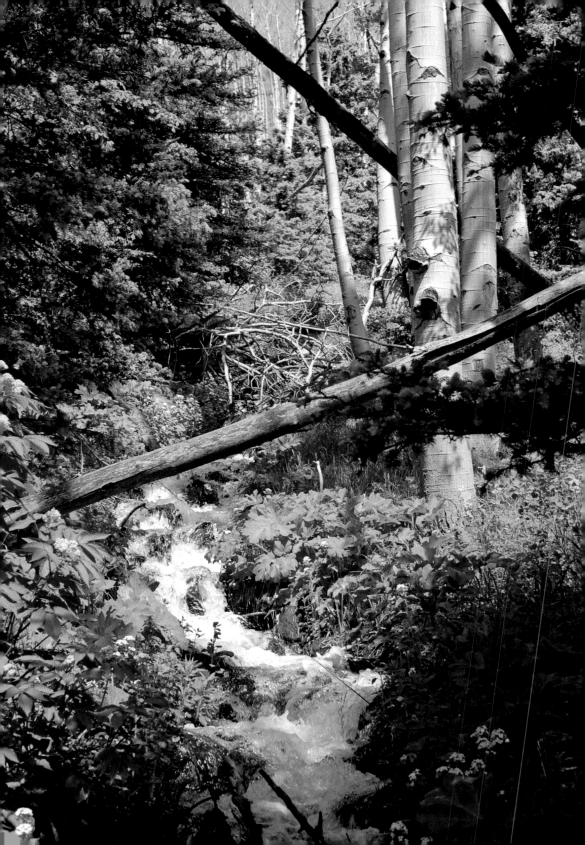

INTRODUCTION

Welcome to the vast world of working with plants for medicine. This book contains an array of medicinal plants known throughout the greater Southwest region for their remarkable healing properties. Most of these herbs have been used for thousands of years here in the Southwest; others were brought to this continent over the past 500 years and have become integrated into the local ecology and folk medicine practice. Lifetimes of knowledge are embedded within this collective wisdom still being passed down and continually reinvented through our intimate and loving relationships with wild plants. This book may introduce a whole new generation of those seeking to answer the call to know the plants once again, or to reacquaint those who have lost track of this knowledge, perhaps bridging the gap between what remains and what has been lost to time and neglect.

The first section of this chapter will describe the various habitats we have throughout the Southwest, preparing the reader for what they may find on their own sojourns into the wild. We are fortunate to have endless realms to explore, from deserts to lush conifer forests and canyons.

OUR REGIONAL HABITATS

The Southwest bioregion is exceptionally diverse, spanning 8 states and covering roughly 470,000 square miles from the deserts of southern California eastward to the South Texas Plains, up along the Balcones Escarpment, and up into the cross timbers, great plains, and high plains ecozones of western Oklahoma. This volume seeks to encapsulate an ecological region that is independent of specific political boundaries. Although entire states are encompassed (Arizona, New Mexico), many partial states are included (California, Nevada, Utah, Colorado, Texas, and Oklahoma). This is meant to provide continuity for the reader as well as encompass the general ecologies and plant communities that are present throughout our Southwest bioregion.

Although several interpretations are in existence, I've decided to use some rather basic habitat (or ecozone) definitions to assist beginners in their understanding of our region. Those of you familiar with more exacting definitions of habitat variations will begin to see overlap as well as subtle differences among the various categories provided here. Please note that these categories are not meant to be adhered to rigidly; rather, they are to be utilized as a general guideline for locating the plants you're seeking, or getting a general idea of what you may find when entering a particular habitat.

Keep in mind, too, that these habitat types may be so close in proximity that one could conceivably weave in and out of them along a half-mile hike, in some areas. Alternatively, one could walk for days on end, in some areas, without leaving a particular habitat type (such as high-elevation conifer forests, or the Hill Country). What follows is a listing and brief description of each habitat featured in this book.

Desert, Desert Grasslands, Cactus Forests

This habitat makes up the majority of our western half and is largely absent from our eastern third. Cactus forests predominate in the lower Sonoran desert bioregion (below 5,000 feet) intermingled with desert grasslands. Moving into southern California, or eastward into the Chihuahuan desert of New Mexico and western Texas, there are no columnar cacti, and grasslands are less common: inappropriate grazing and cropland development have removed much of the historic grasslands. This is the hottest and

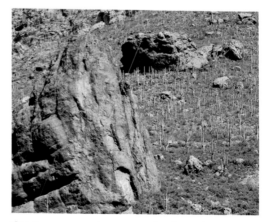

Giant saguaros reign over rocky slopes in cactus forests interspersed by desert grasslands.

driest part of our region, where temperatures may exceed 120F in summer and barely reach freezing in winter. Rainfall is 2–15 inches annually. This area is characterized by such medicinal plants as rhatany, prickly pear, wild tobacco, and brittlebush.

Disturbed Areas, Gardens, Trailsides, Clearings

This section is a bit of a catchall that covers a wide elevation range and includes many nonnative and landscaped plants, some of which may be naturalized. We may find sow thistle, for example, in winter parking lots, gardens, and roadsides from Tucson to Palm Springs, yet find it along the trail or in a campground in July at high elevation in southwestern Colorado. The conditions are roughly similar but juxtaposed across wildly different times of the year. A traveling wildcrafter with a trained eye will begin to see these patterns across the entire Southwest over a year's cycle of changing seasons. Additional plants one is likely to see in this habitat include curly dock, plantain, fanpetals, and mallow.

High Desert

From the western tip of the Oklahoma panhandle to the high desert surrounding Las Vegas, Nevada, this habitat weaves in and out with high plains, conifer forest, and canyonlands. It is distinct from our low deserts, with relatively fewer and smaller cacti and an abundance of drought-tolerant conifers,

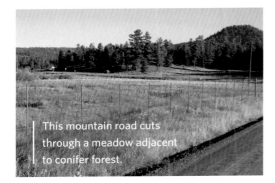

This mountain road cuts through a meadow adjacent to conifer forest.

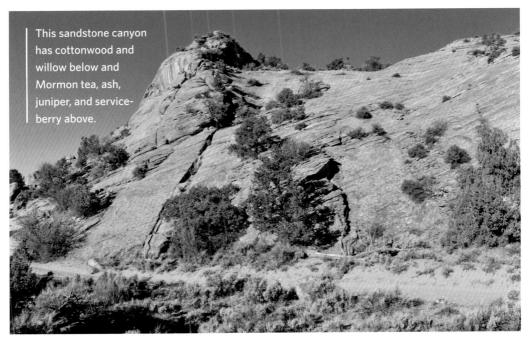

This sandstone canyon has cottonwood and willow below and Mormon tea, ash, juniper, and serviceberry above.

such as juniper and piñon; floral diversity is significantly lower here than in our cactus forest and desert grasslands. These rocky hills and mountains, dense low-growing forests, and sand dunes are home to Mormon tea, snakeweed, and thistle.

High-Elevation Conifer Forest

This lush zone ranges from approximately 5,000 feet in shaded mid-elevation canyons to over 12,000 feet at some of our highest mountain forests. Here winters are quiet, often with several months of snow-covered ground. Late spring brings a flurry of unfolding wildflowers, and the autumn is cool and sunny as the last nuts and fruits ripen. Ponderosa pines often predominate in sunny, exposed areas. Douglas fir, Englemann spruce, and aspen cover shaded, north-facing hillsides; oshá inhabits forest clearings and semi-shaded spots throughout the forested mountains.

High Plains

Ranging from eastern New Mexico through the Texas and Oklahoma panhandles and up into a small section of southeastern Colorado, this area may also be called the shortgrass prairie and includes the "rolling plains." Once the domain of the Comanche and Apache, this habitat has largely been turned over to cattle grazing and some agriculture. Although the floral diversity is limited, in special locations you will find desert willow, chokecherry, echinacea, buttonbush, queen's root, and several oak species.

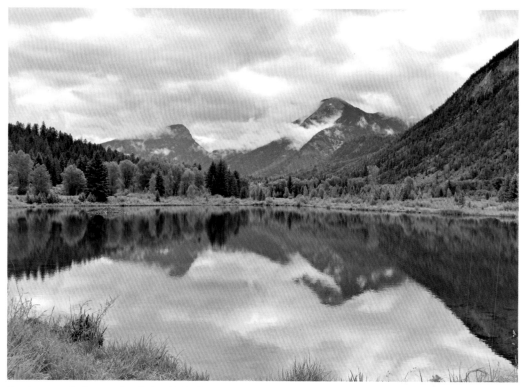

As above, so below . . . A pristine high-elevation lake beckons us to reflect on what moves within and around us.

Hill Country

One of the smaller sections among our various habitats, this area is unique to the Edwards Plateau of central Texas and known for its tremendous wildflower displays each spring. The limestone substrate that rises up from the Balcones Escarpment to the east sits atop the Edwards Aquifer, giving rise to numerous springs and streams throughout the area. Cutting through San Antonio and rising toward Austin, this region has seen a dramatic rise in population and many new land practices over the last century, including excessive grazing and fire suppression. Although Ashe's juniper has come to dominate much of this botanically rich ecozone, we'll still find abundant algerita, silk tassel, hop tree, sage, and skullcap throughout.

Oak Woodlands

This ecozone overlaps with several others, including the Hill Country, conifer forests, high desert, prairies, cactus forests, and desert grasslands. As the national tree of the United States, oaks are found throughout the country but are particularly diverse in the Southwest, with at least 24 species represented. In these woodlands we'll also find bricklebush, red root, cáscara sagrada, tickseed, and manzanita. Oak woodlands are significant in nearly every area of our region and have been held with reverence and closely stewarded throughout the ages.

Prairie: North-Central Texas and Oklahoma

Heading north from Austin, through Dallas, and up into the forested areas of south and western Oklahoma, we encounter a transitional habitat that is generally more humid than much of the Southwest (more than twice the rainfall, on average, than Santa Fe, for example) but that still holds much in

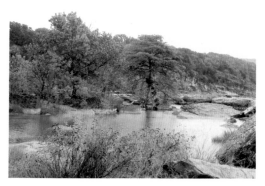

The Pedernales River running through the Texas Hill Country in spring.

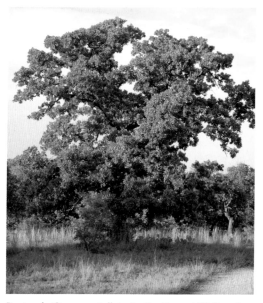

Post oak, *Quercus stellata*, in the Texas Hill Country.

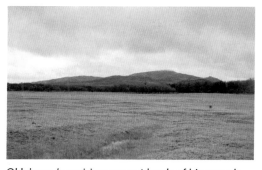

Oklahoma's prairies support herds of bison and boast many species of medicinal plants.

common with other plant communities of our region. It includes the blackland prairie and cross timbers regions. Here, among various species of oak, cottonwood, elm, walnut, and sumac, we also find estafiate, cholla, and prickly pear.

Rivers and Canyons

Ranging from near sea level to over 8,000 feet in elevation, this is another ecozone that stretches across our region. These areas may have perennial water or be seasonally dry; they are particularly significant in such places as the high plains, where the sudden appearance of a deep canyon presents a whole new variety of flora to explore. This contrast of ecosystems occurs throughout our high desert and desert grasslands. Many of our rivers find their beginnings at springs tucked into the lush hillsides of our

high-elevation conifer forests. Rivers and canyons present an opportunity to explore a diversity where edges meet—where prickly pear grows beside elder, or buttonbush and yerba santa thrive a short distance from desert lavender.

South Texas Plains

Sharing much in common with our desert grassland and cactus forest areas, this often hot and dry ecozone is characterized by a diversity of thorny vegetation. Bordered by the subtropical Rio Grande Valley to the south and the grasslands of the Gulf Coast to the east, its variable rainfall can produce huge wildflower blooms alternating with long-standing drought. Just south of San Antonio, we'll begin to find goatbush, kidneywood, puncture vine, flor de tierra, and prickly poppy.

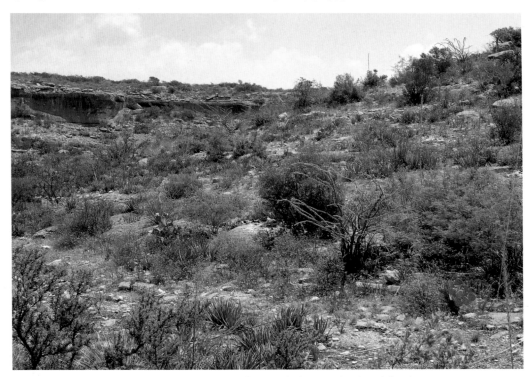

The South Texas Plains possesses some unique flora, including goatbush and flor de tierra.

The value of this book is relative to the reader's experience of spending time in Nature, observing. So before you read any further, make sure the scent of the forest, the feel of the desert's texture and heat, and the taste of wild water is within you. Then come back to sit with this book and digest the words as a supplement to what you have gathered through your senses. This book is not explicit direction on what you have to do, or should do; it is a collection of knowledge from the field as well as a guide to developing one's senses, developing one's true knowledge through the direct and discerning experience of Nature herself. As you walk into the forest, across the desert floor, or into the matrix of a juniper grove, open your senses and surrender yourself to the gifts available before you and within you. Open your heart to the healing that is present in the trees themselves, conveyed to you as you walk openly among them, humbly and confidently. This is true medicine. Our medicine.

Scientific names

Although the plant profiles in this book are organized by common name, each plant is attributed a scientific binomial. This serves the purpose of organizing plant names to a (supposedly) fixed and universal name. Different common names can be applied to the same plant, causing confusion, or the same common name can be applied to entirely different plants, causing not only confusion but potentially serious injury when plants are mixed up as a consequence. As advice is passed across cultural boundaries in which similar names are ascribed to different plants, or a plant is marketed according to a common name that represents a different plant where the raw material is actually being gathered for

market, serious mistakes can ensue. Scientific names do change. Plants are even placed in new families, based upon changing perspectives, or the development of DNA analysis, for example. This is challenging, to say the least, and we are in flux for the time being. All the more reason to be diversified in one's knowledge, both "field literate" and well versed with the literature, for when one knows the plant itself, one cannot be fooled.

When a plant profile covers a genus generally (e.g., prickly pear, *Opuntia* species), this is meant to identify those situations where there are far more similarities than differences between separate species with regard to our interest as herbalists—an important differentiation from the specifics of botany (they don't always cross over). Undoubtedly, differences between closely related plants can and do occur. That is to say, a stand of hawthorn growing in north-central Texas may have unique energetics compared to a stand found along a mountain stream in southern Colorado, or central Arizona. These

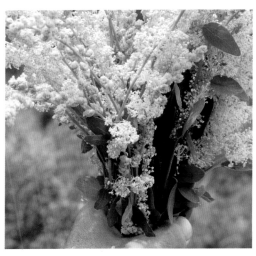

Ceanothus integerrimus, one of several species of red root.

subtleties are discovered through experience and intimate relationship with plants. This is the subtle power latent within intimate relationship with plants, a power that knows nothing of scientific nomenclature. Botany is a tool, which as herbalists we can employ to learn more about cross-cultural usage and international research.

How to identify

Plants are often unfamiliar to you—until they are not. Take the time necessary to look closely at plants as perhaps you've never done before, or at least since you were a small child. There is no rush to identify, classify, and gather. Identification is easily taken for granted when someone simply tells you the name of a plant. Spending time to get to know a plant involves much greater nuance, calling upon our deeper reserves of sensitivity and insight.

Where, when, and how to wildcraft

This section of each plant profile attempts to place into context potentially broad concepts stretched across our vast terrain. You may not find rhatany in your local stretch of desert grassland or cactus forest. This doesn't mean the book is inadequate or that your local ecozone need be reclassified. It's simply an example of the great diversity latent within the broad concepts of habitat offered in this section. When to wildcraft ranges from a highly nuanced to a simple

and straightforward matter. Perceiving the annual fluctuations in seasonal shifts in your area is as important as any information offered in this book.

Medicinal uses

I've attempted both to arrange a simplified look at the medicinal properties of each plant and to lend key insights gained through my personal experience and from speaking to other herbalists firsthand about their medicinal applications. Within several profiles, I've also endeavored to paint a picture of the plant's nature, such that the reader can interpret according to a unique situation that may arise, rather than just "it's good for xyz." I've utilized notes from nearly 20 years of study, the books of other herbalists, and the available ethnobotanical literature for our region. A reader may very well find new uses for each plant listed in this book, or find that some of the uses listed don't work. It is true. Herbs don't always work, through no fault of their own; each "failure" is an opportunity to learn more about the plant and the person who has taken it for medicine.

Future harvests

In this section of each profile, I briefly discuss options to help steward the plant under discussion. Whether through transplanting, seed scattering, or an approach to gathering, we can interact with wild plants in many potentially productive ways.

To move towards the landscape with an open heart and a watchful reverence, you will be absolutely amazed at what it will reveal to you. Landscape isn't just matter, but is actually alive. Landscape recalls one to a mindful mode of stillness, solitude, and silence where you can truly receive time.

Irish poet, John O'Donohue

⚠ Caution

Any necessary information about potentially injurious effects an herb may have on an individual will be conveyed here. Yes, any herb can cause injury, most often under extreme or unusual circumstances. By simply following the guidelines for gathering, preparing, and ingesting the medicinal plants listed in this book, most potentially unsafe scenarios will be avoided. When you begin to make your own medicines, start simply and safely, and use that experience to ask questions and set up a broad foundation of experiential knowledge for yourself. Rare and unusual responses to plants do occur,

so always start slowly when trying new plant medicines.

One truth that has been borne out for me over my years of working with plants and attempting to convey this information to students is that there are *no absolutes*. Apparent contradiction and paradox is the rule, the further and deeper one explores. To adhere to dogma or rigid thinking simply blinds one to the inevitable contradiction lying in wait. Thus, I take all rigid systems of categorization and classification with a grain of salt. This goes for scientific nomenclature and herbal energetics as well. To see clearly what is before one's eyes and within one's heart is the ultimate science.

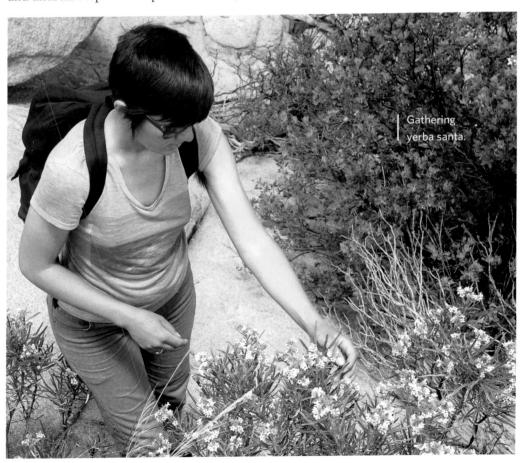

Gathering yerba santa.

BECOMING A BIOREGIONAL HERBALIST

Becoming a bioregional herbalist, in my opinion, is developing relationships with the totality of life in the world around you. This includes the basic elements of Nature, and all aspects of the natural world, even if our particular focus is working with plants for healing. As we seek to find our place within the natural world, we practice listening, feeling our way through. In this endeavor, there are no right answers; there is simply to be.

Gathering plants from the wild can be an exciting endeavor. One never quite knows what's lurking around the corner, thus each outing is an adventure. It is also a responsibility. To gather a plant is to take a lifeform, or a portion thereof. Once that act is done, it is the responsibility of the gatherer to treat the herb with respect and apply it as expressed, or intended. Contemplating what one needs a plant for and what one intends to do with it *before* gathering it is an essential step for the competent and responsible bioregional herbalist. The plants are here to help us. If we give a moment's thought as to how we desire to proceed, express this need and a bit of gratitude for what is to be offered, it can go a long way in supporting our endeavors. The three fundamental ethics of an integrated bioregional herbalist are gratitude, honor, and respect. Should we unfailingly keep these principles in our hearts and minds, we will be supporting harmony in our world and making it more beautiful in the process.

A wonderful first step toward developing a bioregional perspective is to go for a walk—and do so consistently. And observe. Observe. Patient observation and self-reflection are the two greatest teachers. When you first feel compelled to begin gathering herbs, stop for a moment and reflect. "Is this necessary?" "How do I intend to apply this medicine?"

"Am I prepared to treat this herb with honor and respect while gathering it?" If you can provide clear answers to these questions, and the way before you is open, you will next need to be prepared for the gathering, handling, and processing of certain plants.

Relationship through listening

At an herbal conference in the Rocky Mountains several years ago, I led an herb walk. At the end of the walk we stopped at the plant fireweed. I asked everyone to stop, sit down, connect to their breath, feel the Earth beneath their seat, and release their preconceived ideas about the world around them. As the group settled in, the energy shifted around us. The world became something new, and what we felt suddenly became pertinent, relevant, and important. I guided them to connect with the plant before us, without identifying it and without giving any information about usage. We were going to enjoy this experience unfettered by bias or any knowing which we'd brought with us that afternoon. In moments like these, significant knowledge may arrive immediately like a swift breeze in a moment of pure stillness. I heard . . . "courage . . . adeptness . . . erection . . . male reproductive system." These bits of information were unlike anything that I had previously "known" about this plant, and, despite having innumerable experiences like this before, I was still a bit reluctant to believe what I had heard. The following morning, as I was out on my walk amongst the verdancy of high summer at 10,000 feet, I stopped before a patch of fireweed, squatted down and nibbled a leaf in quiet contemplation. There was little of the previous day's experience fresh in my mind at the moment. As I stood up and walked across the patch I heard a voice whisper, "aromatase". Did I just make that up? I thought. Driven by an even greater curiosity now, I sat before my computer and typed "Epilobium + aromatase" into the search engine. Sure enough, a study from almost 20 years ago had demonstrated fireweed's ability to inhibit aromatase thereby improving conditions such as prostatitis or benign prostatic hypertrophy (BPH).

This is the approach of a modern-day bioregional herbalist: bridging the gap between the heart-mind and the intellectual-mind. I experienced the plant openly and directly in its natural habitat. I combined that with my previous experiences with the plant as well as my broader knowledge about physiology, plant energetics, botany and ethnobotany. Trusting in the unfolding of

the process, I was brought to a specific bit of knowledge. Had I learned this information in a book or a classroom, I would be much less likely to retain it as knowledge, apart from being a simple fact memorized. The walk of the bioregional herbalist is to begin to pull from all sources within the Circle of Life, one by one, compiling a personal story of inter-relationship with the living world, Mother Nature, the Elements, and the Plants as our guides.

Basic tools and equipment for the wildcrafter

Personally, I often carry as little as possible. I love the feeling of being in Nature with little or nothing to carry. But there are certain items which, when available, may make your work, both in gathering and transporting any

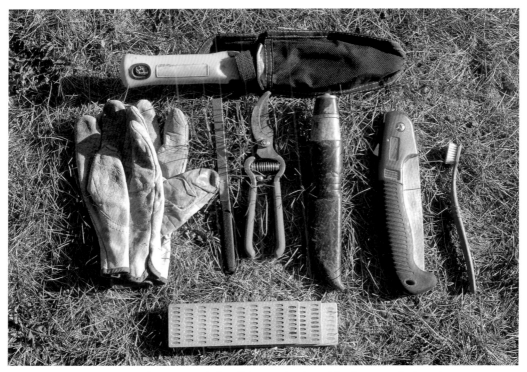

This small assortment of tools can provide for all the needs of a wildcrafter on a day's gathering journey. The blue-handled file can be used to sharpen bypass pruners quickly without disassembling the blade.

herbs you encounter, much easier. I'm all for trying to make use of what you have available, but if you're interested in procuring some useful tools, then consider obtaining the following items to outfit your wildcrafting kit.

Pruners. Simple bypass pruners will suffice for gathering the majority of aboveground plant parts, those with a diameter of ½ inch or less. Pinching or breaking off by hand is also an option with a great number of plants. When purchasing pruners, choose something above the mid-range in price, as it will often be made of more durable materials and of better quality overall. Keep a range of file grits on hand to sharpen the edge before

and after each use. Long-handled pruning shears (aka loppers) work great for removing branches 1–2 inches in diameter.

Pruning Saw. A pruning saw is essential for severing tree limbs up to 4 inches in diameter. Be sure to carry a lightweight, folding pruning saw in your daypack whenever you venture out into the backcountry or head out on a road trip.

Shovel/Digging Stick. A short-handled or folding shovel can be very handy when hiking into wild areas. A hori hori is a versatile Japanese digging tool with a sharp cutting edge on each side, one of which is serrated; it's easily tossed in a bag or worn on a belt.

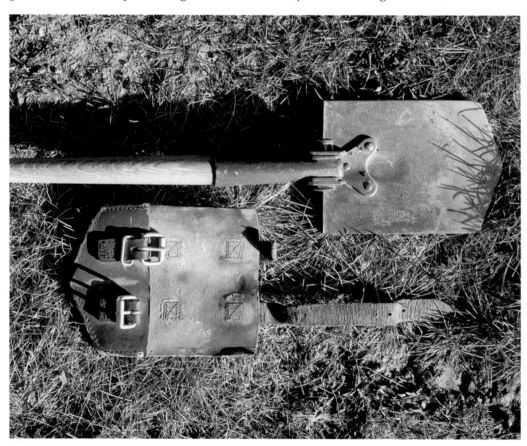

Folding shovel.

Knife. A sharp knife can handle a good number of tasks that the wildcrafter encounters. It is particularly well suited to stripping bark but can be used to cut stems from trees and cut herbaceous plants. If large enough, it can chop large, leafy plants as well.

Gathering Bags. Bags of cloth, paper, or other woven natural materials are preferred for gathering herbs; something with straps will keep your hands free, especially when hiking in. Some prefer to use baskets for more fragile items, such as flowers or ripe fruits. Bed sheets come in handy for long plants, such as nettle or horseweed, both of which are irritating to the skin; laying them on a sheet with gloved hands while gathering helps to reduce skin irritations.

Sharpening Stones. Diamond sharpening stones and honing files can now be purchased inexpensively. These tools help to keep your sharp edges refined and ready to cut.

Where to wildharvest

The world around us has become largely compartmentalized and segmented through our approach to life. When we walk out of doors into the world around us, what do we see? We could begin wildharvesting right in our own yard, neighborhood, local parks. The questions regarding legality are another matter. I believe it is our right to participate with the natural world around us. Acknowledging private ownership is an aspect of recognizing that mutual right. Some public lands prohibit gathering of anything whatsoever; some are open to gathering various plant parts for personal use. Check with local authorities about their current policies, but above all, conduct yourself with honor and respect with regard to the plants and always offer your gratitude.

The United Plant Savers is a non-profit association dedicated to fostering awareness of plant species loss in North America. In the Southwest, a few species are of limited concern, largely due to habitat loss. Identify threatened or at-risk plants within your area and work to learn more about their ecology. You will be better prepared to protect them, if necessary.

Gathering, processing, storing

There are some basic points to remember when gathering and processing herbs. Some herbs (elder, ocotillo flowers) will mold quickly, whereas creosote bush and other plants can sit in a bag for 3 days before being spread out to dry. Before gathering, be sure that you have ample space that is shaded and relatively dry. With a little planning and ingenuity, this can be accomplished on a road trip or while camping. Nearly all herbs should be dried in the shade, but darker roots can be dried in the sun. Drying screens or repurposed window screens can be stacked to allow for air flow, which expedites drying and thereby reduces the potential for mold. Bringing herbs into an air-conditioned home (where moisture is reduced) may help prevent spoilage in humid areas. Occasionally, when the weather is particularly cold and/or damp, a dehydrator may be necessary for heavy, moist herbs.

Upon gathering, inspect your herbs to clean out any foreign debris, and shake or wash off any excessive dirt. Fresh herbs can be processed by hand or with the tools listed earlier. Upon drying, they can be broken down by hand or powdered using a kitchen appliance with a blade assembly, or with a traditional mortar and pestle. Even though it adds time to the project, every step in the process is layered with the intention to heal.

Whenever possible, store dry leaves whole, especially those of aromatic plants. This will help maintain freshness and viability for many years. Keep away from heat and

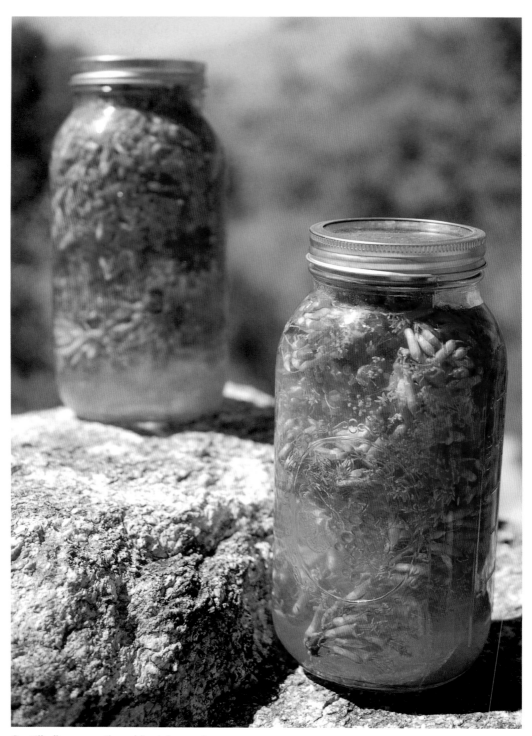

Ocotillo flowers, gathered fresh for sun tea.

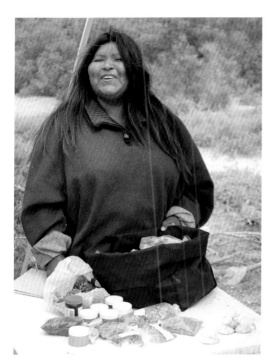

Seri (Comcáac) herbalist Maria Luisa Molino Martinez of Punta Chueca, Sonora, stores her herbs in plastic, too.

light to whatever extent possible. I have used herbs stored in plastic bags, away from sun, that were still potent medicine although they were gathered 12 years previously.

Gathering Tree Medicine. How we approach gathering tree medicine impacts both the health of the tree and the potency and vitality of our medicine. Several trees in this book are really worth getting to know for their medicine, but it's important that we gather from them properly. Due to the differences in tree and shrub species within our region, these instructions may need be followed with some accommodation in order to achieve an optimal outcome.

Recognizing that life force flows through trees differently at different times of the year (as well as at different times of the day and lunar cycle) will aid us in gathering optimal medicine. As a tree rests over winter, much of its vital force is held within its roots (even evergreens). As spring begins in early February, the sap held within the roots begins to move more freely up through the inner bark. The tree's bark is full of potency throughout the spring and summer. Gathering bark in autumn is also beneficial as the tree is often finished producing seeds by this time (if not much earlier). During the late autumn, the bark's vibrancy diminishes somewhat, as the tree's vital force slowly returns to its roots.

Be on the lookout for recently downed trees or fallen branches from high winds. Branches loosed from the tree will make great medicine, and there's no need to cut into the tree. When cutting a branch is necessary, select one that is no more than 2 inches thick, with smooth bark. Seek out branches that will soon be shaded by larger branches, or areas of the tree where branch production is thickest. Cut the branch just above where it attaches to the larger limb. If the tree produces sap, collect some and cover the scar to reduce pathogenic infiltration. Remove twigs and smaller branches, which may be used whole for medicine. To remove the bark from relatively straight, smooth-barked branches (ash, aspen), score the bark around with a knife every 12 inches or so, then make long cuts in between these circumferential scores. Pry underneath the bark strips and pull off. Dry the strips on a cloth or gather them loosely in a paper bag. Some branches, especially when gathered during drought conditions, may require stripping with a knife, as the bark does not readily come off in strips. In a humid climate, these strips may need to be pierced and hung in order to dry properly.

Some bark is well suited to fresh tincturing (pine, kidneywood) and other barks are best dried before tincturing (chokecherry, aspen). Bark can be broken down into small pieces to store more easily. Grinding down to a powder, however, will cause the bark's constituents to degrade more rapidly.

Digging Roots. When performed with awareness, digging wild roots can be a deeply moving experience for the wildcrafter. These instructions are meant to assure optimal potency of the medicine one gathers, to support the health of the stand, and to fully engage one's heart and mind in the act of unearthing this medicine from the underworld.

As always, when wildharvesting medicine, first ask permission and blessings from the plants, and from the guardians of place where you gather. Offer something of value (e.g., tobacco, water), perhaps something of ourselves (e.g., a lock of hair), or words of gratitude, to express respect and appreciation for what is being offered, to set the stage for a beneficial outcome of the endeavor, and to allow the healing to unfold before us.

When digging up plants for medicine, some prefer not to use metal tools out of respect for the plants, instead choosing "softer" materials such as wood, bone, or stone, as our ancestors did. Whatever your choice, remember that some plants may require digging a hole large enough to bury a sink. Others (e.g., cholla) may require only prying up around the perimeter; in sufficiently wet soil, some may be uprooted simply by pulling up on their base (e.g., filaree). A digging stick or pickax (aka mattock) works well for prying up distal rhizomes; the mattock, when paired with a spade shovel, is very effective for excavating big holes. Other digging tools not yet mentioned include a trowel, a San Angelo bar (best for hardpan caliche soil), or, of course, one's hands. Which tools are chosen may depend on personal

preference and the circumstances of the gathering location. Hauling in a San Angelo bar and mattock pick on a 4-mile round-trip hike is not so fun. A short-handled shovel or a hori hori and a digging stick may be all that is needed for such backcountry jaunts.

There are various things to consider when identifying which plant to dig. In large, mature stands of oshá and other relatively long-lived perennials, I often gather from the perimeter of the stand, where the newest growth tends to be. When the stand appears to be at a climax, I dig from within its center; the digging and perturbation serves as a healthy and stimulating intervention for the stand, and regrowth will occur. Developing relationship with the location and the movement of the seasons and their recent effects on the local ecosystem and the plants you're considering, will all play a significant role in deciding where and how to dig. Often, simply engaging in active listening leads to a clear-headed and practical decision. This approach to digging is not necessarily the most efficient, although it will foster a deeper respect for and understanding of the plants one works with. *Remember*: it is often an important and wise decision *to not harvest anything*. You simply need to be in tune with the needs of the local ecosystem.

When beginning to dig, look around for sensitive plants in the vicinity and, if encountered, either choose a different spot, carefully replant them, or if possible utilize them in your harvest. Clear away any mulch from the top and set it off to the side; retrieve it to cover up the soil when refilling the hole to help maintain integrity within the ecosystem and preserve moisture under the soil's surface.

Loose, damp, sandy soil is often the best digging substrate in our region. In such a soil, you can pull out roots that are still buried several inches simply by rocking the plant back

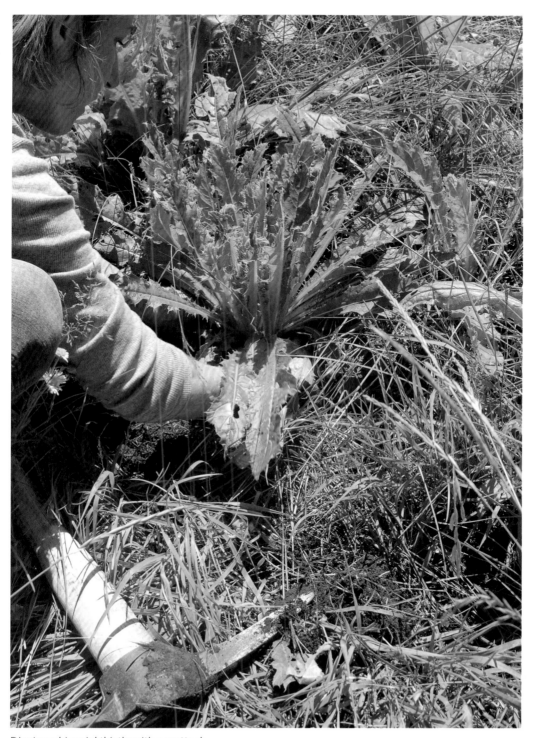

Digging a biennial thistle with a mattock.

and forth several times as the soil loosens around them. Challenging locations include rocky areas (e.g., nettle root weaving through boulders in a wash); zones interpenetrated by tree roots (aspen groves); or dry soil with a relatively high clay content, which can bend thinner metal tools that attempt penetration.

Once an optimal location for digging has been identified, take into account the size of the roots you are gathering. This can vary greatly from one plant to the next, and often bears no relation to the size of the plant's aboveground parts. If making a tincture for personal use, a half-pound of root should be plenty. Refrain from gathering more than is necessary, especially on the first time gathering a plant. Wait until you have a better feel for the plant and its usage before gathering more. Roots are powerful medicine, and a little often goes a long way.

As a general rule of thumb, for every foot of depth, dig 1½–2 feet out from the center of the plant, in all directions. In some cases, you may be able to extract a large root by digging up 180–270 degrees of the plant's circumference; the shorter the arc, the less likely you are to chop off roots that may be difficult to find later. Some plants may resprout if root pieces are left in the soil, but that is not always the case. Experiment with replanting root crowns of perennial plants after the distal portions have been harvested, and mark those locations to come back the following season, or year, to see if they have resprouted. Some roots (e.g., oshá) require delicate handling to keep intact while harvesting, but if broken off from the root crown, they may possibly sprout again.

Keep your roots from dehydrating too quickly by keeping them in a cloth bag in the shade while in the field. If you intend to dry what you gather, there are several ways to approach it. Primarily, roots are dried in the

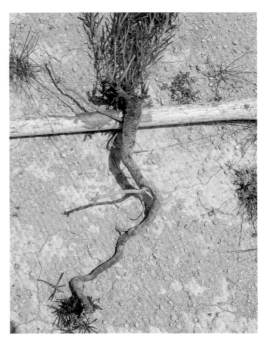

Queen's root, unearthed.

shade, but oshá and other darker roots can be dried in the sun to hasten drying, if necessary. Some roots (algerita, red root) dry so hard that they must be chopped prior to drying.

Once finished digging, push the extracted soil and rocks back into the hole you dug. Re-situate plants that needed to be dug up in hopes they will survive the replanting. If on a slope, attempt to make a small berm on contour to allow for some water catchment at the digging spot. This is also an opportunity to plant seeds, especially if you're digging in the fall (or perhaps you've brought seeds from the previous season to sow after digging). Many may think this is "Nature's job"; however, we as stewards can make our wild medicinal plant gardens more robust and beautiful through thoughtful and intentional involvement with the stands we interact with. This is the legacy of the ancient ones who once cultivated abundantly fruitful wild plant gardens throughout the Americas.

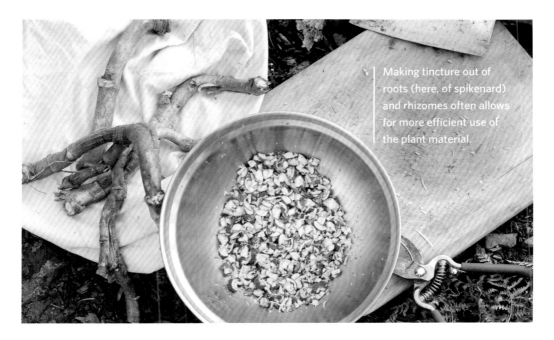

Making tincture out of roots (here, of spikenard) and rhizomes often allows for more efficient use of the plant material.

THE ART AND SCIENCE OF HERBAL MEDICINE MAKING

Concocting healing creations to imbibe for our health and wellness is a sacred rite as much as it is the right of every human on this planet. The wisdom of how to heal with the help of wild plants was once passed down from generation to generation. Alive and fluid, it was an integral part of all cultures across the globe. To reclaim this right is to embrace what it is to be human, to answer the call from within and from the world around us. Always remember, there is at least as much art in the co-creative endeavor of herbal medicine making as there is science.

Variability is the rule when it comes to plants and healing. Once we tune in to the world around us, we can see that change is the general rule of Nature. It's inevitable. Yes, the climate is changing, and the world is changing around us. To adapt to change, to become resilient in the presence of major shifts and alterations in our environment,

despite the severity, despite the degree of adversity—despite the particular virulence of the microorganism—is the epitome of what our ancestors recognized as vitality.

Turning to the wild plants growing around us for our medicine and developing a sensorial relationship with them carries tremendous power and healing potential for our physical, mental, and emotional ills.

In this section, I'm going to share with you a variety of traditional herbal preparations that can be easily prepared at home, or in the field, by the beginner. We'll explore some of the "whys," including some of the scientific principles behind the methods we use as herbalists. As I introduce you to these concepts (or refresh your memories, as the case may be), I'll be encouraging you to follow your inspiration within these relatively loose guidelines. May your new skills help you to forge a deep, loving relationship with the

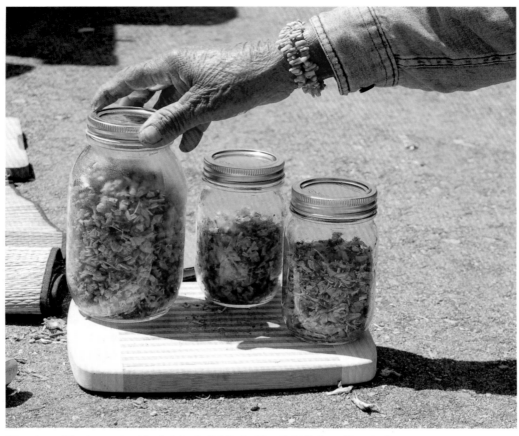

Glass jars of tincture set out by folk herbalist Doña Olga Ruíz Cañez of Imuris, Sonora.

vibrant plant communities with whom we share our Southwest home.

Please remember that these instructions are meant to be *guidelines*. Exceptional and endless variability exists within the plant kingdom, despite our best efforts to compartmentalize and categorize it. As a result, you may find different and/or better ways to extract the herbs you're working with; utilize these guiding principles to get you started and get your footing, then build from that foundation as your experience and confidence grows. Pay close attention to what you observe, and follow your intuition. Beautiful and powerful medicine goes well beyond the realm of reductive reason.

Dosage Considerations

- ~50 drops of tincture = 1ml
- 3ml = 1 teaspoon
- ~150 drops = 1 teaspoon
- 75 drops = ½ teaspoon
- 3 teaspoons = 1 tablespoon

Poultices

Aside from eating plants, poulticing is one of the simplest ways to use plants as medicine. Chew up a plantain leaf, place it upon a bee sting, burn, or fresh wound, and witness the pain diminish rapidly. A fresh plant poultice can provide immediate relief in a variety of situations. Simply gather up a small quantity of fresh herb and roll it around in the palm of your hand. Place it directly over the affected area and hold the poultice in place with a bandage, a bandana, a T-shirt, a belt, or even other plant material. Change frequently if bleeding is an issue, or leave on for several hours, or until the pain-relieving benefits have worn off. A dry plant poultice can be prepared with powdered plants. Either sprinkle the powdered plant directly onto a wound, or blend with powdered chia seed to help the poultice stick together. Scoop it onto a sheet of plastic wrap or a piece of cloth, then cover the affected area. Remove and replace, as needed.

Water extractions

Decoction. If you want to extract medicine from bark, roots, twigs, seeds, and pods, you will generally want to use the method of decoction, which refers to the simmering of plant material in water. Decoctions extract all water-soluble constituents from an herb. The continued application of heat allows for the structural cell walls of the plant matter to be broken down most efficiently, thus allowing the plant constituents to become readily soluble in the water.

The ratio for a standard decoction is 1:32—one part plant material by weight (1 ounce) and 32 parts solvent (water) by volume (32 fluid ounces).

First, combine the water and the herbs in a stainless steel, glass, or ceramic pot—these materials have the least reactive potential with the plant material (aluminum and Teflon-coated pots should be avoided). Bring to a rolling boil, then turn the heat down to a low simmer. Leave the pot covered for at least 20 minutes while simmering. Then turn the heat off and leave the pot covered where it was cooking for another 15–20 minutes

before pouring through a strainer. Pour enough water back through the herb to obtain the original volume of water. Drink the tea as advised. Make enough tea for 1–2 days' worth.

For optimal extraction of minerals, slowly decoct mineral-rich herbs over low heat for several hours or overnight.

The remnant herbs, or marc, can be utilized again in most cases. For acute cases, replenish with fresh herb stock before making another preparation to gain the fullest potential from your tea. For chronic cases, or regular nourishing and balancing support, reuse the herbs until there is no more taste left in the tea. Since the medicinal potency decreases with each subsequent batch, this is not recommended for acute infections.

A strong decoction is made by simmering 1 ounce of herb in 16 ounces of water (1:16), medicinally twice as strong as a standard decoction. Simmer the herb for 30–60 minutes, then let sit covered for 20–30 minutes before straining. Pour enough fresh water through the herb to regain the 16 fluid ounces you started with. The tea can be reheated before drinking.

A weak decoction uses half the amount of herb as a standard decoction—½ ounce of herb to 32 ounces of water (1:64); it is otherwise prepared the same way. This preparation is most often used for stronger herbs, for the elderly, or for children.

Fomentations (aka compresses) are generally made from decoctions. A fomentation is made by soaking a piece of cloth in a hot or cold tea and applying it directly to the body. When applied hot, it is often advisable to cover the fomentation with a dry towel to hold the heat in. Leave it on until the heat dissipates, and repeat if needed. A fomentation is a valuable remedy for cold, stiff, achy conditions.

A steam inhalation is yet another healing method derived from the decoction. The exact ratio is not as important, but it should generally be made as a strong decoction, or stronger. Boil the herb for 10–15 minutes, then remove from heat or place on low. With a towel spread overhead, lower your face carefully over the steaming pot and gently inhale the warm vapors. This can also be done in the bathtub as a full body bath, or in a sweathouse or sauna, if available. This is another ancient healing method with so many applications.

A sitz bath is commonly utilized postpartum to help heal the vaginal tissues and prevent uterine infections and postpartum fever. Decoct the available herbs and add the liquid to the tub before drawing the bath. Herbs most appropriate for infusion (e.g., desert lavender) can be added once the heat has been turned off and allowed to sit for at least 30 minutes. The tea can also be added to a small tub in which the patient can comfortably sit, a method useful for a variety of genitourinary complaints. An intermediate step is to place a steaming pot of aromatic herbs, prior to straining, directly beneath a perforated or open seat. The patient, male or female, sits and takes in the healing aromatic steam directly on the genitalia and anus. This is useful for a variety of conditions, including those requiring enhanced circulation to the area.

Infusion. Most delicate plant parts—leaves, stems, and flowers—are preferably made as an infusion (aka tisane), which is made by pouring boiling hot water over dry herbs. Dry herbs are preferred over fresh herbs as they are more soluble and readily give up their constituents in water. What is generally referred to as a "tea" is, in fact, an infusion—"tea" being a specific plant, *Camellia sinensis*, the source of both black and green tea.

A standard infusion is generally understood to mean a ratio of 1 part herb, by weight, to 32 parts water, by volume (1:32). Add 1 ounce of herbs to 32 ounces of boiled water. Let sit, covered, for 20–30 minutes. Strain and drink.

For a strong infusion, cut the ratio in half (1:16). A stronger preparation method maximizes the therapeutic effectiveness of the herb for immediate benefit.

Another type of preparation is the cold infusion. Cold infusions are a superior preparation method for herbs that contain mucilages, aromatic oils, or bitter principles. Begin with 1 part herb by weight and thoroughly moisten it with cool to room-temperature water. Place the herb in a muslin tea bag and suspend it in a jar in 32 parts of room-temperature water overnight. Squeeze the herb out into the tea in the morning and return the total volume to 32 parts by adding water.

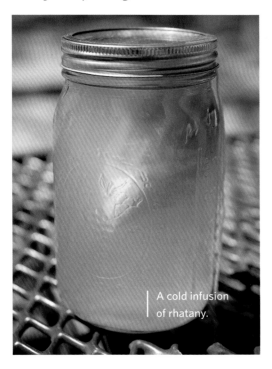

A cold infusion of rhatany.

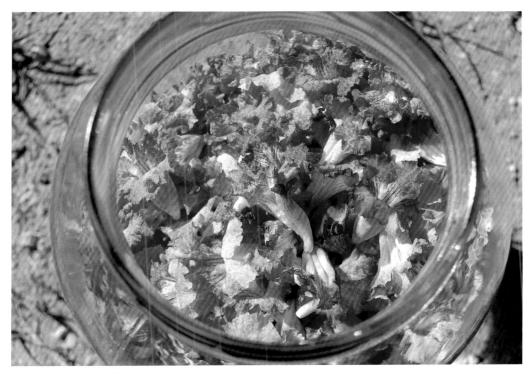
A sun tea of desert willow flowers.

Sun teas are yet another sort of infusion. Exposed to direct sunshine for 3–5 hours, the vibrancy and warmth of the sun's rays permeate the herbs and the water, uniquely energizing this preparation.

Tinctures

A tincture is a solution of plant material within a menstruum, or solvent, such as ethanol (e.g., grain, cane, or grape alcohol). Tinctures are valued for their convenience, portability, and potency. They are also one of our primary way of safeguarding certain plant medicines that may otherwise be overused. Some at-risk plants can be taken as low-dose tinctures thus requiring a minimal amount of herb per dose. Herbal tinctures have been part of medical practice in North America since the early 1800s and go even farther back in Europe and elsewhere.

Whenever any plant part is covered in a menstruum and allowed to sit for some time, a tincture is made. The alcohol is the means and method of extraction in itself. It is hydrophilic (Greek for "water-loving); it sucks water and therefore dehydrates the plant. Through this process of dehydration, the plant relinquishes a variety of its constituents into the menstruum. Certain plant constituents are more soluble in alcohol (e.g., essential oils, phenolic compounds, terpenoids, phytosterols); other constituents are more soluble in water. Most plants, fortunately, have a good mix of alcohol- and water-soluble constituents. Herbalist and chemist Lisa Ganora writes, "Highly polar compounds tend to dissolve in highly polar solvents (e.g., water); compounds with low overall polarity tend to dissolve in low-polarity solvents (e.g., ethanol). Solvents

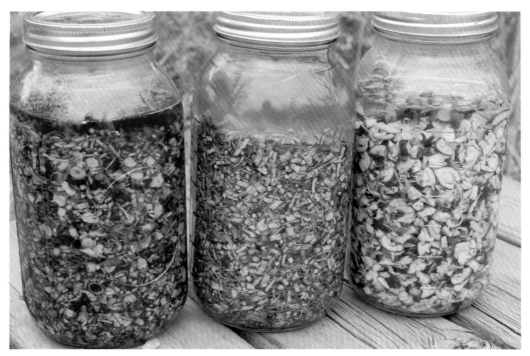

Root tinctures macerating. Left to right: *Ceanothus, Urtica, Aralia.*

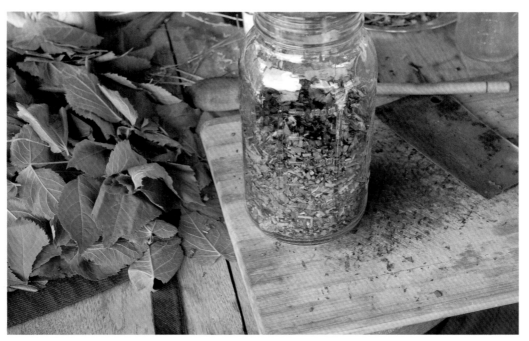

Always prepare tinctures (here, of fresh spikenard leaf) in glass or other nonreactive containers, which have zero potential to pollute the extraction.

with similar polarities to one another will mix (e.g., ethanol and water); solvents with very different polarities will not mix (e.g., oil and water)." The general principle? Like dissolves like.

Vinegar and vegetable glycerin are often used as solvents to avoid the use of alcohol for ethical, psychological, or physiological reasons; however, these two solvents are generally inferior. In most cases, they don't extract the plant's constituents nearly as well as water or alcohol. The relatively low pH of acetums, or vinegar solutions, lends itself to alkaloid and mineral extraction but not many other plant constituents; acetums can be made according to the same methods as the fresh and dry plant tinctures. Glycerin has a higher polarity than alcohol and may be used to your advantage in cases where that is desirable (e.g., polysaccharide extraction).

Tinctures are made from both fresh and dry plant matter. Using a dry plant can have several benefits. The drying process may render any toxic substances inert, and having dried plant material offers easy accessibility to a plant's medicinal components if the plant is not in season. For many plants, whenever you have access to them is when you can make tincture from them; others need to be harvested in the season they are available in order to prepare them fresh.

Some plant parts (roots, bark, woody fruits) can be left in the menstruum for years with no problem. But fresh, leafy plants will need to be pressed within a short period, often within a few days. Searching for a means to extract every last bit of medicine from your menstruum may be an expensive endeavor. Heavy-duty plant presses are more efficient but rather costly for the home user. What one can do with their hands and a little ingenuity goes a long way toward getting a tincture strained with little waste. A used fruit press may provide increased efficiency at an affordable price.

There is no one way to make herbal tinctures, but there are safer and more effective ways. The overall approach should be a familiarity with the particular plant rather than any dogmatic approach to tincture-making. That said, let's look at a detailed approach to making fresh and dry plant tinctures.

Fresh Plant Tincture. Ratio 1:2. Items needed:

- 1 quart canning jar with clean lid (plastic or metal)
- 10 ounces fresh, chopped herb
- 20 fluid ounces organic cane alcohol (95%)

Thoroughly chop the herb to break the cell walls of the plant and to increase the surface area exposed to the solvent. Chop to less than ¼ inch for fresh, leafy plants. Larger pieces occupy too much volume when the jar is filled, disrupting the intended 1:2 ratio. Lightly pack a quart canning jar with the 10 ounces of finely chopped herb. Then pour the 20 ounces of alcohol over the herb. Poke the herb

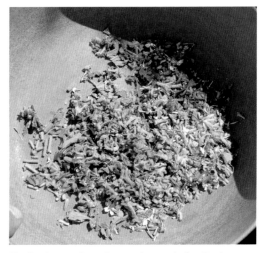

Finely chopped mock vervain, ready for tincture.

repeatedly with a chopstick, or something of similar shape and size, with an up and down motion for several minutes. This helps release any air trapped within the liquid and prevents mold growth within the tincture.

Watch as the color recedes from the herb over the following days. Fresh, leafy herbs such as mock vervain should be pressed out within 4–7 days. Most barks, roots, fruits, and some drier, leathery leaves can be left to macerate for several weeks to several months. A good rule of thumb is to taste your tincture weekly to ascertain how the maceration is developing over time. Some tinctures, for instance, may be serviceable in a month but reach a greater potency and fullness of extraction after 2–4 months. There is no need to shake fresh plant

tinctures as they macerate. The extraction process is facilitated by dehydration from the alcohol. However, if you observe a substantial amount of solvent not touching the herb (most often the case with heavier herbs), shake the tincture jar to redistribute the solvent.

A simple method for pressing out tinctures that have finished macerating is to place a metal sieve over a glass or metal bowl, leaving some space below the strainer to accommodate a volume of tincture. Place a muslin cloth, bandana, or some similar weave over the sieve (cheesecloth may be too porous for finer materials). Pour the tincture out onto the cloth, scooping out the herb from the jar as needed. Wrap the bundle up by pinching the corners together tightly,

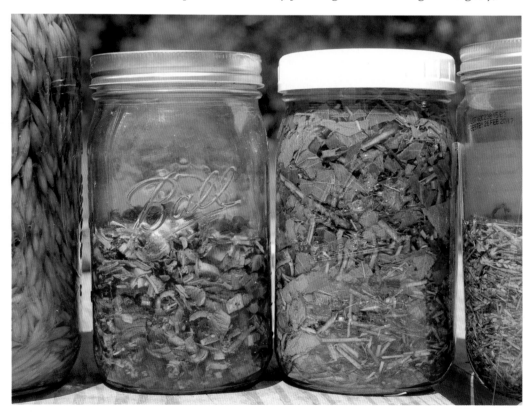
Making fresh plant tinctures in the field.

twisting the excess material down to the bundle of herb. Squeeze vigorously with your hands, wringing out as much of the solvent as possible. The remnant herbs, or marc, may be composted. The remaining liquid is your tincture. Keep it in dark, clearly labeled, glass bottles and store away from heat and light. Properly stored tinctures can last a decade a more. Only very rarely does a tincture lose its potency within a few years.

Dry Plant Tincture. Ratio 1:5. Items needed:

- 1 quart canning jar with clean lid (plastic or metal)
- 5 ounces dry, chopped herb
- 12.5 ounces spring water
- 12.5 ounces organic cane alcohol (95%)

Dry plant tinctures are simple to prepare, given that the herb has already been fully processed. Both water and alcohol are used in all dry plant preparations. As a general rule, the herb:solvent ratio is 1:5 (5 ounces of herb to 25 total ounces of solvent). A solvent that is half water, half alcohol is a safe bet, although some preparations may benefit from a slightly higher ratio of alcohol to water. We generally use half water and half alcohol, dividing the 25 total ounces of solvent by 2, or 12.5 ounces each of water and alcohol.

Cut or crush the herb into a coarse powder to optimize total surface area exposed to the dehydrating effects of the alcohol. You don't want a fine powder, as this will tend to clump and decrease solubility. Weigh out 5 ounces of dry herb, then add to the quart jar.

Measure out 12.5 ounces of water and 12.5 ounces of 95% alcohol, and combine in one vessel to produce 25 total ounces of solvent. Mix together and pour directly over the dry herb, filling the jar. Shake the maceration on a daily basis in order to fully incorporate the herb with the solvent if the level of the solvent reaches well above the level of the herb, facilitating an equal and optimal extraction.

Allow 4–6 weeks for a full extraction, then press as described for a fresh plant tincture. Dense, dry herbal material (roots, bark) will yield much less from mechanical pressing than fresh herbs.

Honey infusions

Fresh flowers, thoroughly chopped roots, and some leaves make excellent honey infusions. Always use wildflower or other high-quality organic honey for honey infusions. Begin by measuring the herb and honey; in general, 1:4 is an adequate ratio. Add some of the herb (2 ounces) to a glass jar, then pour some honey on top (8 ounces). Alternate the two until the jar is full, or all the herb has been used. If the herb has a high water content, the infusion may need to be strained within 4–7 days; roots and many flowers can sit for 4–12 months with no concerns. Many flower infusions are ready within 2 months. Roots should macerate for 4 months to develop a richer flavor profile. These honeys are used therapeutically and may also be used in preparing food.

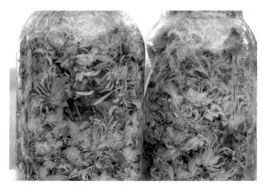

Wild oregano honey infusion.

Oxymels

An oxymel is an ancient preparation dating back millennia. Its name refers to its sharp (*oxy*) and sweet (*mel*) flavors from the two main ingredients: vinegar and honey. With these two ingredients alone, this preparation is considered a respiratory and digestive tonic, but in combination with herbs, an oxymel can stimulate a great variety of effects. (See the entries on oxymels under various plant profiles.) One option is to simmer the herbs in apple cider vinegar (1:16), strain the herbs out, and add about ½ part honey to the vinegar, or the herbs can be decocted in water (1:10), or a combination of water and vinegar (1:16). Honey is then added at an equal amount to the tea after straining (vinegar is added along with the honey for a water decoction). Simmer to the desired consistency. Tinctures may be added to the oxymel once removed from the heat. Oxymels are usually taken in cool water during hot weather, or in hot water in cold weather.

Syrups

A syrup can be obtained by making a strong decoction and adding honey to the strained tea at 75–150% of the final tea volume. The more honey added, the sweeter, of course, but the shelf stability will increase. Refrigerated syrup should last at least a year with a minimum concentration of 75% honey by volume of tea.

Oil infusions

Alcohol Intermediate Oil Infusions. This method, our preferred method for oil infusions, has been in use since the 19th century (if not much longer); it allows for the optimal extraction of a wide array of constituents. The alcohol initiates the extraction process, and the oil finishes it. Items needed:

* dry herb
* 95% alcohol
* organic extra virgin olive oil
* blender
* scale, bowl, measuring cups

Grind the dry herb to a roughly uniform coarse material; if using a blender or high-powered kitchen appliance, add only a small amount of herb at a time, as such devices are designed primarily for liquids. Weigh out the desired amount of herb and transfer it to a large glass, ceramic, or stainless steel bowl. Add the alcohol; the amount to use is normally 50–100%, by volume, of the given herb's weight. Begin by adding 50% and gradually add more, until the herb is properly moistened. Cover and let sit for 12–24 hours. The alcohol will begin acting as a solvent on the crucial medicinal constituents of the plant. Only use high % alcohol for this (75% or greater). After the time has passed, add the herb to a blender along with at least 5 ounces of olive oil for every ounce of herb (be careful not to overfill). Turn it on and blend until the sides of the blender become warm. At this point, you can either strain out the plant debris and collect your finished oil, or pour the oily slop into a glass jar and place it in a warm place (on top of the fridge or water heater; in a paper bag in the sun) for a few more days. This may result in a slightly better extraction, but a perfectly serviceable oil results straight out of the blender, thanks chiefly to the preliminary alcohol extraction. Most herbs work best with this method.

Fresh Plant Oil Infusions. Although fresh plant oil infusions are common, the risk for molding is much greater, and the finished product is often inferior to what the alcohol intermediate can accomplish. The amount of water and resins in a fresh plant may be influential factors. Fresh plant oil infusions need to be subjected to consistent heat and must be watched carefully to identify any fermentation, or subsequent mold invasion. Keeping the oil slurry well ventilated allows the plant moisture to evaporate. Items needed:

- fresh herb
- organic extra virgin olive oil
- serrated knife, pruners, or utility scissors
- cutting board
- scale, bowl, measuring cups

Finely chop the fresh herb with a serrated knife, bypass pruners, or utility scissors. Add the herb and the olive oil to the jar, alternating each, layer by layer, softly stuffing the herb as you go along. Once all the herb is in the jar, finish by fully covering the herb with olive oil. Close the lid and set it in a warm place for at least 4 days. During warm, sunny weather, place it in direct sun in a paper bag, and it may be ready in as little as 3 days. When ready to press (as described for a fresh plant tincture), be careful not to extract water from the plant into your oil—that is to say, don't squeeze too hard. You may feel as if you are sacrificing some of your oil, but you are preventing it from going rancid by keeping the water out. If you do notice water patches in your oil, you can slowly heat it on the stove top at the lowest temperature, or in our hot and dry climate it can be left out in a shallow pan to allow the water to evaporate.

Why not use alcohol in all preparations in order to extract the best medicine? Applying alcohol to a dry herb at a 1:2 ratio will often yield a nicely moistened herb; adding much more alcohol than that is excessive and will create a soup. Dry herbs readily absorb alcohol, whereas fresh herbs do not absorb alcohol. Rather, they become dehydrated by alcohol, leeching their water out into the alcohol, leading to fluid accumulation in the oil, making it susceptible to mold infestation. Heat, to some degree, must take the place of alcohol in a fresh plant extraction. Certain herbs simply turn out better as fresh plant oil infusions.

Salves

A salve is the combination of an herbal infused oil (or animal fat) and beeswax. The greatest utility of a salve is in its protective effects and its ability to act locally. Salves work as a mechanical barrier on open wounds or dry, irritated skin; they are also convenient, allowing the individual to apply the therapy at any time, without having to prepare an infusion, decoction, or poultice.

Herbal oils are the primary ingredients of salves. Salves can be made up of a combination of plants. Mix all the crude herbs and prepare the oil as a formulation, or pour the individual pre-made oils together at the time of making your salve. There is no difference in outcome. It's your choice. Items needed:

- herbal oil infusions
- beeswax
- double boiler
- heat-resistant spatula
- scale, glass bowl, Pyrex measuring cup
- containers for finished salve

Place the glass bowl in the freezer. This will be used to weigh the beeswax. Make space to arrange open salve jars so they are ready to receive the liquid salve; the edge of the table may work best. Begin heating the double boiler. Measure and combine the oil infusions in the double boiler to heat them. Use 1 ounce of beeswax for every 5 ounces of oil infusion for a medium-density salve; use less for a softer salve, more for a harder salve. Measure the beeswax in the glass bowl from the freezer, and add the beeswax to the hot oil when ready (beeswax melts quickly at 160F). Using the spatula, stir in the beeswax until melted. Once fully integrated, pour the oil/beeswax mixture into the Pyrex cup, and quickly but carefully pour the liquid salve into the containers. Place your salve in the freezer for 5 minutes to harden it, so you can test the consistency. If you find it too soft, then you can add more beeswax. If it's too hard, add more oil. Salves remain effective for many years away from heat and light.

Herbal energetics

This is a vast subject, but I will endeavor here to introduce some of the basics. Various advanced systems of healing from around the globe have evolved around knowledge of the fundamental building blocks of Nature. Although this varies somewhat from culture to culture, there are some basic universal concepts. The most basic may be deemed the 4 Qualities of cold, hot, moist, and dry. Additionally, 3, 4, or 5 Humours, or Elements, may be seen as the basic building blocks of all life in the universe. For example, in Ayurvedic medicine, the 3 Humours are *Phlegm*, *Bile*, and *Wind*. These 3 humours are present in all things, thus are manifest in plants, places, and humans alike, in a myriad of combinations. We, too, can perceive the Humours as they

present themselves throughout the seasons with variability, yet in a fluid, emerging pattern. Thus, the effects of herbs can be witnessed within the triad of reflection occurring at any given time between the person, place, and plant.

4 Basic Qualities

Cold

Hot

Moist

Dry

Humours

Ayurvedic Humours

Phlegm

Bile

Wind

Galenic Humours

Phlegm

Blood

Yellow Bile

Black Bile

Flavors

Ayurvedic Rasa

Sweet—heavy, cold

Acid—heavy, hot

Salty—heavy, hot

Acrid—light, hot

Bitter—light, cold

Astringent—light, cold

Additionally, herbs can be viewed as having affinities for certain organs. Thus, their energetics are generally directed toward those organs, or are likely to affect those organs. More advanced herbal pairing takes into consideration these organ affinities alongside the prominent qualities, humours, and flavors present in each herb. Tasting herbs and spending time with them in their native habitat can teach us so much about the energetics of plants.

Safety concerns

Nothing is entirely safe in this world, so why should herbs be any different? Knowledge of plant usage since ancient times is extensive across the globe. Although we are emerging from a relative Dark Age of herbalism, many are present among us to guide the way. Following the example of experienced herbalists, asking elders within your community, consulting local plant experts, and reviewing the ethnobotanical literature is due diligence toward reestablishing a healthy and vibrant personal relationship with plants. Be sure of what you are gathering and—always—begin by consuming a very small amount. Toxic plants do exist, but the vast majority of plant poisonings are due to negligence and carelessness that ignored reason, common sense, and basic awareness. Take your time. There are abundant safe herbs available for us, and relatively few toxic plants. Rather than emphasize what is toxic in this book (as nearly every herbal does), I will emphasize following a path of awareness and sound reason. Although its 112 plant profiles may be enough for many to begin gathering, *this book is not a direct invitation to gather herbs*. Rather, it is an invitation to develop a relationship with your home landscape through stillness, listening, and continued observation. As we open our awareness once again to the stories Mother Nature has to tell us, we become educated in her expressions of fluidity and her subtle and unexpected commands.

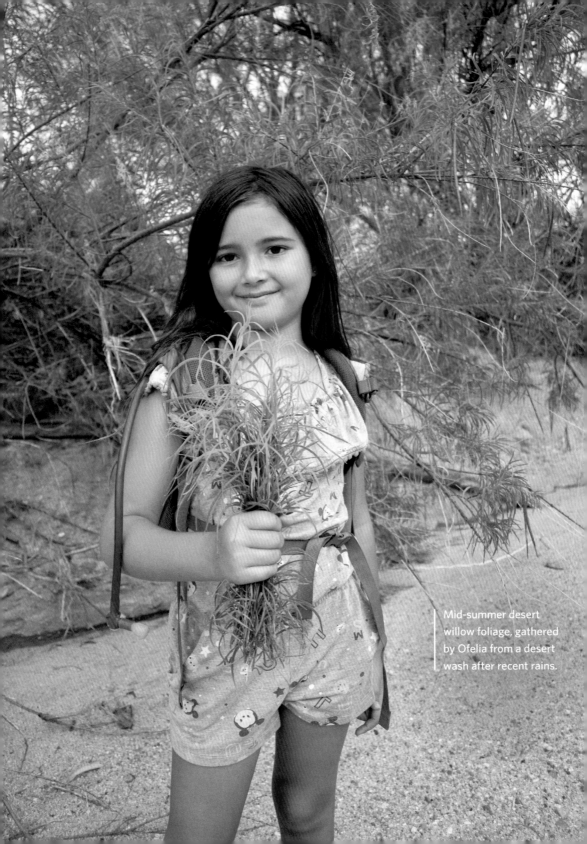

Mid-summer desert willow foliage, gathered by Ofelia from a desert wash after recent rains.

WILDHARVESTING WITH THE SEASONS

Each season engenders a particular feeling within each of us—its own memories, smells, desires, and dreams. These sensations are all indicative of the medicine within a season, or, in turn, our own tendencies toward illness. Seasons can be viewed as a collection of elements continually presenting themselves to us in a consistent pattern, albeit in infinite subtle variations. Spending time observing the plants through the seasons imparts in us a sense of wholeness through a fluid continuum of this expression of life.

I'd like to frame the seasons in a particular way for you to follow throughout your experience of this book. In our culture, seasons are often seen as beginning on a certain date on the calendar; however approximately accurate that may be, I'd like to reframe it. The conventional way we view the beginning of a season is, in fact, the height of that season. For instance, when we say the "beginning of spring" is 20 March (or whenever the vernal equinox falls in a given year), we are actually witnessing the *height* of spring. For spring begins roughly 7 weeks before that, halfway between winter solstice and the vernal equinox—a time my Irish ancestors referred to as Imbolc (1 or 2 February), which was marked by the calving season and the reappearance of sheep's milk in the local diet. In turn, the beginning of summer would occur around May Day (1 May) or the feast of Bealtaine, as spring began its quiet retreat and summer's heat increased with lengthening days. The full flowering of summer then heralded the fruits of late summer and early autumn. Thus, we experience an overlapping presence of seasons in a dance, an ebb and flow, which speaks to the tremendous variety and vitality present in all Nature, present within ourselves.

Some may say the Southwest possesses no seasons, but in the Sonoran desert, for example, we recognize 5 distinct seasons. These seasons are distinctly, or slightly, different as one moves across our region's landscape.

Throughout the Southwest, winter is relatively cold and damp. The higher the elevation, and the further north you go, the greater the likelihood of snow. The southernmost, lowest deserts experience very little freezing temperatures, but the longer nights grow considerably colder. Spring emerges in stages, again continuing northward and up in elevation as the months move on. The late spring is exceptionally humid in central Texas, but grows drier and hotter from the Chihuahuan desert westward, all the way to the southern California deserts. High-elevation conifer forests are often moist throughout the year, relying upon snowmelt during the relatively dry late spring weather. Monsoon rains grace the Sonoran and Chihuahuan deserts roughly June through October, whereas the southern California desert generally remains dry throughout this period. From north-central Texas up into Oklahoma, the tendency is for drier winters with more rainfall in the warmer months (particularly April–June), but rainfall is possible any time of the year.

In short, moisture can be found somewhere in the Southwest at any time of the year; but due to occasional drought conditions, nearly the entire region can experience dry spells simultaneously.

As you spend time in your local environment walking the land, observing, and feeling, you will be developing an internal catalog of experiences, an individualized and intimate language that will forever serve you in your continually deepening awareness and progression of knowledge. To understand plants in a strictly literal context—excluding their natural state of being and the elements that surround and create them, season by season—is a very limited understanding. As you begin to feel the seasons within you and become familiar with their emerging characteristics, you will be awakening to the language of our ancestors, still alive within you and all around you in the natural world, thus accessing the subtler knowledge of *how* plants heal. Nature as a whole conspires to bring us back to a state of harmony, continually calling us back to this state, season by season, blossom by blossom, carrying us to the ocean of our belonging, to the greatness of emerging creation itself.

Note: in the seasonal lists that follow, unless a specific plant part is mentioned, presume that all parts of the plant listed in its profile may be gathered at this time.

WINTER

We now celebrate our New Year in the heart of the winter season. In past ages, many of our ancestors viewed this as a midpoint, a gathering of energies, a time of great potency. The sun reaches its lowest point on the horizon during the winter solstice, and the days grow longer over the next 6 months. The further north you go, the more noticeable the difference. We experience varying degrees of winter in the Southwest, from several feet of snow on the ground for months at high-elevation conifer forests, to only a handful of freezing nights at the lowest sunbelt elevations. Illustrating the significant difference between these two life zones, one can find the same annual plants growing at high elevations in the summer that grow at lower elevations during the winter. As always, habitat observation is key in discovering what the area around your home offers. Gathering of medicinal plants in the

Southwest can continue well into the winter season; however, wildharvesting is most often curtailed from late November to mid-January (even longer at the higher elevations) throughout our region.

Winter begins as the nights grow cold and noticeably long and dark. This is the time my Irish ancestors knew as Samhain, from which the modern holiday of Halloween is derived. This time is associated with the process of beginning the descent into quiet tranquility within oneself. As we look at the natural world around us, we can see something similar occurring: many plants become senescent and drop what is no longer necessary (their leaves), drawing their life force deeper into their root system within the Earth. A quiet stillness ensues.

Seeking to harmonize with this particular season, we seek the quiet stillness of our own bedroom, or the cozy couch beside the fireplace at night. This is a time of beginning. Walking through the desert, mountains, or river grove, we hear the stillness present around us. Our world becomes smaller, our focus more internal, our senses more attuned to the steady rising of the breath as the cool, crisp air of winter strikes the surface of our lungs, bracing us and perking us up. Trees and shrubs become identifiable by their buds, twig and bark patterns, or perhaps the persistent fruits left behind to nourish overwintering cardinals or the stalwart squirrels of the conifer belt.

In winter, contemplate all that you have witnessed throughout the preceding seasons, and meditate on what you seek to create and experience in the coming half of the year. Take note of the new plant friends you have made, and visit their graves in the dead of winter, paying homage to their lives while bidding them return once again as their season comes into fruition.

Winter plants by habitat

Desert, Desert Grasslands, Cactus Forests

canyon bursage root
cottonwood leaf bud
desert lavender
desert willow bark
goatbush stem
golden smoke
hopbush leaf
ocotillo bark
queen's root
rhatany root

Disturbed Areas, Gardens, Trailsides, Clearings

chickweed
curly dock leaf
desert willow bark
evening primrose leaf, root
filaree
mallow leaf, root
nettle leaf
shepherd's purse
sow thistle leaf, root
thistle root

High Plains

cottonwood leaf bud
desert willow bark

Hill Country

curly dock leaf
nettle leaf
thistle root
yucca root

Oak Woodlands

dandelion
manzanita leaf
yucca root

Prairie: North-Central Texas
and Oklahoma

  chickweed
  cottonwood leaf bud
  dandelion
  evening primrose leaf, root

Rivers and Canyons

  cottonwood leaf bud
  dandelion
  desert willow bark
  evening primrose leaf, root
  filaree
  monkey flower
  thistle

South Texas Plains

  goatbush stem
  nettle leaf
  thistle

SPRING

Observing my local habitat, I've discovered numerous events that indicate spring has begun. In addition to the initial wafts of warm breezes arriving on the morning air, desert anemone blossoms may begin to open along with the dangly male (staminate) flowers of jojoba and the tiny cream-colored hopbush flowers, tinged with magenta.

A bursting forth of vibrancy across the landscape is characteristic of spring. I'm sure the reader has felt this very same thing, deep within. As irrepressible life re-emerges, reclaiming the right to grow up and out across the landscape, herbalists are enticed to partake of Nature's succulent offerings, re-enacting an ancient and sacred rite. Spring's verdancy is resplendent in myriad ways—even in the desert Southwest. Down in the desert washes, male and female flower

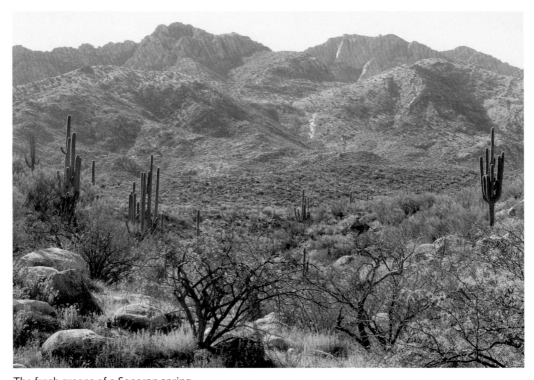

The fresh greens of a Sonoran spring.

buds of cottonwood often open at the full moon of mid- to late February. As the landscape reawakens, there's a singing and dancing among the insects, birds, and mammals. The presence of the creative force of Nature becomes apparent once again across the land. As the calendar moves into May, spring extends up the mountainsides to higher elevations when tree buds such as aspen and oak begin to open.

Within our own bodies, the liver and gall bladder respond to the spring season most actively. Their harmonious activity is responsible for our own foresight, initiative, and impulse to grow and create across the landscape. Distributing our nutrients and moving our blood throughout the body, they spur us toward courageous action. When excessive, these actions breed disharmony within us. Proper equilibrium is maintained through thoughtful contemplation and clear vision, leading to the benefit of all through this natural expression of the self. Through quiet observation of our local environment, we begin to harmonize with it. We can see its qualities reflected back to us, bringing insights to our state of health.

Spring plants by habitat

Desert, Desert Grasslands, Cactus Forests

- algerita
- anemone
- ash leaf
- bricklebush
- brittlebush
- California poppy
- canyon bursage leaf
- cáscara sagrada bark
- chia
- cholla
- copperleaf (southern California)
- desert cotton
- desert lavender
- desert willow
- elder leaf, flower
- estafiate
- evening primrose leaf, root
- filaree
- flor de tierra
- globemallow
- golden smoke
- hackberry
- jojoba
- kidneywood bark
- manzanita leaf
- mock vervain
- monkey flower
- Mormon tea
- mulberry leaf, fruit
- ocotillo
- oreganillo
- plantain
- prickly pear flower
- red root
- rhatany
- sage
- thistle
- wild buckwheat
- wild tobacco
- yerba santa
- yucca

Disturbed Areas, Gardens, Trailsides, Clearings

- Bermudagrass
- chickweed
- curly dock
- dandelion
- desert willow
- evening primrose leaf, root
- filaree
- globemallow
- mallow
- Mexican palo verde

mock vervain
mullein root
nettle leaf
oat (milky seed)
plantain
prickly pear flower
shepherd's purse
Siberian elm
sow thistle
sweet clover
thistle
tree of heaven bark
wild tobacco
yerba santa

High Desert

algerita
bricklebush
cholla
curly dock
desert willow flower
estafiate
evening primrose leaf, root
filaree
monkey flower
Mormon tea
pine inner bark
queen's root
rhatany
Siberian elm
thistle
wild buckwheat
yucca root

High-Elevation Conifer Forest

alder leaf, stem
anemone
Arizona cypress
aspen catkin
betony
cow parsnip root
elder leaf
evening primrose leaf, root
filaree
fireweed
globemallow
horsetail
mallow
mock vervain
monkey flower
mullein root
nettle leaf
pine inner bark
plantain
red root
thistle
violet
wild buckwheat
yucca

High Plains

algerita root, fruit
bricklebush
curly dock
desert willow bark, leaf,
  flower
estafiate
globemallow
mock vervain
plantain
prickly pear flower
rhatany
thistle
yucca

Hill Country

alder leaf, stem
algerita root, fruit
anemone
ash leaf
beebalm
blazing star
bricklebush
camphorweed
cáscara sagrada bark
curly dock
elder leaf, flower
estafiate
fanpetals
flor de tierra
globemallow
goldenrod
hackberry
hawthorn
hop tree leaf
horsetail
inmortál
kidneywood bark
mock vervain
mulberry leaf, fruit
nettle leaf
plantain
prickly ash bark, leaf
prickly pear flower
prickly poppy
queen's root
rhatany
sage
silk tassel
skullcap
sweet clover
thistle
walnut leaf
violet
yarrow
yucca

Oak Woodlands

algerita root, fruit
anemone
bricklebush
cáscara sagrada bark
cholla
estafiate
evening primrose leaf, root
filaree
flor de tierra
globemallow
goldenrod
inmortál
manzanita leaf
mock vervain
monkey flower
mulberry leaf, fruit
nettle leaf
pine inner bark
plantain
prickly pear flower
red root
rhatany
sage
silk tassel
skullcap
thistle
violet
wild buckwheat
yerba santa
yucca

Prairie: North-Central Texas and Oklahoma

anemone
ash leaf
beebalm
blazing star
bricklebush
cáscara sagrada bark
chickweed
curly dock leaf
dandelion
elder leaf, flower
estafiate
goldenrod
golden smoke
hackberry
hawthorn
mock vervain
mulberry leaf, fruit
mullein root
plantain
prickly poppy
queen's root
rhatany
sage
yarrow

Rivers and Canyons

alder leaf, stem
Arizona cypress
ash leaf
bricklebush
curly dock
dandelion
desert willow leaf, flower
elder leaf, flower
estafiate
evening primrose leaf, root
filaree

goldenrod
hackberry
hawthorn
hop tree leaf
horsetail
mock vervain
monkey flower
nettle leaf
oat
oreganillo
plantain
silk tassel
skullcap
thistle
walnut leaf
wild tobacco
willow bark
yerba mansa

South Texas Plains

algerita fruit
ash leaf
beebalm
blazing star
cáscara sagrada bark
estafiate
fanpetals
golden smoke
mock vervain
nettle leaf
plantain
prickly pear flower
prickly poppy
sage
skullcap
thistle
yarrow

SUMMER

There are two summers in the Southwest, a dry summer and a wet summer. In the central part of our region, the wet summer follows the dry summer, often beginning late June or early July. Conversely, from central Texas northward, the dry summer follows the wet summer. In southern California's desert region, rains cease around April and don't return until late autumn, early winter. Given elevation changes from below sea level to over 12,000 feet, our region offers a floral variety that rivals most of the continent. In the warmest and wettest areas of the Southwest, this results in seasonally tropical habitats—and summer is the time to explore this variety.

The dryness of the desert is akin to the proverbial clean slate. When the rains appear once again, baptizing the earth with their life-giving magic, seeds begin to sprout and perennial plants come alive again. This dynamic is tempered by the long, hot days of summer, challenging our bodies to stay cool and keep our internal organs properly moistened and nourished amid the searing temperatures. Inactivity, a form of hibernation, is often the best way to deal with this heat. Upon the first indications of autumn's arrival in early August, our bodies feel a sense of relief; however, it will be a couple more months of heat before the nights are consistently cool enough to begin recharging our batteries.

Exposing our bare skin to the sun is necessary for our well-being, but if we are overexposed we can suffer. Just as in winter, moderation is more challenging in summer.

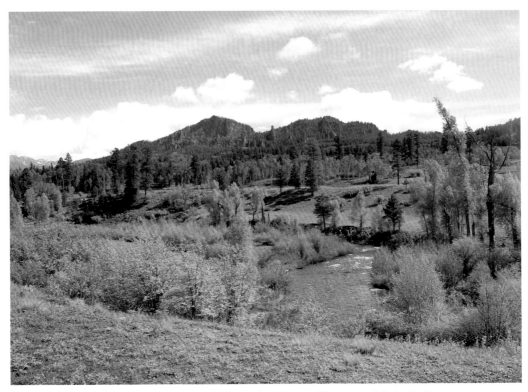

Spending time near water, tall trees, and moist earth is essential for our well-being in the summer.

Observe the habits of indigenous peoples and the creatures native to your area to better understand how to moderate the effects of the extreme seasons.

As the *chubascos* (monsoon rains) drench the desert and pour down from the mountains, rivers and streams swell. A fullness is experienced by the landscape and the animals alike. Damp conditions become prominent and are exacerbated within those who carry dampness, or who dwell in more humid locations. Look to drying and cooling herbs (curly dock, Mormon tea, creosote bush) for topical and internal use when hot, damp weather aggravates skin conditions, respiratory problems, autoimmune conditions, or digestive disorders. Observe the effects of the weather patterns on your physical body, mental body, or emotional body. Noticing and acknowledging what is present before you lends a subtle power to your well-being. Your ability to make sound choices in advance of illness or harm, a skill that is rarely developed or communicated within our current cultural framework, will expand and grow in complexity.

The long days of summer can be spent exploring new terrain, gathering an abundance of herbal material, and processing robust and powerful medicines to store away for the seasons to come.

Summer plants by habitat

Desert, Desert Grasslands, Cactus Forests

algerita leaf, fruit
bricklebush leaf
brittlebush leaf, sap
buttonbush
camphorweed
cholla
cleavers
copperleaf

creosote bush
cudweed
desert lavender
desert willow leaf
elder berry
estafiate
evening primrose flower
fanpetals
prickly poppy
red root stem, flower
snakeweed

Disturbed Areas, Gardens, Trailsides, Clearings

agrimony
Arizona cypress leaf
beebalm
Bermudagrass
camphorweed
chaste tree
chickweed
cleavers
copperleaf
cudweed
curly dock leaf
desert willow leaf
evening primrose flower
fanpetals
gumweed
horseweed
mullein flower
oxeye daisy
pearly everlasting
puncture vine
self-heal
sweet clover
tickseed

High Desert

algerita leaf, fruit
blazing star flower
bricklebush
camphorweed
cleavers

cudweed
desert willow leaf, flower
elder
estafiate
evening primrose leaf, flower
filaree
globemallow
goldenrod
gumweed
horseweed
monkey flower
plantain
prickly pear
prickly poppy
rosemary mint
sage
snakeweed
thistle
yucca

High-Elevation Conifer Forest

agrimony
alder leaf, stem, catkin
algerita leaf, fruit
Arizona cypress leaf
aspen bark
beebalm
betony
bricklebush
chickweed
chokecherry fruit
cleavers
copperleaf
cow parsnip seed
cranesbill
cudweed
curly dock leaf
elder
evening primrose flower
figwort
fireweed
golden smoke
horsetail
horseweed
mullein flower
oshá root
pearly everlasting
red root stem, flower
sage
skullcap
spikenard leaf, fruit
wild mint
yarrow

High Plains

algerita leaf, fruit
beebalm
blazing star
bricklebush
buttonbush
camphorweed
chickweed
copperleaf
cranesbill
curly dock leaf
desert willow leaf
estafiate
golden smoke
gumweed
horseweed
snakeweed
yarrow

Hill Country

- alder catkin
- algerita leaf
- anemone
- beebalm
- blazing star
- bricklebush
- buttonbush
- camphorweed
- chaste tree berry
- chickweed
- cleavers
- copperleaf
- cranesbill
- cudweed
- curly dock leaf
- elder berry
- estafiate
- fanpetals
- gumweed
- horsetail
- horseweed
- passionflower
- thistle
- tickseed
- walnut hull
- yarrow

Oak Woodlands

- algerita leaf, fruit
- beebalm
- betony
- bricklebush
- cleavers
- copperleaf
- cranesbill
- cudweed
- curly dock leaf
- estafiate
- evening primrose flower
- horseweed
- passionflower
- plantain
- red root stem, flower
- tickseed
- wild oregano

Prairie: North-Central Texas and Oklahoma

- agrimony
- alder leaf, stem, catkin
- beebalm
- blazing star flower
- bricklebush leaf
- buttonbush
- chickweed
- chokecherry fruit
  (late summer)
- cleavers
- cranesbill
- cudweed
- elder
- estafiate
- figwort
- gumweed
- horseweed
- lobelia
- snakeweed

Rivers and Canyons

- agrimony
- alder leaf, stem
- Bermudagrass
- bricklebush
- buttonbush
- camphorweed
- chokecherry fruit
- cleavers
- copperleaf
- cudweed
- curly dock leaf
- desert willow leaf
- elder
- estafiate
- evening primrose leaf, flower
- horsetail
- horseweed
- lobelia
- Mormon tea
- passionflower
- self-heal
- tickseed
- walnut hull
- wild mint

South Texas Plains

- algerita leaf, fruit
- beebalm
- blazing star flower
- camphorweed
- cleavers
- copperleaf
- cranesbill
- creosote bush leaf, stem,
  flower
- cudweed
- estafiate
- fanpetals
- goatbush fruit
- horseweed
- passionflower

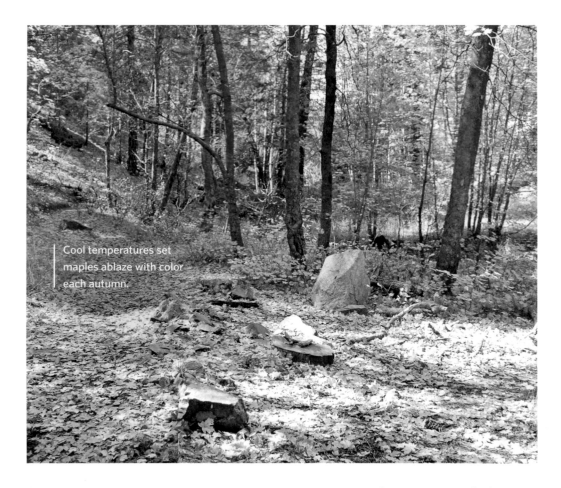

Cool temperatures set maples ablaze with color each autumn.

AUTUMN

In the desert Southwest, the first hint of autumn comes on the cool, dry breezes of the early morning air at the beginning of August. By mid-autumn, at the autumnal equinox, the nights may show their first hint of cool crispness, yet they are still followed by warm, dry days. These days may be interspersed by heavy rains from offshore hurricanes, or chilly, damp weather that heralds the winter season to come. On either side of these wet spells, a warm, dry "mini spring" occurs in mid- to late autumn (mid-September to mid-October); perennial plants may put out new growth just as they would in spring, annual plants germinate, and some plants may attempt to flower once more before the arrival of winter and its shorter days of limited light.

In southern California, the rainy season begins by late autumn; in the eastern portion of our region, the summer rains continue through autumn and into winter again.

Autumn is a time of scaling back our energy output and gathering what has come to fruition. A time to begin reflecting on what we have endeavored to create and where we have ventured over the previous two seasons of expansion, while we appreciate the fruits of our labor. It is a time of richness in the fat of the land, and a time for appreciating all that we have been given.

Wild animals move about the land gathering up winter provisions to be stored within their bodies, in the earth, or in tree trunks. Many tiny life forms begin to transition, leaving their carcasses behind to replenish the soil which will nourish the new life to come.

As herbalists, our attention may shift toward root, seed, and bark medicines as some of the last flowers of the year make their appearance and transition into seed. Some medicines may come from our gardens, while others can be found only in the wild. These stands must be protected, looked after, and our deep gratitude continually offered to show our appreciation and encourage growth and renewal. The concentrated energy in root and seed is made into medicine as tincture, honey, or oil infusion, or dried for tea. Roots macerate on the shelf in a dark corner, slowly imbuing the solvent with their medicine, drop by drop.

The essence of these wild medicines will one day provide relief to those in need. The beauty of this circle of life is experienced in the form of healing by the humble plant friends we have come to know throughout the seasons.

Autumn plants by habitat

Desert, Desert Grasslands, Cactus Forests

algerita root
ash bark
canyon bursage root
cáscara sagrada bark
cholla root
creosote bush
desert lavender
desert willow bark, leaf
elder leaf
estafiate
evening primrose flower, root, seed
fanpetals

ocotillo bark
oreganillo
pecan fruit
prickly pear fruit
thistle root

Disturbed Areas, Gardens, Trailsides, Clearings

American licorice
Bermudagrass
curly dock root
desert willow leaf
evening primrose flower, root, seed
fanpetals
mallow
nettle seed
plantain
prickly pear fruit
sow thistle
thistle root

High Desert

algerita root
American licorice
blazing star root
cholla root
curly dock root
estafiate
evening primrose root, seed
juniper berry
prickly pear fruit
thistle root

High-Elevation Conifer Forest

alder bark
algerita root
aspen bark
chokecherry bark
evening primrose root, seed
juniper berry
mallow root
nettle root, seed
oshá root
plantain

spikenard root
thistle root
violet
yarrow root

High Plains

blazing star root
cholla root
curly dock root
desert willow leaf
   (uncommon)
echinacea root
estafiate
prickly pear fruit
thistle root

Hill Country

algerita root
alder bark
ash bark
blazing star root
cáscara sagrada bark
curly dock root
elder leaf
estafiate
fanpetals
hop tree bark
inmortál
juniper berry
nettle seed
pecan fruit
plantain
prickly ash fruit
prickly pear fruit
thistle root
violet

Oak Woodlands

algerita root
American licorice
   (southern Utah and
   southwestern Colorado)
cáscara sagrada bark
cholla root
estafiate
evening primrose
inmortál
juniper berry
monkey flower
nettle seed
prickly pear fruit
thistle root
violet

Prairie: North-Central Texas and Oklahoma

ash bark
blazing star root
cáscara sagrada bark
chokecherry bark
curly dock root
echinacea root
estafiate
juniper berry
mallow
plantain
thistle root
violet

Rivers and Canyons

American licorice
alder bark
ash bark
Bermudagrass
chokecherry bark
cottonwood bark
curly dock leaf, root
desert willow leaf
elder leaf
estafiate
evening primrose
hop tree bark
juniper berry
monkey flower
nettle seed
oreganillo
pecan
thistle root

South Texas Plains

algerita root
ash bark
blazing star root
cáscara sagrada bark
creosote bush
estafiate
fanpetals
nettle seed
prickly pear fruit
thistle root

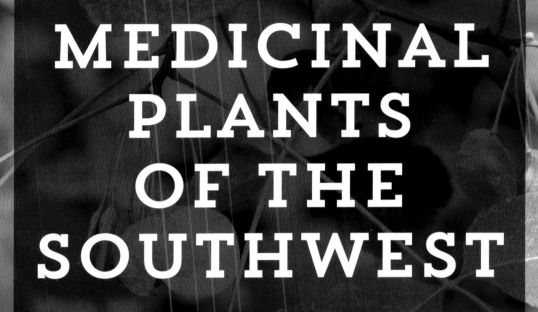

MEDICINAL PLANTS OF THE SOUTHWEST

agrimony

Agrimonia striata
PARTS USED aerial

Agrimony soothes and relaxes where tension breeds anxiety and frustration. Relaxing the liver, it brings warmth, through increased circulation, throughout the body.

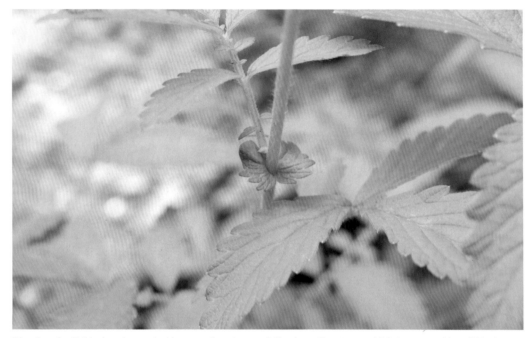

The deeply divided and serrated leaves of agrimony fully clasp the stem, which is covered in stiff hairs.

How to identify

This herbaceous perennial has alternate leaves with serrated margins; the 7–13 oddly pinnate leaflets of each leaf are softly fuzzy on the underside. When first emerging, agrimony can be difficult to distinguish from *Potentilla* species (such that even herbarium specimens are frequently incorrect), so wait until the terminal flowering raceme begins to emerge, which clearly distinguishes agrimony from *Potentilla* and other high-elevation rose family relatives; nonetheless, the uses between *Agrimonia* and *Potentilla* are thought to be interchangeable (Wood 1997). Maturing at 20–40 inches tall, agrimony stands out amongst the surrounding lush vegetation once its tiny, 5-petaled yellow flowers begin to open. These are followed by small, round achenes with stiff burrs upon maturity.

Where, when, and how to wildcraft

Agrimony occurs abundantly in our high-elevation conifer forests. Look to shaded, moist areas, often alongside mountain

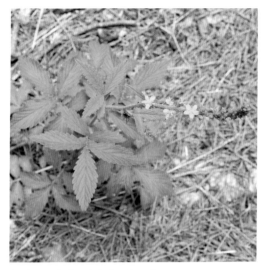

Agrimony's 5-petaled yellow flowers appear on terminal spikes by mid-summer.

streams. It can also be found (along with *Agrimonia parviflora*) in shaded areas of the plains of Oklahoma. Flowering begins mid-summer and continues into late summer. Gather the flowering stems and process fresh for tincture, if desired, or dry loosely in the shade for tea, or dry plant tincture.

Medicinal uses

All the species within our region have been used for medicine. Traditionally, agrimony has been used as an infusion to treat fever, build the blood, help soothe and limit vaginal discharge or diarrhea, and address various digestive complaints. Drink the hot infusion daily to improve leaky gut. It has been snuffed for nosebleeds and employed as an anti-emetic and, conversely, an emetic. In my own experience, I find it to be warming and relaxing, and a bit drying. Increasing the circulation initially, it brings a sensation of warmth throughout the body, which may relieve musculoskeletal pain or anxiety (particularly in cold, deficient states). The experience of increased blood flow links agrimony to the liver, further relating it to the female reproductive system, digestive complaints, and traditional applications of having "too much gall." From an Ayurvedic perspective, this plant calms wind and enhances the fluidity of the bile humour. In Chinese medicine, it is used to reduce liver and gall bladder heat/constriction. It's also astringent to the urinary tract, and it's specific for kidney ailments as well as pain in the lumbar region passing through to the abdomen. Try agrimony for restricted breathing, tension headaches, or migraine. As a Bach flower remedy, agrimony is used when one hides their true feelings behind a cheerful facade. Applying the tea or tincture for tense, aggravated states will also prove beneficial.

Future harvests

Modest gathering practices (2 of every 10 flowering stems) will support the longevity of this plant in areas where it is already established. Consider digging up rhizomes in the autumn to replant in suitable locations.

HERBAL PREPARATIONS

Herb Tea
Standard Infusion
Drink 4–8 ounces, up to 3 times per day.

Flower/Leaf/Stem Tincture
1 part fresh herb, by weight
2 parts menstruum (95% alcohol),
   by volume
or
1 part dry herb, by weight
5 parts menstruum (50% alcohol,
   50% spring water), by volume
Take 25 drops to 3ml, up to 5 times per day.

alder

Alnus incana ssp. *tenuifolia*, *A. oblongifolia*
alamillo
PARTS USED bark, leaf, stem, catkin

This age-old remedy offers a mild flavor and an array of medicinal applications. Apply in cases of skin rashes, chronic infections, swellings, sore joints, leaky gut, and much more.

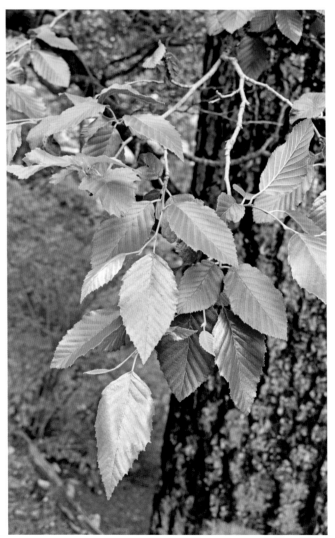

All alders have alternate leaves with doubly serrated margins.

How to identify

Alder grows in two basic forms within our region—a tall tree (30–160 feet high) with a single trunk, or a shrubby tree (no more than 25 feet tall) with multiple thin trunks. All *Alnus* species have alternate leaves that are doubly serrated (the teeth have teeth). *Alnus incana* ssp. *tenuifolia* has narrower leaves, which are often rounded and lobed at the base; the leaves of *A. oblongifolia* are elliptic, oblong, or lance-shaped. The longer male catkins and cone-like female catkins occur on the same tree and appear in late autumn; they remain on the tree until they open in spring. The female catkins linger on the tree through summer and are brick-red upon maturity. The bark is dark gray and smooth, breaking up into oddly shaped flat plates as the tree ages. When elk and deer scratch their growing, itching antlers against an alder in the spring, they may reveal the bright reddish orange inner bark beneath.

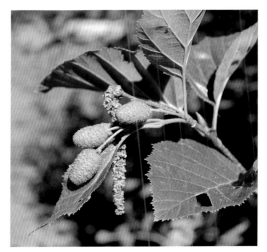
Alder inflorescences appear in late autumn and open the following spring.

Where, when, and how to wildcraft

This noble tree grows near water. Look streamside at mid- to high elevations in the central portion of our region. *Alnus serrulata* and *A. maritima* are occasionally found along the eastern edge of our region from Austin northward. The leaves and stems are best gathered in the spring; the catkins can be gathered late summer. For direction on harvesting bark, see "Gathering Tree Medicine" (page 25).

Medicinal uses

Alder has been used medicinally all over the world for centuries, if not millennia. Internally, it's been used to alleviate allergies, diarrhea, constipation, urinary tract infections (UTIs), rheumatism, colds, asthma, cough, tuberculosis, muscle spasms, anemia, fever, and the pains of childbirth. Topically, it alleviates joint pain and pain from sprains, strains, and bruises; helps heal ulcers, skin rashes and infections, burns, and wounds; and is used as a wash for sore eyes or the skin irritations of a sensitive baby, including thrush.

Clinically, we can apply it to stimulate lymphatic movement, address stagnation in the liver (hepatic steatosis, jaundice), or help resolve mycobacterial infections. As a relaxing astringent with anti-inflammatory and wound-healing properties, consider combining it with agrimony, horseweed, and estafiate for leaky gut.

Due to the presence of diarylheptanoids throughout the genus, researchers are looking into the various anticancer actions of alder bark preparations. Interestingly, this research has unveiled alder bark's ability to protect the body's healthy cells during chemotherapy. The bark is slightly bitter and astringent as a tea, but combines well with other herbs and mushrooms. Include demulcent herbs (mallow) or aromatic spices (ginger, cinnamon, fennel) for flavor and effect. It is safe for regular long-term use.

Future harvests

Gather with care. Trim only young branches, or seek out recently fallen branches after a storm.

HERBAL PREPARATIONS

Bark Tea
Standard Decoction
Drink 2–4 ounces, up to 3 times per day; apply topically, as needed.

Leaf/Stem Tea
Standard Infusion
Drink 2–4 ounces, up to 3 times per day; apply topically, as needed.

Leaf/Stem/Catkin Tincture
1 part fresh herb, by weight
2 parts menstruum (95% alcohol),
   by volume
Take 10–30 drops, up to 4 times per day.

Mahonia species (*Berberis* species)
agarita, palo amarillo, yerba de la sangre, desert barberry, grape root
PARTS USED leaf, stem, root, fruit

This cooling, bitter remedy is useful for infections of the skin and digestive system and excellent for premenstrual bloating and discomfort.

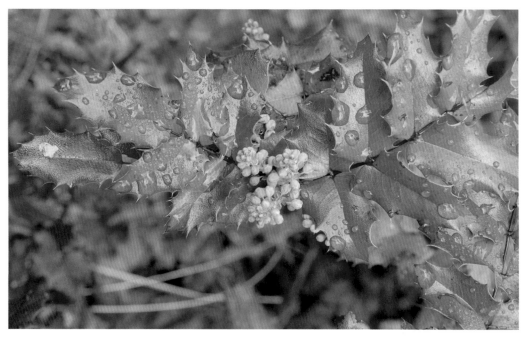

The pinnately compound, serrated leaves of *Mahonia wilcoxii* often turn blood-red from winter into spring as the plant begins to flower; its ripe fruits are light blue.

How to identify

Thick, leathery leaves with sharply toothed margins help identify our *Mahonia* species, which occur in a wide range of ecosystems and in various forms. The low-growing *M. repens* often occupies pine and fir forests at mid- to high elevations. *Mahonia wilcoxii*, a variably creeping to very tall, spindly forest understory plant, is confined to the Sky Islands of southeastern Arizona and southwestern New Mexico at middle elevations.

The larger, bushy (4–15 feet tall) species, *M. fremontii*, *M. haematocarpa*, and *M. trifoliolata*, prefer sun exposure. The spiny leaves are pinnately compound, with 3–9 leaflets depending on the species, and may be rather square or elongated in shape; they may turn a deep burnt orange or red in winter, *M. repens* in particular (hence *yerba de la sangre*, "herb of the blood"). Clusters of bright yellow 6-petaled flowers appear from the leaf axils from late winter to mid-spring. Algerita's

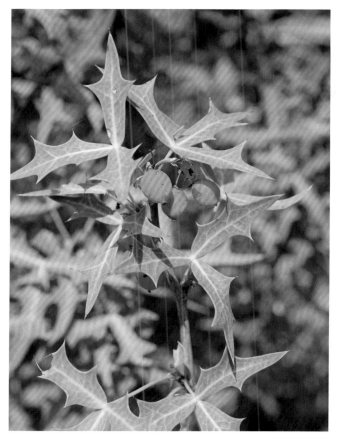

Mahonia trifoliolata's juicy berries ripen to a bright red.

encountered at the right time as they don't remain on the plant for very long—they're consumed quickly by critters. The berries ripen from late spring to mid-summer, depending upon the species and location. The roots may be gathered at any time of the year, but the optimal time would be early autumn to early winter, after the fruits have fully ripened and fallen off the bush. Early spring, pre-flowering, is another optimal time to gather the roots. Depending on the species and the particular growing conditions, lower stems can also be used in addition to the roots. Occasionally, one may derive medicine from brightly colored stems alone. Generally, it is not necessary to dig up the entire plant. For shrubby types, simply probe the ground 2–5 feet from the plant's base, moving in a circle around it. Once a distal root is encountered, begin to pull it up back to the base of the plant and cut it off near the root crown. Depending on the size of the plant, and its current vitality, one can sustainably gather 1–5 root pieces this way. For creeping types (*M. repens*, *M. wilcoxii*), select a plant and dig around it, loosening the root crown and surrounding rhizomes from the soil. Pull it up and out of the soil until another plant is reached and cut within 10 inches of its end. Chop the root pieces while still fresh, as they will dry very hard.

wood, particularly its roots, is tinged light to bright yellow, almost orange when fresh, indicating the presence of berberine in the plant. The berries may be semi-solid or hollow, depending on the species; they range from yellow, red, and purplish red to dark blue or purple in color.

Where, when, and how to wildcraft

One *Mahonia* species or another can be found scattered throughout our region, including desert grasslands, cactus forests, oak woodlands, high desert, conifer forests, and canyon edges, but it is absent from Oklahoma and most of the high plains. The leaves can be gathered at any time, but the berries must be

Medicinal uses

Our Southwest *Mahonia* species offer a wide variety of medicinal applications. Apply

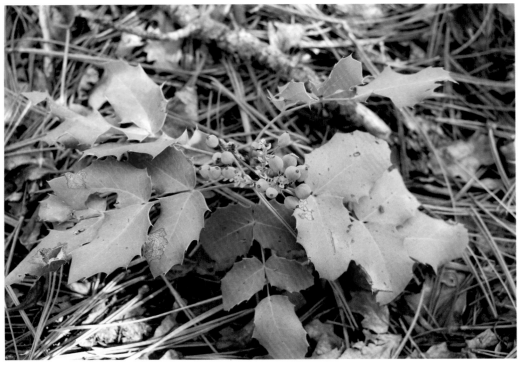

Mahonia repens, grape root, is our low-growing species often occupying pine and fir forests, as pictured in this photo.

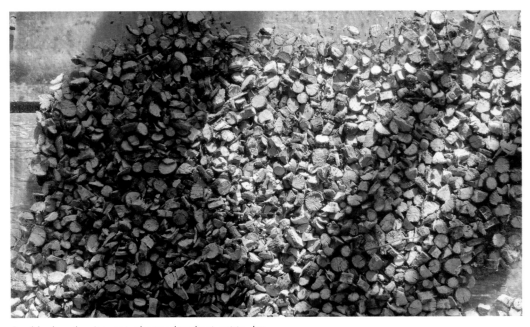

Freshly dug algerita root, chopped and set out to dry.

algerita in damp, hot conditions, topically and internally. These conditions may be of the skin, digestive tract, reproductive system, or urinary tract, for example, and are likely to be acute in nature. Specific examples include sores, bites, stings, boils, cellulitis, intestinal infections causing diarrhea, strep throat, certain UTIs, or PMS with bloating. Combine algerita tea or tincture with goatbush, tree of heaven, or creosote bush for parasitic gut infections.

Used internally, algerita tincture may help to relieve sensations of cold at the extremities, gradually, when this is caused by a deficient type of congestion in the liver (algerita has a stimulating effect on the liver). Indications include difficulty sleeping through the night, pain in the ribs, intense frustration, frontal headaches with nausea, a bitter taste in the mouth, or pain and bloating with a slow to start menses. This condition may be exacerbated by food intolerances present in the diet and/or a chronic viral infection, such as hepatitis. Conversely, prolonged use (several months) of algerita for the purpose of stimulating digestive secretions, may provoke an opposite effect and induce sensations of cold for individuals with otherwise healthy circulation.

Algerita is an excellent remedy for hot, irritated skin conditions (eczema, psoriasis, rosacea) both as a topical and internal remedy. The berries, as well as the leaf or root tea, can be applied topically in such conditions.

Algerita root tea is traditionally drunk to "build the blood." This remedy may serve those who feel weak or fatigued, perhaps with low blood pressure.

Algerita leaf tincture is recommended to relieve nausea (Coffman 2014). Also, algerita can be taken along with antibiotics to improve their efficacy.

Future harvests

Follow the earlier instructions for root coppicing of shrub types or creeping types. Cut out segments of the interconnected rhizome, and replant root crowns. Place ripe berries, if available, in the soil after root digging.

Caution

Just as algerita may potentiate antibiotics, it may also potentiate or inhibit other pharmaceuticals. In such cases, consult a healthcare practitioner before use.

HERBAL PREPARATIONS

Root Tea
Cold Infusion
Drink 1–4 ounces, up to 3 times per day.

Leaf Tincture
1 part fresh leaf, by weight
2 parts menstruum (75% alcohol, 25% spring water), by volume
Take 10–30 drops, as needed.

Root Tincture
1 part dry root, by weight
5 parts menstruum (50% alcohol, 50% spring water), by volume
Take 10–60 drops, up to 4 times per day; root and leaf tincture may also be combined.

Oil Infusion
1 part dry, ground leaf, by weight
5 parts extra virgin olive oil, by volume
Prepare as alcohol intermediate oil infusion (see page 38).

American licorice

Glycyrrhiza lepidota
amolillo, palo dulce
PARTS USED root

This cooling demulcent relieves common respiratory complaints and soothes irritated mucous membranes. It's especially important for its ability to impart a deep sense of strength and calm to a depleted nervous system.

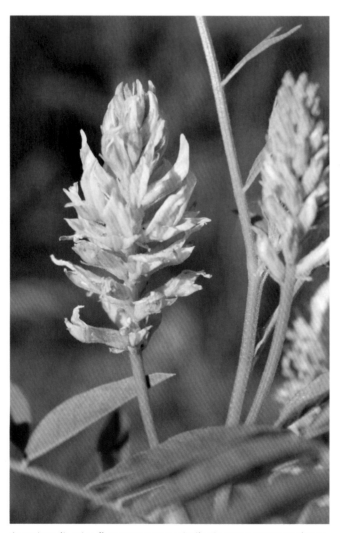

American licorice flowers are very similar in appearance to those of red clover, another pea family member.

How to identify

This herbaceous perennial can occasionally grow to be over 6 feet tall. The alternate, pinnately compound leaves with entire margins can be several inches long; the underside of the leaflets are covered in tiny glands. Its terminal and axillary clusters of white to cream-colored inflorescences are followed by barbed, oblong seedpods, which aid in late summer/early autumn plant identification. The light-colored, musty-smelling root with thin, brown bark is both rhizomatous and taprooted.

Where, when, and how to wildcraft

American licorice exists throughout the northern tier of our region in grasslands, sandy washes, conifer forests, meadows, and along the edges of rivers. It can also be found along the Rio Grande, from southern New Mexico into the Big Bend of Texas. Dig from larger stands, ideally, in the early spring or late summer/early

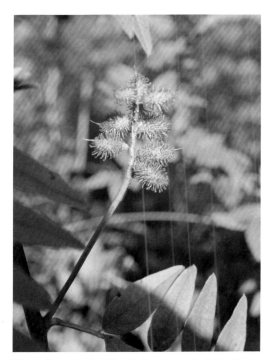

The quintessential identifying characteristic of American licorice is the burred, brick-red seedpod.

of chronic inflammation, chronic infection, mucous membrane irritation, autoimmune conditions, and adrenal depletion. Soothing to an irritated urinary tract, the root tea can also help to break up kidney or bladder stones. American licorice root makes a nice addition to cough syrups and is useful for chronic or acute respiratory complaints.

American licorice, as a tea or tincture, will aid in strengthening the stress response. One can simply chew on the fresh root for the same purpose. It has an anabolic effect on the body, enabling a deeper sense of relaxation while simultaneously imparting a feeling of having energy to spare. This is an excellent remedy, in my opinion, for the average human in our modern world. Taken daily with oatstraw tea or milky oat tincture, it can have a deeply soothing effect on the nervous system. American licorice nourishes the yin aspect of the body, our creative energy, imparting a sense of calm invigoration.

autumn. Stands growing in sandy soil are much easier to dig. Dry for tea or tincture.

Medicinal uses

Native throughout much of North America, American licorice is far less sweet than the licorice of commerce (*Glycyrrhiza glabra*, *G. uralensis*); the saponin glycyrrhizin causes these species to taste sweet, but it is also responsible for slightly raising blood pressure when taken in very large quantities. There is no such potential with American licorice, which lacks glycyrrhizin and is, in fact, rather bitter.

Licorice has dozens of applications and is often included in formulations by herbalists in the East and West, even in very small amounts (less than 5%) as a means to harmonize a formula; we can use American licorice similarly. Include licorice root in cases

Future harvests

Dig only from large stands and spread sections of rhizome (with a stem portion attached) to appropriate habitats.

HERBAL PREPARATIONS

Root Tea
Standard Infusion or Strong Decoction
Apply the decoction to skin infections; drink 2–4 ounces, up to 3 times per day.

Root Tincture
1 part dry root, by weight
5 parts menstruum (50% alcohol,
   50% spring water), by volume
Take 10–60 drops, up to 5 times per day.

anemone

Anemone species
windflower, pasqueflower
PARTS USED aerial

Anemone has a unique ability to change the emotional state quickly, helping one to become grounded or more deeply aware when strong emotions suddenly arise.

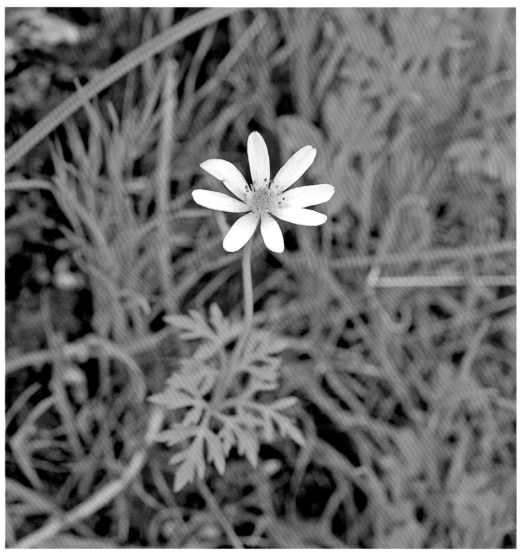

Anemone tuberosa begins flowering around the traditional Celtic festival of Imbolc (1 or 2 February).

How to identify

The Southwest *Anemone* species are herbaceous perennials arising from rhizomes or tubers. The basal leaves often differ from the stem leaves, which are sparse and often lobed, or deeply divided. The terminal inflorescences often occur on long stems, reaching 12 inches or more above the nearest leaves below. *Anemone patens* is often under 12 inches tall. Sepals surround an elongated central hump of a fruiting body that's composed of numerous, tiny petal-less flowers that may be white, pink, blue, green, yellow, or tinged purple, depending on the species. The compressed seedheads, similar to cattail, unfurl and expand, releasing hundreds of plumed seeds into the air. Shortly after going to seed, all traces of anemone disappear from the landscape.

Where, when, and how to wildcraft

In the western half of our region, look to mid-elevation, boulder-strewn hillsides to find *Anemone tuberosa*, desert anemone; it occurs from the Big Bend of Texas all the way to southern Nevada and southern California. *Anemone berlandieri*, tenpetal anemone, is found in clay soils in central Texas, from south of San Antonio northward into Oklahoma. Anemones flower from early February to early May, depending on the species and elevation. Gather the aboveground parts and process fresh for tincture. Process fresh anemone outdoors or with a good cross breeze, as the chopped plant emits volatile and irritating constituents, which can cause dizziness or fainting if breathed within a closed area.

Medicinal uses

Anemone is a first-rate emotional remedy. Taken in small doses (1–15 drops), it allays emotional anxiety for many, as well as

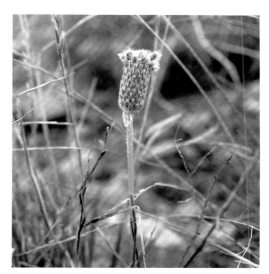

The feathery seed cluster appears shortly after, then unfurls to release the tiny seeds to the wind.

improving depression or insomnia for some. The cause of the emotional upset may be unknown or of a deeply repressed nature. Acute anxiety attacks may benefit from anemone tincture. It relaxes the nervous system, increases circulation to the brain, and can have a beneficial effect on the female reproductive system when circulation is obstructed to the point of causing painful menstrual cramping.

As an emotional heart remedy, anemone offers a tremendous potency of healing as it warms and softens the heart center. The use of the fresh plant tincture, a nibble of fresh plant, sleeping with the pressed plant beneath one's pillow, or meditating with the live plant are all potent methods for delving deep into any past emotional wound that is calling to be tended to.

The tincture is also taken to abort a migraine or tension headache, relieve pain along the spine due to inflammation, rheumatism, or injury, and stimulate peripheral circulation. Applied topically, the fresh plant may be used to resolve boils.

An acrid-tasting tincture is indicative of its potency. Use anemone tincture within 3–4 years.

Future harvests
Gather carefully from large stands in years of abundant flowering (may occur about every 5 years with *Anemone tuberosa*).

⚠ Caution
The tincture is very acrid but is not caustic to the mouth; apply with caution to the skin. Tasting the fresh plant, or tincture, on an empty stomach may cause stomach irritation. Use with caution in very hot conditions; anemone is suited to cold, deficient, chronically obstructed states. A strong release of heat when using anemone is normal.

HERBAL PREPARATIONS

Leaf/Stem/Flower Tincture
1 part fresh herb, by weight
2 parts menstruum (95% alcohol),
  by volume
Take 1–15 drops, as needed; take with food if stomach is sensitive.

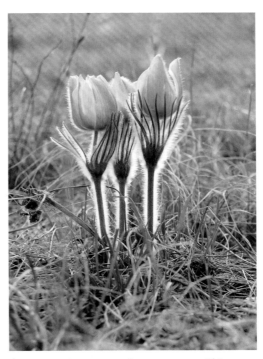

Anemone patens, pasqueflower, occurs within our region at high elevations in northern New Mexico and southern Colorado.

Arizona cypress

Cupressus arizonica
ciprés
PARTS USED leaf, stem

A wonderful remedy for fungal and bacterial infections,
Arizona cypress also lifts the spirit and brings mental clarity.

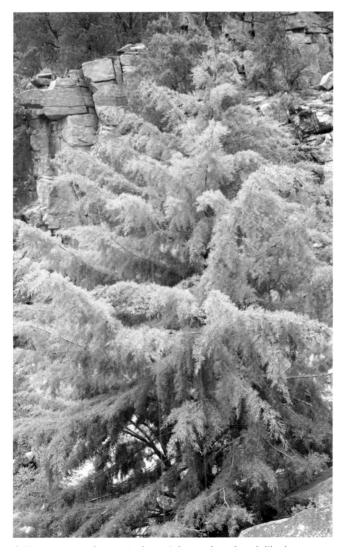

Arizona cypress has a single upright truck and scalelike leaves, which make the branches appear drooping.

How to identify

A large evergreen conifer, approaching heights of 80 feet, this majestic tree favors rocky canyons in mid-elevation mountain ranges and also graces residential landscapes as an ornamental. Its smooth bark is cherry-red or dark brown when young, gray with darker furrows and peeling strips at maturity. The scalelike leaves, showing a diamond pattern outlined in white, are gray-green to blue-green with light specks of resin. Its female cones, with warty spikes and sections that open upon maturation, help to easily distinguish it from *Juniperus* species, with their fleshy "berries." After fires, or as the tree dies, Arizona cypress sheds its bark in long sheets.

Where, when, and how to wildcraft

Naturally occurring in our range from southern Nevada and southern Utah in a southeasterly direction along the mountain ranges into Mexico. Look to canyon bottoms and ascending slopes. It may also

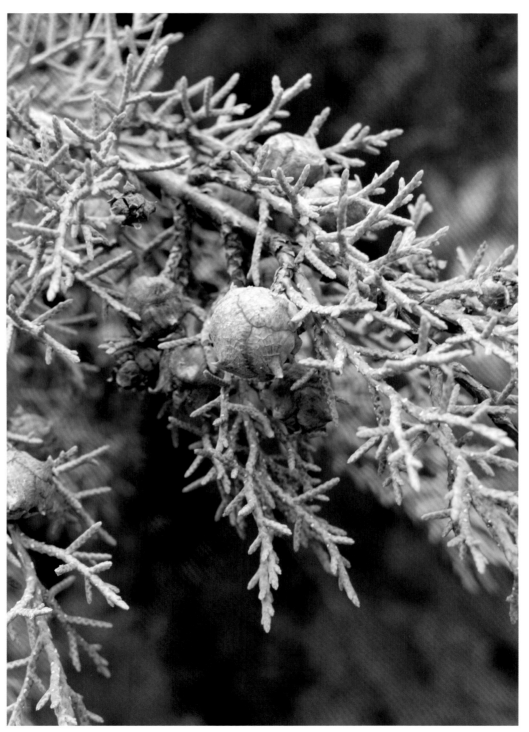

The cones of Arizona cypress separate into sections, each with a warty spike in the middle.

be found scattered throughout New Mexico and the mountains of western Texas, and in central Texas and Oklahoma as an ornamental. Leaves can be gathered any time after sufficient rains, or outside of the flowering season (November–March). Prune back lower stems of particularly tender growth. Seek out young crowded trees in natural environments, or gather from annual prunings of landscape specimens.

Medicinal uses

As part of a family of conifers known for their antifungal effects, Arizona cypress preparations can be used both topically and internally. Use the tincture internally for fungal, viral, or bacterial respiratory infections. A useful immune stimulant, it enlivens a slow digestion and aids in addiction recovery, meditation, and lifting languid depression. A standard infusion of the leaves may help resolve UTIs and astringe intestinal tissue. Drink the hot tea for acute respiratory viruses or rheumatic joint pain. In Chinese medicine, the tea tonifies the spleen, aiding in a variety of damp, boggy, and depressed conditions. Apply the tincture, or tea, topically to any fungal infections, staph infections, or impetigo. Apply an oil infusion, or wash, to the scalp for dandruff.

Future harvests

This tree has suffered in its native habitat over the past decade, and populations are in decline. Prune leaves modestly, and only from abundant, healthy stands of young trees.

⚠ Caution

Extended internal use (more than 3–5 days) of Arizona cypress tea may be irritating to the urinary tract.

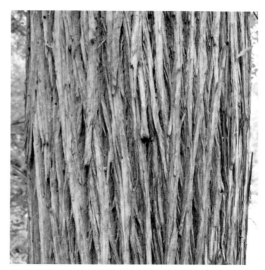

The long strips of Arizona cypress' light gray bark are fibrous with a flat ridge about an inch wide.

HERBAL PREPARATIONS

Herb Tea
Standard Infusion
Drink 4–8 ounces, up to 3 times per day.

Strong Decoction
Apply topically as a wash, fomentation, or soak, as needed.

Leaf Tincture
1 part fresh leaf, by weight
2 parts menstruum (95% alcohol),
   by volume
or
1 part dry leaf, by weight
5 parts menstruum (50% alcohol,
   50% spring water), by volume
Apply directly to the skin; take 5–30 drops, up to 3 times per day, or combine in formulation.

Oil Infusion
1:5
Dry leaves and prepare as alcohol intermediate oil infusion (see page 38).

Fraxinus species
fresno, plumero
PARTS USED bark, leaf, stem

Ash is a cooling, tonifying remedy for digestive complaints, with a mild laxative effect.

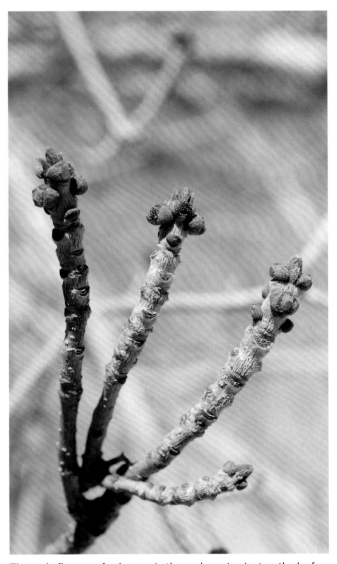

The male flowers of ash open in the early spring just as the leaf buds are opening.

How to identify

This is a deciduous tree, 3–40 feet tall within our range, depending on the species (nearly a dozen within our region) and growing conditions. Two distinct features of (nearly) all ash trees greatly aid in their identification: the leaves and stems are opposite, and the leaves are pinnately compound, with 3–9 leaflets (an exception is *Fraxinus anomala*, single-leaf ash). The leaves are bright green and clearly stand out as the first trees to leaf out in early spring. Generally speaking, its bark is light to dark gray, occasionally reddish brown, scaly with furrows and zigzags; younger bark is smooth and may possess lenticels. Another key feature of ash, a dioecious tree, is the small light yellow samaras (single-seed fruits) shaped like paddles or spear points, which persist on female trees throughout winter.

Where, when, and how to wildcraft

Our *Fraxinus* species occur from one end of our region to the other, over a wide variety

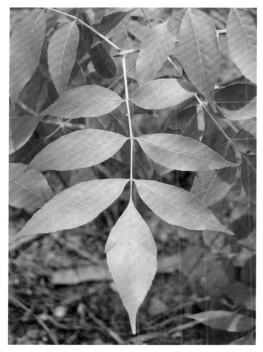

Nearly all *Fraxinus* species have pinnately compound leaves with a single terminal leaflet.

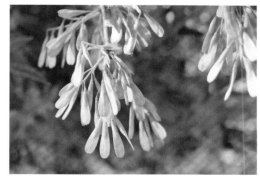

Clusters of paddle-shaped yellow seeds dangle from female ash trees from early autumn on.

of habitats, conifer forests being one place they are absent from. Taller ash trees grow near perennial or seasonal water sources; smaller, shrubby ashes may be found up a hillside from a creek or an arroyo, or on open, exposed sandstone fragments baking in the direct sun (often under 6 feet). The bark is best gathered in late autumn once the leaves have fallen, or late winter/early spring before the leaf buds open. Leaves can be gathered whenever present.

Medicinal uses

Eclectic physicians (physician herbalists of the 19th and early 20th centuries) applied ash bark tincture or tea as a relaxant for digestive disorders and cases of liver obstruction, such as jaundice. We can also combine it with curly dock for skin affections, both topically and internally. Ash leaf tea is mildly bitter and astringent with a mild relaxing effect. In Sonora, a traditional recipe for keeping children cool during the summer is to brew a hot infusion of ash leaves along with elder flowers; strain and add ice and sugar (or other sweetener) before serving. Consider adding ash to an evening tea for disturbed sleep coupled with digestive distress.

Future harvests

Prune only young branches, from late autumn to early spring, choosing those that will be shaded out as the tree grows.

HERBAL PREPARATIONS

Bark/Leaf Tea
Standard or Cold Infusion or Strong
  Decoction
Drink 1–4 ounces, up to 3 times per day.

Bark Tincture
1 part dry bark, by weight
5 parts menstruum (50% alcohol,
  50% spring water), by volume
Take 15–60 drops, up to 3 times per day.

Populus tremuloides
PARTS USED bark, leaf, stem, bud, catkin

As an emotional heart remedy it stands alone, offering relief for emotional trauma, "broken" hearts, PTSD, or linked physical maladies. Aspen is a wonderful digestive tonic with potent effects on the genitourinary system as well.

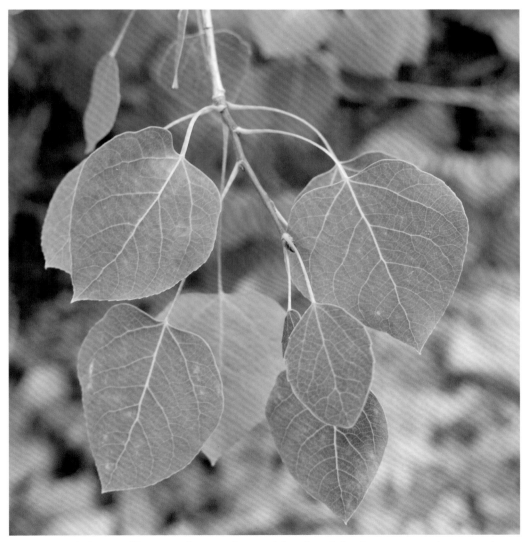

Aspen's rounded, pointed leaves are borne on long petioles; the subtlest breeze causes them to quake and tremble.

How to identify

Aspen is one of the largest living organisms on the planet. It reproduces clonally, covering whole mountainsides as a single entity. The limbs of this tall, slender white-barked tree have black rings and scars, occurring mostly toward the top quarter of the tree. Leafless from late autumn to late spring, male and female catkins unfold by early summer—each on separate trees. Because aspen occurs in clonal colonies, all plants within a colony will be either male or female. Early summer flowering is followed by the unfurling of heart-shaped leaves with flattened stems. The leaves flutter readily in the breeze (hence "quaking" aspen). In early autumn, leaves of entire colonies turn bright yellow, burnt red, and orange, creating one of the most spectacular sights in nature.

Where, when, and how to wildcraft

Aspen occurs in high-elevation conifer forests in the western half of our region, from southwestern Texas northward. Gather the flower buds or opening flowers in early summer, or the leaves and stems throughout the summer. Look for fallen trunks after summer storms in order to peel and harvest the bark. The bark can also be gathered in late autumn; see "Gathering Tree Medicine" (page 25) for more details.

Medicinal uses

Although it shares much in common medicinally with other members of the willow family, aspen possesses some very special attributes. I discovered many years ago its potency as an emotional heart remedy. Maladies such as depression, unexplained emotionality, musculoskeletal pain or dislocations, fears deeply embedded within the body (such as through PTSD), or simply an aching for something lost long, long ago can

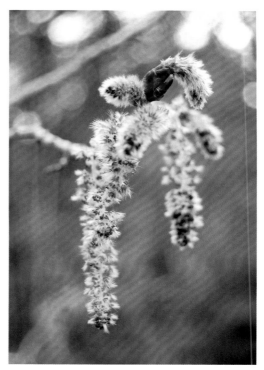

The fuzzy male catkins of aspen open in the early summer.

be allayed, or begin to be healed, through the use of aspen medicine. At times, this calls for nothing more than allowing oneself to become aware, open, and vulnerable to the present moment while in the presence of an aspen grove. Ingesting a bit of the flower tincture (1–5 drops) can also lead one into the mindset of healing these aches.

Traditionally, the leaf/stem tea was viewed as an excellent remedy for urinary hemorrhage, pain, or congestion. It's also useful for prostatic hypertrophy and uterine congestion.

As a digestive aid, aspen bark or leaf/stem tea (or tincture) is excellent. Use alone or in a formula to stimulate appetite or tone up the digestive process; also for diarrhea, constipation, or heartburn. The tincture of the buds can be used as an expectorant, bringing warmth to the lungs and breaking up mucus;

it was traditionally used for pneumonia, coughs, and colds. Aspen bark (tea or syrup) is a phenomenal remedy for long-standing or intermittent fevers once weakness and emaciation set in.

Apply the tea of aspen bark, leaf, or stem to painful joints, fractures, sores, abscesses, or bleeding wounds (powdered bark, as well) for relief.

Future harvests

Follow the guidelines given at "Gathering Tree Medicine" (page 25).

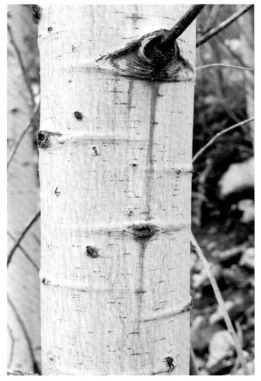

Aspen bark is smooth until much older, and covered with a white chalky substance.

HERBAL PREPARATIONS

Bark Tea
Standard Decoction
Drink 2–4 ounces, up to 3 times per day; apply topically, as needed; convert to a syrup by adding 2 parts wildflower honey to 1 part tea.

Leaf/Stem Tea
Standard Infusion
Drink 4–6 ounces, up to 4 times per day; apply topically, as needed.

Catkin/Bud Tincture
1 part fresh herb, by weight
2 parts menstruum (75% alcohol, 25% spring water), by volume
Take 10–30 drops, up to 4 times per day.

beebalm

Monarda punctata
spotted beebalm, horsemint
PARTS USED aerial

A pungent, warming herb with a flavor reminiscent of peppermint, thyme, and oregano. The relaxing effects of this pleasant-tasting tea soothe nervous tension that's inhibiting digestion.

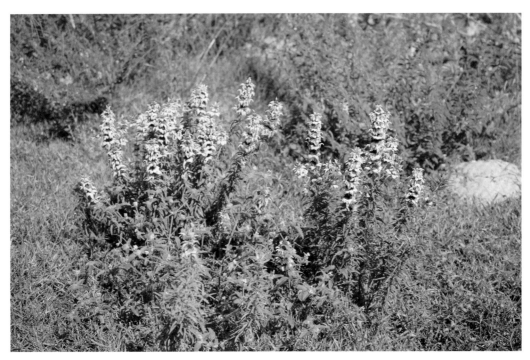
Beebalm occupies disturbed areas throughout Texas and Oklahoma.

How to identify

Long, frosted (to greenish) white or lavender-pink bracts that hang down and come to a point are one of the key traits of this herbaceous perennial mint. Leaves are opposite and may also be frosted white at the base; they are lance-shaped, with sharply toothed margins. Several rounded whorls of spotted, 2-lipped white to creamy yellow flowers, purple-spotted at the throat and packed tightly, surround the square stem at the top of the plant. The upper lip of the corolla is arced into a hood; the lower lip is spotted. The whole plant is aromatic.

Where, when, and how to wildcraft

Common within the eastern third of our region (as var. *lasiodonta*), this species reaches as far as western New Mexico at higher elevations (as var. *occidentalis*). In the

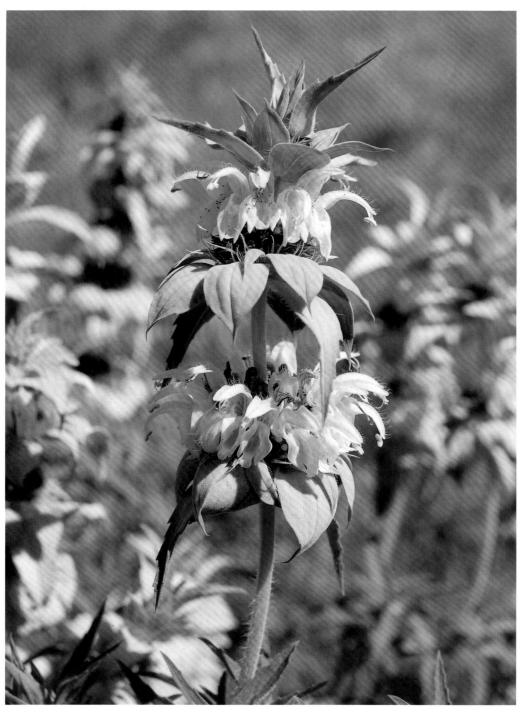

The large colorful bracts of var. *lasiodonta* help differentiate it from var. *occidentalis*, which has a pink hooded corolla with spotted lower lip.

West, look to streams and canyons. Its leaves can be gathered in mid-spring when the plant becomes clearly visible. The flowering period is long, from late spring to late autumn on the eastern edge of our region. Simply snip stems just below their lowest green growth, gathering 2–3 of every 10 stems encountered. Set aside to dry, or tincture fresh.

Medicinal uses

Beebalm is a pleasant-tasting tea that stimulates digestive function and blood flow, thanks to its warming nature. Applied energetically, consider using the tea in any cold, tight, depressed tissue states in order to invigorate functions, deliver more blood flow, and relax tension due to cold obstructions in the body.

A hot tea will reliably promote sweating with a fever, stimulate digestive secretions, and stimulate menses, especially when circulation is poor and the limbs are cold. The tea or tincture enhances circulation to the brain, is noticeably diuretic, and can relieve a variety of arthritic joint pains. It relaxes the nervous system, allaying tension to allow for a restful sleep.

This beauty is worthy of garden cultivation yet possesses numerous useful qualities as a medicinal: vulnerary, antiseptic, anti-inflammatory, oral astringent and antiseptic, mood elevator, digestive tonic, enhances respiration, anodyne, immune stimulant, antiviral, musculoskeletal relaxant, and nervine.

Consider a hot cup of tea at the onset of a cold or whenever cold and dampness have begun to settle into the lungs (combine with yerba santa, gumweed, or cudweed) to help dissolve the phlegm and open the lungs. The tea combined with a bit of cinnamon (or algerita leaf) will help stop vomiting. Gargle the hot tea for a sore throat. Conversely,

drink cool to enhance tissue toning, increase urination, and reduce inflammation. Also, try cold infusions applied as a fomentation or wash to the head and face for a headache.

The honey infusion is soothing and antiseptic to a sore throat or cases of laryngitis.

Future harvests

Gather only from large stands. In late autumn, consider propagating in favorable areas by transplanting the fresh rhizome, with a stem node attached, into moist soil. Scatter seed in disturbed areas or streamsides where it is already growing in the vicinity.

HERBAL PREPARATIONS

Herb Tea
Standard or Cold Infusion
Drink 2–8 ounces, up to 4 times per day, or use as a gargle; apply to the affected area consistently until resolved.

Tincture
1 part fresh herb, by weight
2 parts menstruum (95% alcohol),
  by volume
or
1 part dry herb, by weight
5 parts menstruum (50% alcohol,
  50% spring water), by volume
Take 10–60 drops, as needed.

Honey Infusion
Follow directions on page 37; take ½–1 tablespoon, as needed.

Bermudagrass

Cynodon dactylon
durva, zacate Bermuda
PARTS USED leaf, rhizome

A prime stock feed, an invasive nuisance, a putting green—and a revered medicinal plant in India. Bermudagrass could be our most extraordinary overlooked healing plant.

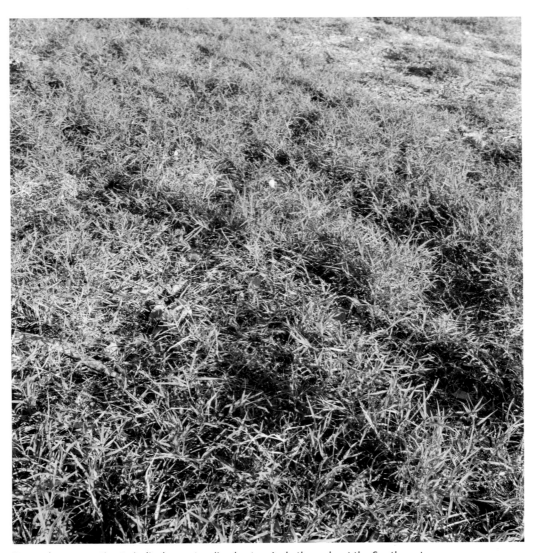

Bermudagrass, native to India, has naturalized extensively throughout the Southwest.

How to identify

This perennial grass grows and spreads from rhizomes, or stolons, that may penetrate 18 inches down into the soil. The creeping stems may reach 4 feet or more when propped upon another plant or thick clusters of its own stems. As it creeps out (up to 50 feet in length!), it will root from the nodes of the grass stem, expanding its terrain throughout an exposed and disturbed area, creating dense mats of tangled stems. Its alternate leaves are flat, short, and narrow. Slender panicles of 2–9 finger-like branches, with spikelets densely packed in 2 rows, form the terminal inflorescences. The stems turn beige with age, similar to the rhizomes.

Where, when, and how to wildcraft

Bermudagrass is found abundantly and commonly throughout our region, generally below 6,000 feet. Look to streambanks as well as vacant lots, roadsides, and alleyways for this naturalized, weedy grass. It is present nearly year-round given sufficient moisture but may die back due to freezing temperatures. Cut back the fresh grass with a curved blade or snip with shears or scissors. Tincture fresh or pound when fresh with a mortar and pestle and apply the juice directly to the skin or emulsify into a lotion. Dig up the entire plant (to the best of your ability) and pass the shovel of soil through a ¼-inch screen. Sift out the soil and cut the rhizomes from the aerial portions. Dry and cut the rhizomes for tea. When selecting your area to harvest from, use caution. Avoid potentially toxic sites where industrial wastes may have accumulated; Bermudagrass has shown bioremediation potential at sites saturated with heavy metals. Do not harvest from areas that have been sprayed with weed-killing agents or irrigated with reclaimed water. There's a lot of suspect Bermudagrass in the Southwest—get to know your area first.

Medicinal uses

In India, durva (as it is known there) is one of the most revered medicinals in the herbal repertoire. Classified as a rasayana (rejuvenative herb), it is juiced by pulverizing the fresh leaves and stems. This juice is taken with sugar to relieve nausea, or applied to the skin along with ghee to heal wounds, treat burns or fever, or relieve inflammation. I once tried juicing the young leaves of thick, lush, post-monsoon-rain Bermudagrass in a juicer, but not a drop was extracted. Smashing handfuls of fresh cut leaves and stems in a mortar and pestle with a bit of added water seems to be the most effective, at-home method to extract the juice. Use the juice to prepare skin lotions. Fresh juice is a particularly potent inhibitor of MRSA and other pathogenic microbes.

Bermudagrass has proven to be effective against cancer cell lines in vitro. In part, this might be attributed to its high quercetin content, as well as an abundance of other antioxidant flavonoids and carotenoids. This rich array of antioxidants may explain its known effectiveness in relieving rheumatoid arthritis, as well as its ability to help manage neurodegenerative diseases. It is traditionally employed in Ayurvedic medicine for Alzheimer's, Parkinson's, and the like. Both the leaf tincture and the tea have demonstrated abundant antioxidant potential.

A decoction of the rhizome, traditionally mixed with sugar, is used to relieve fluid retention and will help reduce bladder stone formation. In Iran, a tea of the rhizomes is applied in cases of heart failure and atherosclerosis.

A variety of animal studies have revealed that a tincture (hydroethanolic extract) of the aerial portions of Bermudagrass is hepatoprotective, cardioprotective, sedating to the nervous system (promoting sleep and relieving pain), antiulcer, and antidiabetic (significantly improving LDL, triglyceride, and fasting glucose levels). Some of these results were also observed with a tea, particularly the antidiabetic effects. Wow. What an incredible plant.

Future harvests
What are we waiting for?

HERBAL PREPARATIONS

Herb Tea
Standard Infusion
Apply topically, as needed; drink 2–8 ounces, up to 4 times per day.

Root Tea
Standard Decoction
Drink 2–8 ounces, up to 3 times per day.

Tincture
1 part fresh herb, by weight
2 parts menstruum (95% alcohol),
  by volume
Take 15–30 drops, up to 4 times per day.

Lotion
Use fresh juice to prepare an emulsified lotion.

Pedicularis species
lousewort, parrot's beak, elephant's head
PARTS USED aerial

This herb is a prime muscle relaxant remedy which also tones digestion and shows significant promise in other areas of health and healing.

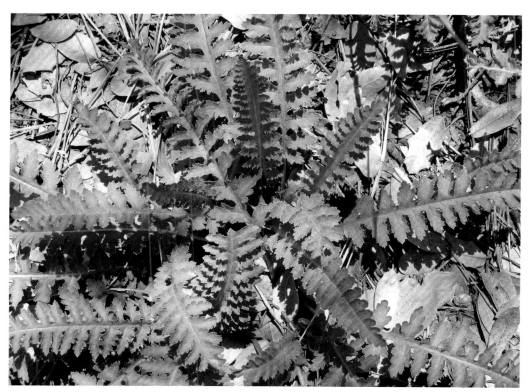

The pinnatifid basal leaves of *Pedicularis centranthera*, dwarf lousewort, appear in the early spring under the cover of oak or piñon-juniper woodlands.

How to identify

Betony is a large genus of hemiparasitic plants; they obtain nutrients from the roots of other plants but also produce energy by photosynthesis. Within our region, they range from low-growing (less than 5 inches tall) to nearly 6 feet in height. The leaves are predominantly basal and may be 3–24 inches long, depending on the species, and are finely divided and fernlike (except *Pedicularis racemosa*, parrot's beak, which has lance-shaped, simple leaves with serrated margins). The terminal spiked inflorescence is generally much shorter in the low-growing species (*P. canadensis*, *P. centranthera*, and *P. groenlandica*) at

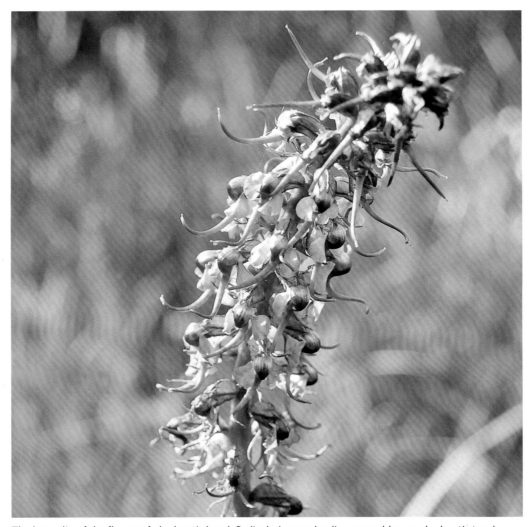

The lower lip of the flower of elephant's head, *Pedicularis groenlandica,* resembles an elephant's trunk.

1–2 inches, but the taller species (*P. procera*, in particular) may produce flowering spikes up to 2 feet long. The bracts of the individual flowers may be longer than the corolla itself. The corolla is highly irregular with the throat enlarging toward the apex. The arched, sometimes twisted upper lip, or hood, may be longer than the lower lip (curving downward then upward like an elephant's trunk in *P. groenlandica*, elephant's head). Corolla colors within our region may be white, yellow, pink, purple, or tinged with red or pink lines. Fruits are capsules containing tiny seeds.

Where, when, and how to wildcraft

Pedicularis species are found exclusively at mid- to high elevations within our region. Only *P. centranthera*, dwarf lousewort, exists in mid-elevation oak woodlands, as well as piñon-juniper and pine woodlands. Overall, betony prefers moist, shady locations above

7,000 feet (occasionally lower) within the western half of our region. *Pedicularis canadensis*, Canadian lousewort, the only betony species native to eastern North America, is found in eastern Texas and Oklahoma but not within the region this text covers. However, it can also be found in the mountains of southern Colorado and northern New Mexico, occasionally in abundance. Gather the aerial portions of dwarf betony mid- to late spring. All other betony species can be gathered from late spring to early autumn depending on the location and the particular year's weather pattern. Only gather aerial portions, and in areas of limited population, only gather the leaves, not the flowering stems. Dry in the shade for tea or tincture, or make a fresh plant tincture.

Medicinal uses

The tea or tincture of betony is an excellent muscle relaxant serving to relieve pain after injury, relax the body after arduous physical activity, or alleviate chronic muscle tension. Commonly, it takes 1–2 teaspoons of the tincture to fully relax from serious injuries or extreme physical labor or exercise. Herbalist Howie Brounstein of Eugene, Oregon, popularized smoking dry *Pedicularis* leaf as a mood-altering muscle relaxant. Studies of Asian *Pedicularis* species (over 500 species worldwide) show the plant's ability to restore the body from fatigue as well as promote vitality.

It is also a mild bitter tonic useful in stimulating digestion. It has also been shown to be protective in stomach and hepatic cancers. Recent scientific trials reveal its hepatoprotective and neuroprotective properties.

The leaves and roots of several species have been used as a food including *Pedicularis canadensis*. In Alaska, Eskimos ferment and freeze the young greens and mix with oil and sugar as a dessert.

Future harvests

Although *Pedicularis* species are hemiparasitic, they do produce seeds. Allow the seedpods to grow to maturity and scatter in appropriate locations from late autumn to early spring.

⚠ Caution

Avoid gathering *Pedicularis* species when growing adjacent to potentially toxic bean family plants (e.g., *Thermopsis*) or *Senecio* species as they may obtain toxic compounds when parasitic on these plants.

HERBAL PREPARATIONS

Leaf Tea
Standard Infusion
Drink 4–8 ounces, up to 4 times per day.

Herb Tincture
1 part fresh herb, by weight
2 parts menstruum (95% alcohol),
  by volume
or
1 part dry herb, by weight
5 parts menstruum (50% alcohol,
  50% spring water), by volume
Take ¼–2 teaspoons, up to 3 times per day;
take 10–30 drops as a bitter tonic.

Liatris species
cachana, button snakeroot, gayfeather
PARTS USED flower, root

A traditional remedy for sore throat, this acrid herb is also used as a diuretic and to reduce swellings and painful rheumatic joints.

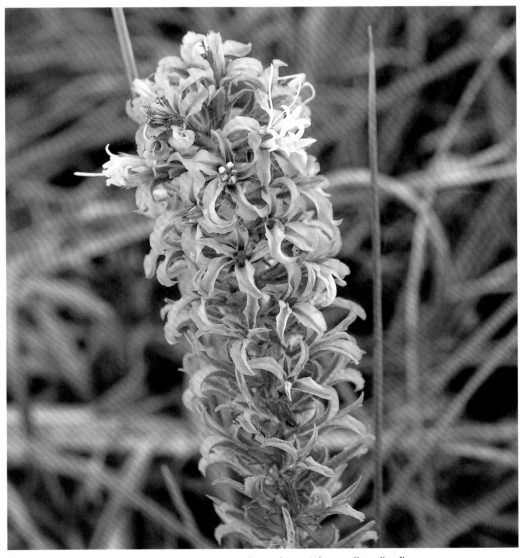

The long inflorescences of *Liatris elegans* may produce white, pink, or yellow disc flowers.

How to identify

This herbaceous perennial herb grows from its root crown as a clump of stems 2–3 feet tall. The mostly smooth thin leaves are erect and linear. The inflorescence is a spike of discoid flower heads, each with a 5-lobed corolla of white, pink, or yellow. The lightweight seeds, which are attached to bristly plumes, take flight upon maturity. The slippery gray flesh of the root is covered in a thin brown bark.

Where, when, and how to wildcraft

Blazing star is spread across the prairies, high plains, piñon-juniper woodlands, Texas Hill Country, and South Texas Plains—from southeastern Colorado to the southern tip of Texas. Gather the flowers when still in bud, because, as is the case with most aster family plants, they turn into a feathery mess upon opening—even after harvesting. Dig the roots in autumn, after the plant has gone to seed.

Medicinal uses

Several *Liatris* species were used in similar fashion by Eclectic physicians of the 19th and early 20th centuries; they employed the root tea or tincture as a diuretic, kidney tonic, and emmenagogue, and for sore throat, dyspepsia, and spasmodic bowel affections of children.

The root and flower teas of *Liatris punctata* were traditionally used for sore throat. For a useful cough syrup, Michael Moore suggests combining equal parts of the fresh, chopped root and honey, blending, then simmering for a half hour before straining. The energetics of the root are warming and drying with an affinity for the lungs, genitourinary tract, and digestive tract.

Traditionally, the fresh root poultice was applied to swellings and rheumatic joints, causing blood to enter the area, transforming the relatively cold and static condition.

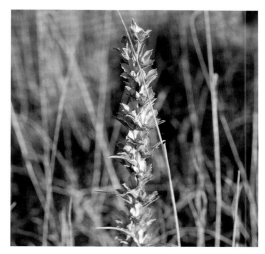

Across the prairies, the dried flower stalks of *Liatris punctata* can be found into the following spring season.

Among the various Plains tribes, springtime roots were roasted over coals and eaten. The roots contain inulin, an indigestible starch.

Future harvests

Scatter the seeds over exposed, disturbed soil in the spring. Blazing star works to stabilize the soil and restore prairie habitat.

HERBAL PREPARATIONS

Root Tea
Strong Decoction
Drink 2-4 ounces, frequently.

Root Poultice
Apply topically, as needed, to swellings, painful joints, rashes, or itchy skin.

bricklebush

Brickellia species
prodigiosa
PARTS USED leaf, stem

A bitter remedy still revered for its effects on the digestive system and for lowering blood sugar. Used topically, it can also relieve arthritic pain.

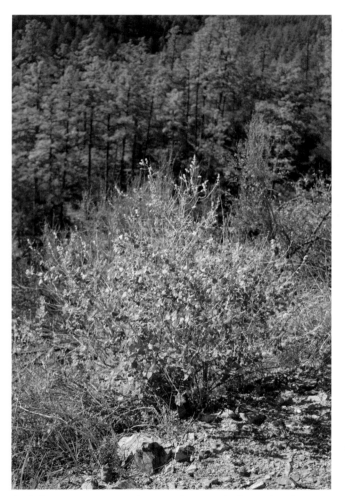

Brickellia species commonly grow along roadsides and at the edges of canyons in disturbed, dry soils.

How to identify

This genus of shrubs and herbaceous perennials presents an array of sizes, forms, and leaf displays and is often quite aromatic and sticky to the touch. The slender, rayless composite inflorescences, with white or cream disc flowers, are subtended by several rows of phyllaries, which may be tinged red, yellow, or purple. Leaves may appear opposite near the growing tips of some *Brickellia* species, confounding identification, but are generally alternate elsewhere on the plant. The ripe seeds are topped with bristly tufts. *Brickellia californica* is found abundantly in the western two-thirds of our region at 2,500–9,000 feet; its leaves are triangular with rounded teeth on the margins that may be tinted red. *Brickellia grandiflora*, tasselflower, is found in the western half of our region at 4,000–10,000 feet; its loose clusters of solitary inflorescences hang down slightly.

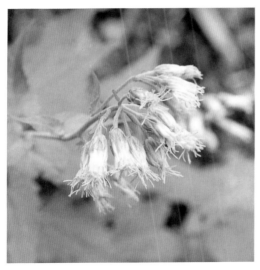

The composite flowers of bricklebush are discoid and often pendulant.

Where, when, and how to wildcraft

Bricklebush is found throughout our region, with the exception of the South Texas Plains, inhabiting mountain roadsides, canyons, and washes as a small understory desert shrub, or on the rocky margins of forests. Local elevation and moisture conditions will dictate where one goes to gather the herb. In dry seasons, seek higher elevation if possible. In early spring or late autumn, seek lower, warmer elevations, particularly in the western half of our region. Otherwise, it is best to gather the stems just before flowering. Simply snip the stems below the lowest green growth; dry stems by spreading them out in the shade or hanging in bundles. Dozens of *Brickellia* species are found throughout our region. Some species can sustain extensive gathering better than others. As medicinal properties can vary among species, please get to know your local plants.

Medicinal uses

This herb is sharply bitter and should be expected to increase appetite and stimulate all digestive secretions. The tea is a traditional remedy for stomachache, gas, bloating, and gall bladder congestion. Avoid using it with active biliary blockage. Take 10–20 drops of the tincture after a particularly fatty or heavy meal to stimulate digestion. A liniment or a decoction of the herb can be used to bathe sores, injuries, or arthritic joints. Decoct it with creosote bush, wild tobacco, and camphorweed to bathe arthritic joints. As a metabolic aid for pre-diabetics or early-stage type 2 diabetes, prepare an oxymel by simmering the herb in apple cider vinegar and cinnamon, and combining with 1 part wildflower honey.

Future harvests

An abundant herb; harvest modestly and it will live on.

Caution

In relatively small amounts (1–4 cups), it can be emetic.

HERBAL PREPARATIONS

Herb Tea
Standard Infusion
Drink 2–4 ounces, 2 times per day, before meals.

Tincture
1 part dry herb, by weight
5 parts menstruum (50% alcohol,
   50% spring water), by volume
Take 30–60 drops, up to 3 times per day.

brittlebush

Encelia farinosa
incienso, yerba del vaso
PARTS USED leaf, flower, sap

Warming, pungent, and slightly bitter, it is decongestant, analgesic, carminative, and relaxing to the nervous system. Also, consider brittlebush for any pain in the head.

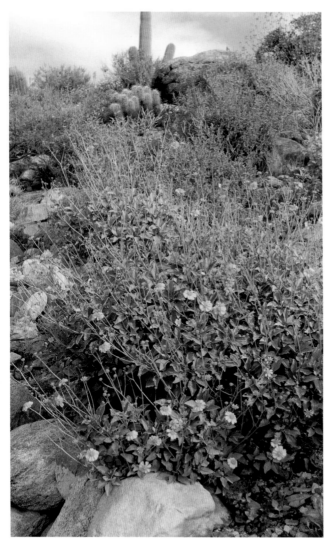

Brittlebush, a common hillside plant throughout the Sonoran and Mojave deserts, begins flowering in early spring.

How to identify

In the early spring, rocky desert hillsides are covered by the golden yellow flowers of this compact deciduous shrub. The ray flowers, each notched at the end, encircle the central orange-yellow disc flowers; a ring of pointed green bracts surrounds each flower head. The fuzzy, silvery green leaves, which are located near the growing tips of the branches, sprout in response to winter rains and again in response to the summer rains (in the Sonoran desert) but fall to the ground in response to freezing temperatures or drought; translucent yellow sap is easily found oozing from stem joints or broken twigs during this time. Before flowering, the plant is often confused with white sage, however, the leaves of white sage are opposite, whereas the leaves of brittlebush are alternate. *Encelia frutescens* and *E. virginensis* have also been used medicinally.

Where, when, and how to wildcraft

Find brittlebush on dry, rocky mountainsides of desert grasslands and cactus forests from southern Arizona to southern California, and up into southern Utah and Nevada, below 3,000 feet. Also found on the edge of desert washes, where it may be accompanied by Mormon tea or desert lavender. Gather the leafy branch tips before flowering to tincture fresh or dry for tea. The flowers are gathered in the spring and used fresh, or dried to make oil infusion.

Medicinal uses

The tea or tincture can be taken for hay fever, sinus or chest congestion, joint pain, or headache. Just as it dries the excessive secretions of hay fever, internal use of the tincture also gradually restores proper lubrication to dry eyes. For all manner of pains and discomforts of the head, consider using brittlebush in one form or another. The pain of toothache, sore gums, cold sores, earache, or eye pain can be relieved by chewing on twigs, inhaling the steam, drinking the hot tea, or holding the tea or tincture in the mouth.

If taken in the evening, the nervine and sedative properties of the tincture help to relax the body and mind. Brittlebush is also able to induce or enhance the mind's ability for keen focus, so I recommend taking small doses of the tincture in preparation for a meditative practice.

The sap is a mild expectorant when eaten fresh, although it takes consider-able effort to gather enough to tincture. A fresh flower poultice can be applied directly to open wounds or sore joints alike, as it is anesthetic, anti-inflammatory, and wound-healing.

Future harvests

Gather after new growth has been put out in response to moisture. Always gather with respect, even if plants are abundant.

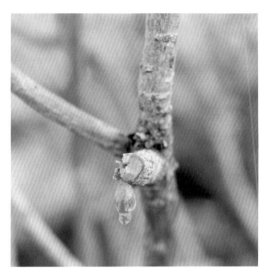

The sap is easiest to find once most of the leaves have dried and fallen off, or a short time after the brittle branches are broken.

HERBAL PREPARATIONS

Herb Tea
Standard Decoction
Drink 2–4 ounces, up to 3 times per day; mouth rinse for sore gums or toothache.

Tincture
1 part fresh herb, by weight
2 parts menstruum (95% alcohol),
 by volume
or
1 part dry herb, by weight
2 parts menstruum (50% alcohol,
 50% spring water), by volume
Take 10–40 drops, up to 4 times per day.

Oil Infusion
Dry flowers and prepare as alcohol intermediate oil infusion (see page 38).

buttonbush

Cephalanthus occidentalis
mimbro
PARTS USED bark, leaf, stem, flower

A bitter tonic traditionally used for fevers and digestive issues, buttonbush can also be used for food poisoning.

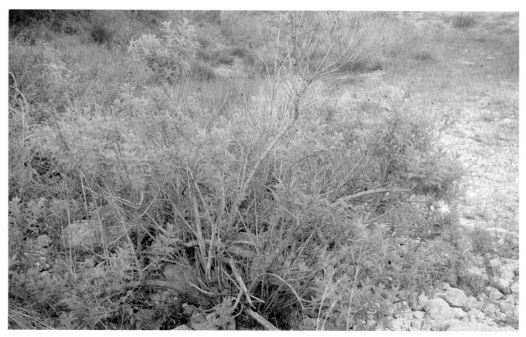

Buttonbush can be found growing right in the river bed in the Texas Hill Country.

How to identify

Buttonbush is a shrubby deciduous tree, generally 6–10 feet tall, occasionally up to 30 feet. The bark is dark gray-brown, and the stout stems enclose a thick pith. Leaves often come to a point and fold up at the midrib. You can see its relationship to coffee (another member of the madder family) in its 2–5 shiny leaves per stem node. Unlike coffee, its flowers occur not at the stem nodes but out at the branch tips. The bright white flowers have exserted stamens, giving the globose inflorescence the appearance of a pincushion. Upon drying, they become reddish brown and harden with age, making autumn through spring identification much easier. *Cephalanthus salicifolius*, Mexican buttonbush, found at the southern tip of Texas, has also been used for medicine, internally.

Where, when, and how to wildcraft

Buttonbush is common in the eastern third of our region near waterways and swampy areas, then hops over to the Sonoran desert along

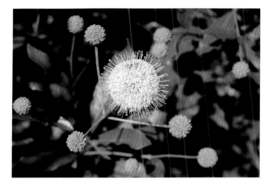

The terminal, globose flower clusters are sweetly fragrant and look something like a pincushion.

mid- to low-elevation arroyos, streams, and riverbanks in among cactus forests, desert grasslands, and canyons. The stems can be gathered any time of year but are best gathered in the spring before flowering. The fresh flowers are gathered from mid-summer to early autumn, but dried flower clusters can be gathered also. Leaves can be gathered whenever present, mid-spring through autumn. The root bark is considered the strongest medicine this plant offers; see "Gathering Tree Medicine" (page 25) for guidelines.

Medicinal uses

Buttonbush is relatively abundant across our continent. A decoction of the flowers, freshly gathered or upon drying, was commonly used by various North American indigenous groups for stomachache and fever. The bark tea was used for dysentery, fevers, headache, toothache (chew the bark), or stomachache, and as a wash for sore eyes. The leaves can also be used topically for rheumatism. Eclectic physicians employed buttonbush for the intermittent fevers characteristic of malarial infections. Due to its effects on the liver and bile release, it was also commonly used to stimulate appetite, improving the digestive process overall. Michael Moore observed that it stimulates endocrine responses between the intestinal, hepatic, and central nervous systems, and that it is indicated when there's a deficiency in liver function. The stem bark was also employed for coughs and colds. Ingestion of any part of the plant in any form provides a reliable stimulation to digestive secretions.

Herbalist Darryl Patton uses the root bark tincture in low doses for food poisoning. In Louisiana, syrup made from the leaves and flowers is a traditional laxative preparation.

Note: concerns expressed in the historic literature regarding buttonbush refer to the injection of an isolated constituent, cephalanthin, not whole plant usage. In fact, cephalanthin has several important medicinal applications (antiangiogenic, protects RBC, stops hemorrhage) when used at the correct dosage. Buttonbush is safe for internal usage.

Future harvests

Gather only from large, established stands. Gather modestly, and these shrubby trees should continue to thrive along with their wet habitat.

HERBAL PREPARATIONS

Flower/Leaf Tea
Standard Infusion
Drink 2–4 ounces, up to 3 times per day, or combine in formulation.

Bark/Twig/Leaf Tincture
1 part fresh plant, by weight
2 parts menstruum (95% alcohol), by volume
or
1 part dry plant, by weight
5 parts menstruum (50% alcohol, 50% spring water), by volume
Take 10–30 drops, up to 3 times per day.

California poppy

Eschscholzia californica
amapolita del monte
PARTS USED whole plant

A gentle sedative and nervine that allays anxiety, it is able to relieve nerve pain both topically and internally. A useful remedy for small children, helping to alleviate discomfort from teething.

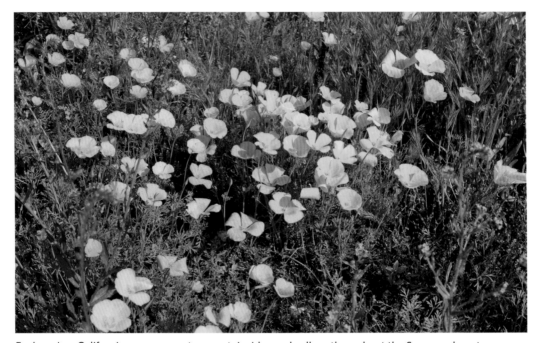

Each spring, California poppy carpets mountainsides and valleys throughout the Sonoran desert.

How to identify
California poppy is predominantly annual within our region. The smooth, blue-green, finely divided, numerous basal leaves may have a lightly frosted look in drier locales. Flowers emerge from an inverted tear-drop-shaped bud on a single stalk, often opening just above the leaves. The 4 petals are commonly yellow or orange (or a combination thereof) but may also be nearly white. The slender ribbed seedpod splits open lengthwise upon maturity, releasing its small, dark seeds. *Eschscholzia parishii*, goldpoppy, found in southern California, has also been used as a topical medicine.

Where, when, and how to wildcraft
California poppy is found predominantly in the western third of our region below 4,000 feet, from southwestern New Mexico to southern Nevada and southern California. It prefers sandy, well-drained soil. It may survive

as a naturalized plant outside of this zone when moisture is abundant and warmth sufficient (e.g., northward along the Pacific coast). This plant may cover entire desert mountainsides in the early to mid-spring. In abundant stands, gather the whole plant when in flower. The root is the most active part. Discard any wilting foliage; chop the fresh plant for tincture, or dry the plant for oil infusion.

Medicinal uses

This herb is perfectly safe and is a wonderful remedy for children despite its relation to opium poppy. Beginning in infancy, the tincture can be rubbed on the gums to allay teething pain. Give to mother to help her relax and to pass the sedative effect onto an irritable baby via breast milk. Drop onto the nipple to be consumed directly. It reliably relieves insomnia due to anxiety. For this purpose, or for nervousness, agitation, or palpitations, pair with desert lavender. Low dosage may be sufficient. Herbalist Christopher Hobbs reports using the tincture to help calm children who are diagnosed with ADHD. The tincture is also recommended for gall bladder or intestinal pain and spasm.

The tincture (the preferred preparation) is also an excellent pain remedy for headache, back pain, or general aches and pains, and it is mildly antispasmodic. It's especially good for nerve pain. Use up to a teaspoon of the tincture in severe pain and anxiety. Nibbling on the flower petals produces similar effects to sipping the tea, but the tea seems to induce grogginess and stupor more readily than does the tincture.

The tea, tincture, or oil infusion can be applied to a variety of pains and spasms, in particular, nerve pain. Prepare the oil infusion from the whole plant.

Topical root preparations were traditionally used to resolve sores and ulcers. Use as a wash when dampness predominates, or the oil when conditions are drier. A decoction of the flowers was traditionally used to cure head lice.

Future harvests

Although seasonally abundant, it can be cultivated in the home landscape or suitable areas in the wild by simply casting the seeds in late autumn.

Caution

Avoid during pregnancy.

HERBAL PREPARATIONS

Flower/Leaf Tea
Standard Infusion
Drink 2–4 ounces, up to 3 times per day; apply topically, as needed.

Whole Plant Tincture
1 part fresh plant, by weight
2 parts menstruum (95% alcohol), by
  volume
or
1 part dry plant, by weight
5 parts menstruum (50% alcohol,
  50% spring water), by volume
Take 15–30 drops, up to 3 times per day; take ¼–1 teaspoon for pain and anxiety.

Oil Infusion
1 part dry plant, by weight
5 parts extra virgin olive oil, by volume
Prepare as alcohol intermediate oil infusion (see page 38).

---

camphorweed

Heterotheca subaxillaris
PARTS USED leaf, flower

*This common summer annual provides pain relief for injuries
and arthritic joints and can be used as an antiseptic wash.*

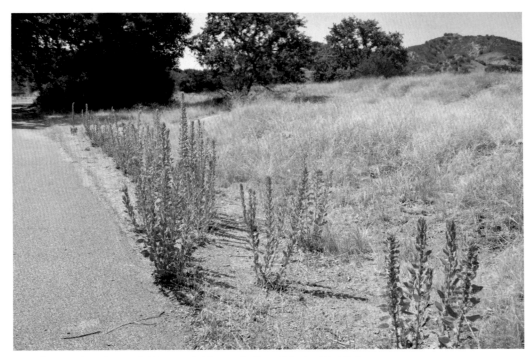

Camphorweed prefers trailsides, roadsides, and other disturbed habitats.

How to identify

This fragrant annual (occasionally biennial) emerges in the early spring, its egg- or
lance-shaped, light green leaves covered
in tiny hairs, making them rough to the
touch. Pointed teeth usually appear along
the wavy leaf margins but are sometimes
absent. Touch the leaf and smell it: it should
have a pungent camphor smell (think Vicks
VapoRub). Panicles of bright yellow composite flowers with 3–4 dozen ray flowers per
head emerge from the leaf axils, just above

clasping leaves. The strong odor persists on
the plant through to the following spring.
Heterotheca villosa, hairy goldenaster, is also
used topically for pain relief.

Where, when, and how to wildcraft

Camphorweed is found in disturbed ground
below 6,000 feet throughout our region,
with limited distribution in the Chihuahuan
desert. Look to roadsides, clearings, and
drainages to find large stands, but you may
also find it growing atop coastal dunes in

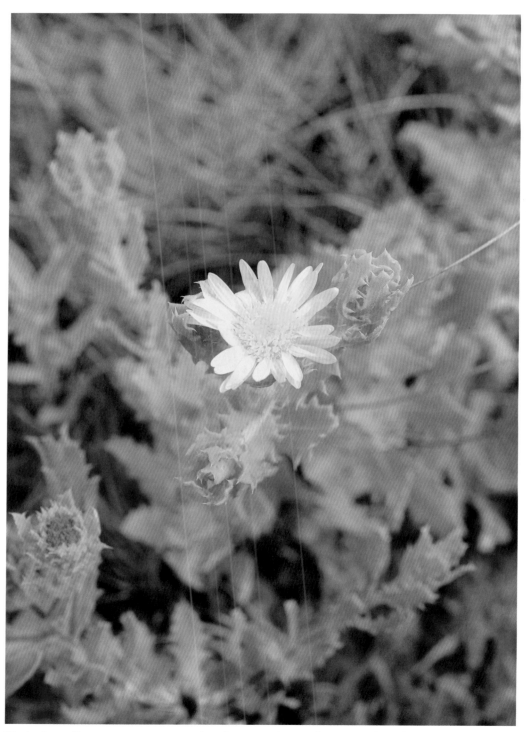

The leaf serrations are more pronounced on these camphorweeds growing along the Gulf Coast of Texas.

south Texas. The basal leaves begin emerging in early spring, with flowering commencing whenever warmth and moisture is sufficient; this tends to be during the summer monsoons in the Sonoran desert and into the late autumn. Gather the aerial parts of the plant for medicine whenever available. Optimally, gather the pre-flowering, erect stalks and dry in the shade. Strip the leaves, flower buds, and small stems from the thickest central stem.

Medicinal uses

Camphorweed is a nice pain reliever. Because it is so prolific and effective, it should be considered one of the Southwest's primary topical pain relief remedies. It can be applied as a fresh plant poultice, tea soak, fomentation, liniment, oil, or salve. The salve is still a popular remedy for joint pain and arthritis in parts of northern Mexico. It's particularly indicated for pain on movement. It has value as a topical antifungal remedy, and the tea can be used as an antiseptic wash for cuts and wounds.

Tea has traditionally been used, internally, for inflammatory conditions of the gut, such as gastritis or acid reflux; however, I feel that other plants are more appropriate for this purpose and so restrict its usage to topical applications only.

Future harvests

Camphorweed does marvelously in regularly disturbed ground. Distribute seed to appropriate areas, and they'll germinate in cool, wet weather.

HERBAL PREPARATIONS

Leaf Tea
Standard Infusion
Apply topically, as needed.

Oil Infusion
1 part dry leaf and flower, by weight
5 parts extra virgin olive oil, by volume
Prepare as alcohol intermediate oil infusion (see page 38).

Poultice
Mash up the fresh plant and apply directly to the body, as needed.

canyon bursage

Ambrosia ambrosioides
chicura, canyon ragweed
PARTS USED leaf, root

The leaf is bitter and astringent, not unlike others in the genus, but its root's warming and stimulating effects on the female reproductive system cause this species to stand out among its relatives.

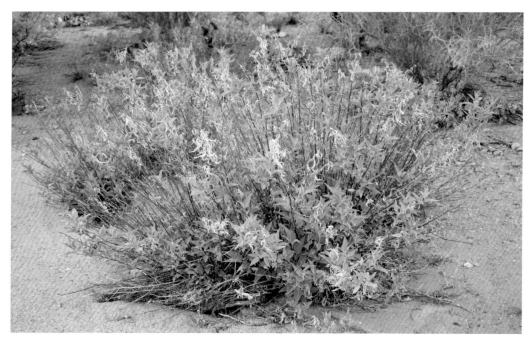

Canyon bursage is common throughout the Sonoran desert, along desert washes or roadsides.

How to identify

The aromatic leaves of this herbaceous perennial are lance-shaped, coarsely toothed, and fuzzy, with yellow veins and an inch-long petiole; they are relatively large and fleshy, becoming curled and crispy and eventually falling off in response to drought. Spikes of male inflorescences are borne terminally in shallow bowl-shaped panicles (very typical of the genus). The female inflorescences appear at the leaf axils; these pistillate heads later become the burred, rusty brown seedpods, which can be found on the plant from summer to winter. New stems arise from the musty-scented beige root in the late winter. Plants will leaf out in response to moisture year-round.

Where, when, and how to wildcraft

This plant is found below 4,000 feet in the Sonoran desert, often colonizing the banks of desert washes, in both sandy and rocky

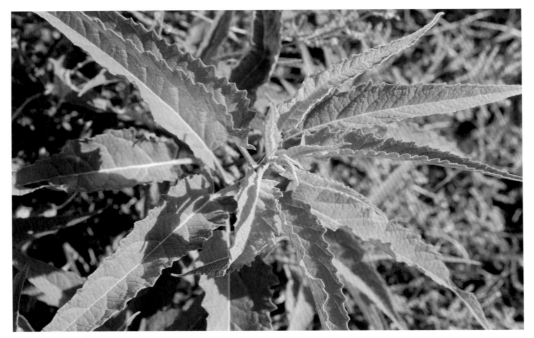

The serrated, lance-shaped leaves of canyon bursage stand out against the relatively sparse desert foliage that surrounds it.

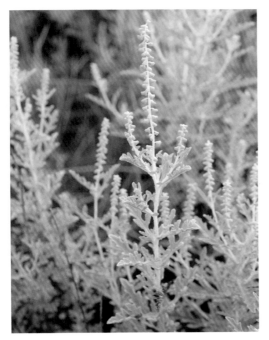

The perennial western ragweed, *Ambrosia psilostachya*, is pictured here on the Texas Gulf Coast.

terrain. Other *Ambrosia* species can be found in nearly every county within our region, but canyon bursage is unique for the medicinal applications of its root. Locate large stands along sandy desert washes from late winter to early spring, or upon the arrival of early winter rains. Dig up plants along the periphery of large stands. Chop the fresh root, and tincture or dry for tea. Gather the sticky, non-flowering leafy stems in late winter or late summer.

Medicinal uses

Any bursage, or ragweed, is particularly helpful at drying up a runny nose from hay fever or seasonal allergies. It's a reliable mucous membrane tonic for its drying action, and it's also a legitimately bitter tonic. The tea and tincture (or a chewed fresh leaf) are wonderful antispasmodics, useful for the cramping associated with dehydration or overexertion;

this is a very valuable remedy in the dry desert Southwest, where leg cramps can bring on sudden severe pain. The root, with its warm, stimulating and dispersing effects, has been used, perhaps for centuries, to address particular concerns of the female reproductive system; it survives today as a well-known postpartum remedy to help "clean out" the uterus, preventing infection and helping to remove any remaining tissue. The root tea or tincture can be used with pain and cramping associated with menses (combine with silk tassel or prickly poppy), particularly when the woman has low libido or is cold and weakened with poor circulation. Among the Seri of northern Mexico, women drink the tea to improve fertility and, once pregnant, to prepare for birthing. Sonoran folk herbalist Doña Olga Ruíz Cañez uses chicura to cure "coldness in the womb," relieve inflammation, and (in combination with *Vitex mollis*, hoja igualama) regulate menstruation. The root also has laxative and diuretic effects.

Future harvests
Follow the instructions just given and refer to "Digging Roots" (page 26).

cáscara sagrada

Frangula (Rhamnus) californica
buckthorn, coffee berry
PARTS USED bark, leaf, fruit

A laxative remedy of repute, cáscara sagrada is also used internally for rheumatic pains and to stimulate liver function.

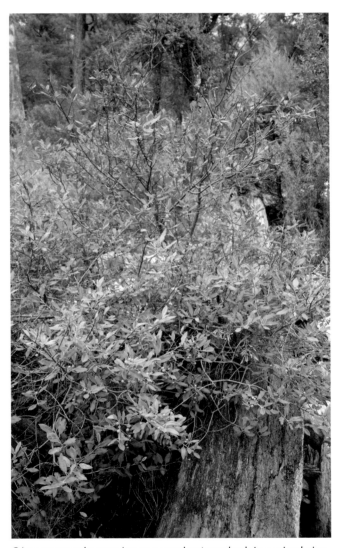

Cáscara sagrada, growing as an understory shrub in a mixed pine and oak woodland at 6,500 feet.

How to identify

This understory evergreen shrub is usually 5–10 feet tall but can reach 15 feet. Its alternate stems are either pinkish red or a soft, fuzzy gray; the mature bark is smooth and dark to reddish brown. The pointed, oval to lance-shaped leaves on short red or yellow petioles are curled under and sometimes wavy at the margins; conspicuous secondary leaf veins run from the central vein straight out to the margins at acute angles. Leaves have a prominent, raised vein on the underside. The small, creamy white to yellow 5-petaled flowers occur in leaf axils in sparse or dense clusters; they are followed by red to purple-black, marble-sized fruits with 2–3 seeds.

Where, when, and how to wildcraft

Cáscara sagrada is scattered throughout our region from middle elevations in the west, to the oak woodlands of the Texas Hill Country and further north. Look for this understory

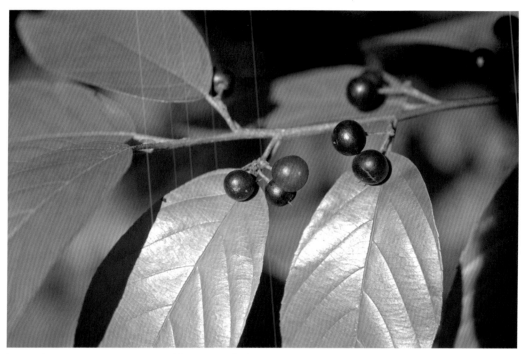

Leaves have conspicuous veins, and fruits ripen by late autumn. *Frangula* (*Rhamnus*) *caroliniana* pictured here.

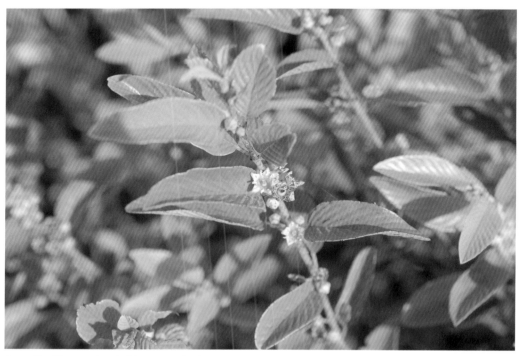

Coyotillo, *Rhamnus humboldtiana*, can be found along the southern rim of Texas, and is also used medicinally.

shrub at the margins of forests or under a full canopy. Coyotillo, *Rhamnus humboldtiana*, found on the South Texas Plains and into the Big Bend area, can be found growing in the open and is used similarly. The bark is best gathered at the end of autumn or late winter/early spring. Age the bark before consuming internally.

Medicinal uses

Cáscara sagrada means "sacred bark" in Spanish. Supposedly, when the indigenous peoples in California had the heart to introduce the suffering Jesuits to this remedy, after their rations of olive oil and red wine had dwindled, they were once again able to relieve themselves. This remedy is used as a laxative to this day. The bark infusion also has a stimulating effect on the kidneys.

The bark must be aged for a year, or heated at a low temperature for several days (sun or low oven) to speed the process. Otherwise, it may provoke vomiting or fervent intestinal griping. Start low and increase the dosage, as needed. The dry bark can be made into tea, tincture, or ground into a powder and encapsulated. When there is a lingering damp heat in the intestines, making certain intestinal illnesses or fungal infections difficult to treat, give 2 "00" capsules in the evening before bed. The bark preparations are also taken internally to relieve rheumatic pains and to stimulate bile secretions. The bark tea can be applied topically to relieve rheumatism or sciatica.

Topically, the berries or leaves have been traditionally used to treat sores, burns, wounds, or to stop bleeding. The tea of the leaves (or bark, mixed with salt) is a traditional remedy for poison ivy rash. An infusion of the wood has been applied for jaundice.

Although some tribes considered the berries poisonous, other groups throughout the West used the berries as food. To this day, many still do.

Future harvests

Gather the bark from pruned peripheral branches, or branches beneath the canopy, and scatter your harvest throughout a large stand. Seeds can be sown in late autumn.

 Caution

Avoid using the fresh bark internally, as it may provoke diarrhea with intense griping. Avoid internal use of the bark preparations with any inflammatory bowel condition, or with diarrhea or loose stools present.

HERBAL PREPARATIONS

Bark Tea
Cold Infusion
Drink 2–6 ounces, in the evening.

Bark Tincture
1 part dry, aged bark, by weight
5 parts menstruum (50% alcohol,
  50% spring water), by volume
Take ¼–1 teaspoon in the evening for laxative effect; use 30–60 drops for hepatic effects and joint pain relief.

Leaf/Berry Poultice
Apply topically, as needed, to swellings, painful joints, sores, burns, or to stop bleeding.

Vitex agnus-castus
PARTS USED leaf, stem, berry

This bitter, pungent plant helps ease restriction in the liver and modulates hormones, allaying symptoms of PMS and providing relief for perimenopausal women. It may also serve as a fertility aid for women.

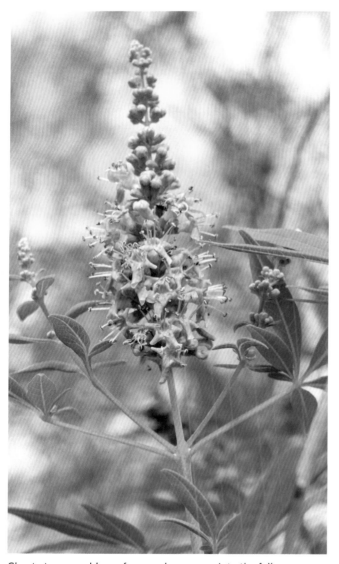

Chaste tree may bloom from early summer into the fall.

How to identify

This deciduous shrub or small tree often reaches 15–20 feet in height. Its mature trunk is light gray to dark brown, the bark furrowing and forming irregularly shaped plates with age. Leaves emerge from rounded leaf scars; they are opposite and palmate, with 5–9 lance-shaped leaflets. The leaflets have smooth margins, and their underside is lighter gray-green; the central leaflet is usually the longest. The inflorescence is a terminal raceme of tiny, 2-lipped lavender corollas enclosed in a cup-shaped, frosted calyx with short teeth. The clusters of round fruits mature from green to purplish brown.

Where, when, and how to wildcraft

This plant is now naturalized throughout lower desert urban areas in the western half of our region. It escapes cultivation more easily in the moist climates along the eastern edge of our region. Here, one may also find *Vitex negundo*, Chinese chaste berry, which can be used

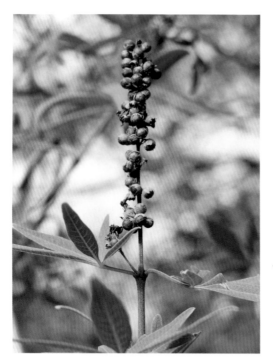

The fruits turn brown upon ripening.

similarly. Gather the leaves and stems prior to flowering or post-flowering. The aromatic berries are gathered upon maturing, from late summer into autumn.

Medicinal uses

Chaste tree is a primary remedy for the female reproductive system. Many consider the berry to be a hormone-modulator and dopaminergic in its action. By increasing dopamine, it inhibit prolactins, and the lowering of prolactin levels has a diminishing effect on follicle-stimulating hormone (FSH), as well as estrogen and testosterone (chaste tree was once thought to enhance estrogen, but it does not). It appears to improve progesterone and enhance the building actions that occur during the luteal phase of menses (post-ovulation). Taken as a tincture, each morning, from ovulation to menses, it relieves many common symptoms of PMS

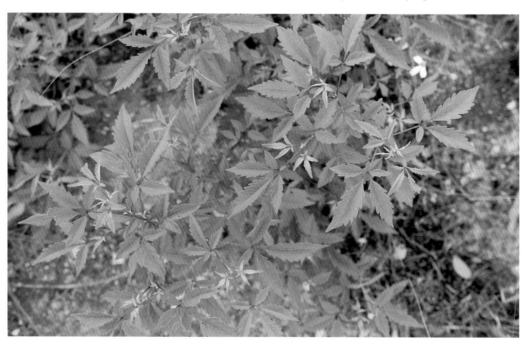

Vitex negundo, mu jing, a native of China, has become naturalized in parts of central Texas. It can be used similarly to chaste tree.

(breast tenderness and swelling, painful cramping, headaches, anxiety, depression). Traditionally, it was considered an anaphrodisiac (hence the "chaste," in reference to monks). However, the energetics of this herb may help to release stored or stagnant energy in the liver, enhancing blood flow and thus increasing libido in individuals of both sexes.

Its ability to resolve restrictions within the liver ameliorates abdominal blood stagnancy and improves the conditions that might lead to PMS symptoms. Combine with estafiate, algerita, and other herbs that relax liver constriction and promote the flow of liver chi, particularly during the second half of the cycle. Be sure to include chaste tree when the onset of menses is accompanied by acne, skin rashes, headache/migraine, frustration, anger, or impatience.

Although some consider it best to avoid chaste tree when depression is present, many others have experienced an alleviation of PMS symptoms with concurrent depression. I believe this relates directly to its ability to relax liver constriction. Some also use it to great effect for severe mood swings and anxiety during perimenopause. It is indicated for a lack of menses (amenorrhea) or excessive (or irregular) discharge of milk, semen, or vaginal fluids.

Used daily, chaste tree can improve fertility. Employed throughout the first trimester, it helps ensure the fetus is carried to term (especially indicated with previous miscarriages). It can improve lactation whenever liver constriction is present, often indicated by concurrent frustration, anger, or impatience. It's also indicated for polycystic ovarian syndrome (PCOS) accompanied by abdominal obesity and insulin resistance.

The leaf and stem tea can be taken to reduce phlegm buildup that provokes coughing. It can also be drunk to relieve painful joints or indigestion due to corresponding accumulated dampness in those tissues; apply the tincture topically as a liniment.

Future harvests

To encourage fruit production, prune branches in the autumn. To increase young leafing branches (and likely reduce seed production), prune branches in spring.

Caution

Avoid in the second and third trimesters of pregnancy, or when taking dopamine-related medications, hormone replacement therapy, or birth control pills.

HERBAL PREPARATIONS

Leaf and Stem Tea
Standard Infusion
Drink 2–4 ounces, up to 4 times per day.

Leaf and Stem Tincture
1 part fresh leaf and stem, by weight
2 parts menstruum (95% alcohol),
  by volume
Take 30–60 drops, up to 4 times per day; apply topically as a liniment to sore joints, muscle pain, and injuries.

Berry Tincture
1 part fresh berry, by weight
2 parts menstruum (95% alcohol),
  by volume
or
1 part dry berry, by weight
3 parts menstruum (65% alcohol,
  35% spring water), by volume
Take 10–30 drops, once in the morning; to improve fertility, take 30–90 drops, 2-4 times per day.

Salvia columbariae
PARTS USED whole plant

Although chia seeds provide substantial nourishment and are also used medicinally, the whole plant has profound effects on the cardiovascular system.

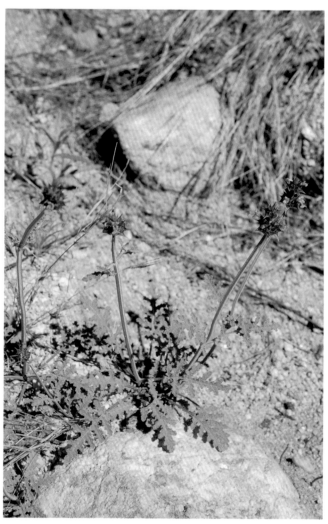

Chia prefers seasonal drainages such as roadsides, the edges of desert washes, floodplains, or rocky canyon hillsides.

How to identify

Chia is an herbaceous annual with deeply and irregularly lobed (often all the way to the midrib) leaves. Leaves are slightly hairy, crinkly in appearance, and (most significantly) pungently aromatic, somewhat reminiscent of skunk. A square stem arising from the basal leaves produces whorls of tiny blue flowers, emerging from sharply pointed green to purple bracts at the opposite leaf nodes. The whole plant turns beige and dies back by early summer, disappearing from the landscape.

Where, when, and how to wildcraft

Chia inhabits low-elevation deserts within the western third of our region, occurring on gradual slopes and in sandy, gravelly washes below 4,000 feet. Gather the whole plant in flower, and seed, by mid- to late spring. Tincture the whole plant fresh. The dry leaves and seeds can also be used as a tea and poultice.

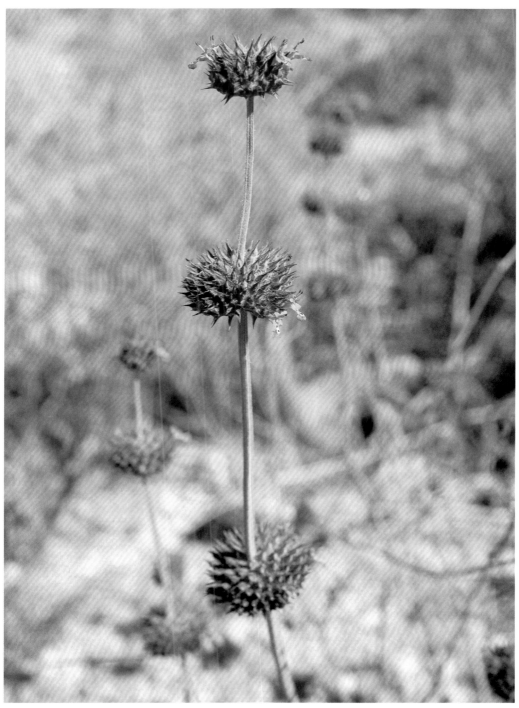

Whorled clusters of flowers occur as interrupted spikes along the stem. Note the lower lip of the 2-lipped corolla is longer and has purple dots along the throat.

Medicinal uses

Known traditional applications of this aromatic bitter herb are limited. A tea of the herb can be taken internally for digestive ailments, although the seeds were more commonly used as both food and medicine. It shares qualtities with sage, which is in the same genus. The moistened mucilaginous seeds were applied topically to sores or infections; placed dry, directly in the eye, to help remove foreign objects; and consumed by runners on long desert runs as pinole, a moistened gruel, for enhanced strength and stamina. Consuming the seeds helped these runners ward off heat exhaustion by protecting their internal organs and preserving the essential moisture barrier, thus preventing overheating.

This warming, aromatic herb also possesses a unique affinity for the heart. It has quite recently been discovered to be the plant that Chumash healers once applied to "wake the dead." Tanshinones, extracted from the root of *Salvia miltiorrhiza*, are compounds used in China as IV injection therapy to help stroke patients recover quickly; chia has about twice as many active tanshinones as *S. miltiorrhiza*. These compounds are known to prevent clotting and dilate the vasculature; they are anti-inflammatory, neuroprotective, and antioxidant. Although a root extract was studied, I've observed that individuals respond well to the cardiac effects from whole plant tinctures. Daily use of the tincture can be an effective remedy for palpitations.

Future harvests

Scatter chia seeds in the late autumn in disturbed ground or where floodwater accumulates.

HERBAL PREPARATIONS

Leaf Tea
Standard Infusion
Drink 2–4 ounces, up to 3 times per day.

Whole Plant Tincture
1 part fresh plant, by weight
2 parts menstruum (95% alcohol),
  by volume
Take 10–30 drops (if root tincture, 5–20 drops), up to 5 times per day.

---

chickweed

Stellaria media
PARTS USED whole plant

A wonderfully soothing demulcent that relieves itchy skin, bites, burns, and slow-to-heal ulcers when used as a fresh plant poultice, tea, powder, or salve. Chickweed is a highly nutritious herb, rich in iron, B vitamins, and vitamin C.

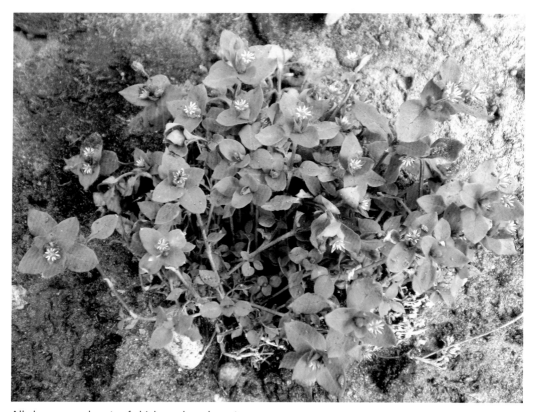
All aboveground parts of chickweed can be eaten.

How to identify

This spreading, low-growing annual possesses rounded, fleshy, simple opposite leaves with entire margins. The terminal white flowers have 5 deeply cleft, nearly heart-shaped petals with 5 pointed, green sepals extending out from just below the petals. A thin line of small white hairs grows along the green to reddish stems. The ethnobotany of our several native *Stellaria* species is unknown, although it appears they have some related qualities. Yet none of them grow to be as lush as *S. media*.

Where, when, and how to wildcraft

This little introduced annual likes moist areas in disturbed ground or shady woodlands.

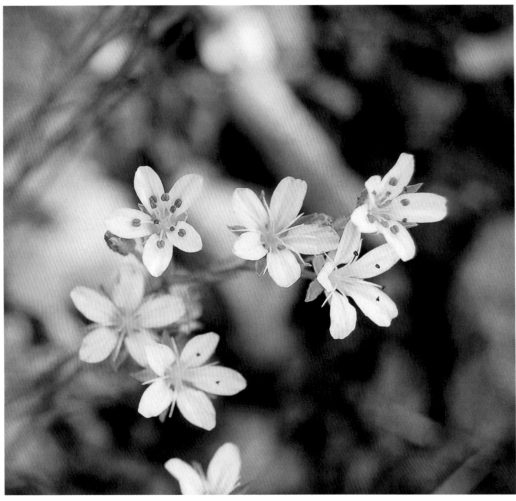

Although not the preferred species for medicine, *Stellaria longipes*, longstalk starwort, a native rhizomatous perennial, can be used topically the same as chickweed.

Look to old ranches, lodges, and ditches or otherwise rich, moist soils along the eastern edge of our region; in the western half, it is sparsely scattered at mid- to high elevations, up to 8,000 feet. Gather the whole plant when in flower (or prior) as a food or to dry for tea. Process fresh for tincture, or tincture shortly after drying. The fresh juice of the plant can also be preserved for topical and internal use with 25% alcohol added to the juice, or simply freeze upon juicing.

Medicinal uses

Chickweed is a classic topical emollient and demulcent herb, bringing relief to abraded, sore, inflamed tissues when applied as a fresh plant poultice, fresh juice, salve, or wash. It's particularly good at relieving itchiness. Place a poultice of the bruised plant over the eyes for conjunctivitis to cool and soothe. The heated fresh plant poultices are a traditional remedy for rheumatic joints and deep, aching bone pain. A strong infusion of chickweed can be applied topically to skin rash, eczema, and other inflammatory skin conditions.

Chickweed tea has a relatively high content of iron and therefore helps reverse iron-deficient anemia. The tea or tincture is also used to treat bronchitis, cough, arthritis, or inflammation of the digestive tract. It is used as a postpartum tonic, emmenagogue, and to enhance lactation. Much of the medicinal values of chickweed can be obtained by eating it fresh or cooked. Chickweed is high enough in vitamin C to have been used to treat scurvy.

Future harvests
This plant is a naturalized visitor from Europe, so think twice before introducing it anywhere other than your own garden.

HERBAL PREPARATIONS

Herb Tea
Standard Infusion
Drink 1–4 cups, daily; infuse overnight to enhance micronutrient content.

Fresh Juice
Smash the herb with a bit of water in a mortar and pestle, or run through a juicer. Use fresh, or preserve with 25% alcohol and store refrigerated or freeze.

Whole Plant Tincture
1 part fresh plant, by weight
2 parts menstruum (75% alcohol,
    25% spring water), by volume
or
1 part recently dry plant, by weight
5 parts menstruum (50% alcohol,
    50% spring water), by volume
Take 30–60 drops, up to 5 times per day.

chokecherry

Prunus virginiana
capulín, black cherry, bitter cherry
PARTS USED bark, fruit

This sweet remedy deepens the breath and calms coughs through its relaxing effects.

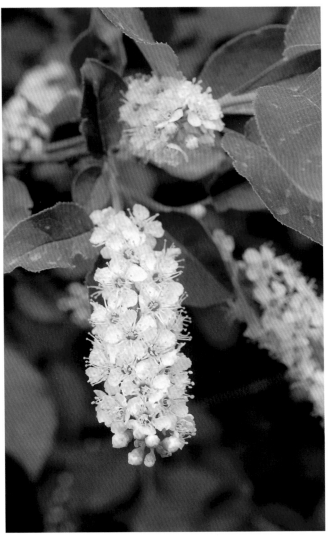

The long, terminal racemes of chokecherry appear after the leaf buds have opened.

How to identify

Ranging in form from a large, multi-trunked or thicket-forming shrub to a single-trunked tree, chokecherry's key feature is its smooth gray to reddish brown bark marked by corky, horizontal lenticels. Also, look for the leaf buds with their many overlapping scales in winter. Leaves are twice as long as they are wide, bright or dark green, and smooth or fuzzy (underside or both sides), with small, pointed serrations lining the margin. White, 5-petaled flowers with yellow stamens are in long, terminal racemes. Bright to dark red to black cherries, or drupes, mature by late summer on long pedicels.

Where, when, and how to wildcraft

Look to desert canyons and mid- to high-elevation conifer forests in the western half of our region. Chokecherry is limited in its distribution in our eastern portion, being sparse in the high plains and prairies, and absent from the South Texas Plains. Begin gathering

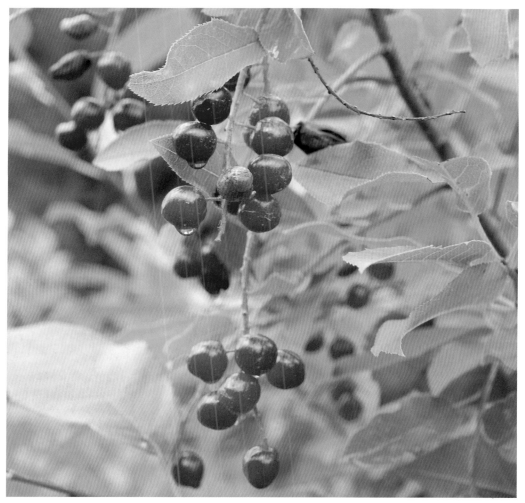

Chokecherry fruits range from bright red to almost black.

bark after mid-summer; see "Gathering Tree Medicine" (page 25). Look for downed trunks and limbs after thunderstorms. *Prunus americana*, found in moist mid-elevation streambeds, can be used similarly.

Medicinal uses

As a centuries-old traditional medicine, tea and syrup preparations of chokecherry bark can be used by both adults and children. Able to alleviate a cough and calm an over-worked body that's attempting to recover from illness, chokecherry is applicable to any respiratory illness, including those with a fever. The bark tea has also been used to stop lung hemorrhage, pain in the chest with cough, and diarrhea; it eases labor pains. Topically, it is used as a wash for sores, eczema, and ulcers (both on the skin and in the mouth). As a tonic to digestion, it aids in convalescence by relaxing the patient while keeping the digestive system well tuned and able to absorb and assimilate the nutrients necessary for recovery. Fruits can be applied

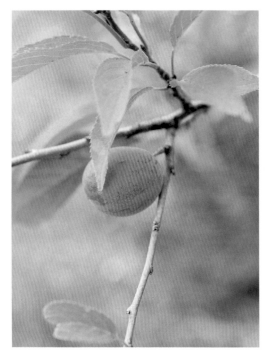

The fruits of American plum, *Prunus americana*, are much larger than chokecherry and the serrated leaves are wider toward the base.

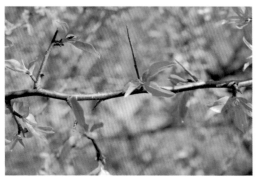

Chickasaw plum, *Prunus angustifolia*, can be found throughout the northeast section of our region. Note the spine-like branches.

⚠ Caution

Do not gather bark before mid-summer: potentially harmful glycosides may be present. Also, avoid using with low blood pressure.

similarly, or combined with the bark preparations, although they are more mild in action.

Decoct chokecherry bark with oshá, spikenard root, cow parsnip root, and gumweed for a potent cough syrup. Add honey once finished.

Future harvests

Prune plants sparingly to encourage growth. Gather no more than a third of the berries from a stand.

HERBAL PREPARATIONS

Bark/Fruit Tea
Cold Infusion
Drink 2–6 ounces, up to 3 times per day, or gargle; apply to the affected area consistently until resolved.

Bark Tincture
1 part dry bark, by weight
5 parts menstruum (60% alcohol,
    30% spring water, 10% glycerin),
    by volume
Take 30–90 drops, up to 4 times per day.

Cylindropuntia species
siviri, chainfruit cholla
PARTS USED stem, root, fruit, sap

This stalwart cactus provides ample relief from the pricks, cuts, burns, and overheating that can happen when spending time in the desert. Drink the root tea to prevent kidney and bladder stones and to find relief from UTIs.

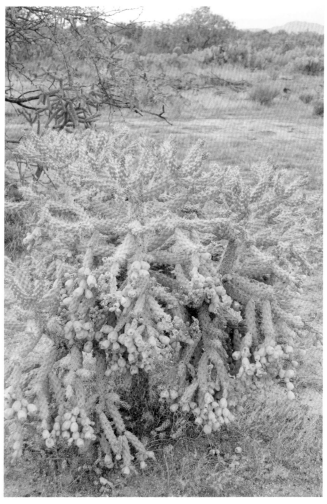

This relatively young and small chainfruit cholla, *Cylindropuntia fulgida,* could sustain 1–2 distal root prunings.

How to identify

This perennial cactus takes on a variety of forms, but its slender stems are always cylindrical. The various species are 1–15 feet tall and often as wide. The green stems are covered in tubercles (rounded and elongated lumps) in an alternating pattern. Each tubercle possesses a light-colored aereole, from which the glochids and spines may emerge. The stems of some species branch at right angles (*Cylindropuntia leptocaulis*, Christmas cholla); others branch at acute angles (*C. versicolor*, staghorn cholla). Some stems are bright or pale green; others have a hint of red, some yellow, or dark brown (*C. bigelovii*, teddybear cholla). Green outer tepals enclose the flower buds, which open to reveal yellow, pink, or red inner tepals and numerous stamens at the center. The fruits that follow may be green, yellow, pink, scarlet, or a combination thereof, with yellowish green flesh and tan or gray

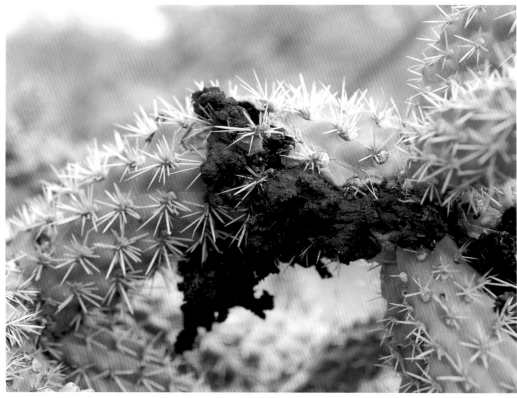
Black sap coming out of a broken stem of *Cylindropuntia spinosior,* cane cholla.

seeds inside. Fruit remains on some cholla species throughout the winter and into the following seasons.

Where, when, and how to wildcraft

Found throughout our region, cholla species inhabit desert grasslands, cactus forests, oak woodlands, high desert, high plains, and the South Texas Plains and Hill Country. The stems can be used for medicine year-round. Gather flowers that have dried upon the plant in late spring. Roots are best gathered in early spring following rains, or in late autumn; see the sidebar for details.

Medicinal uses

Cholla is an amazing plant, seemingly unfazed by drought or frost. Its overall energy is cooling and soothing, as many cactus remedies are. The stems are a traditional topical remedy, dried and powdered and placed on sores, wounds, and boils. The Seri of northern Mexico employ the boiled pulp of the stems as a "heart medicine" and use the fruits as a remedy for diarrhea and shortness of breath; I learned firsthand from them how the fruit pulp, eaten fresh, can prevent imminent heatstroke and have employed it several times since.

Raíz de cholla (cholla root) is a well-known and respected urinary tract remedy throughout northern Mexico. It is diuretic, soothing to irritated mucous membranes of the genitourinary tract, mildly antiseptic, and helps to reduce the formation of calcium oxalate stones—a common malady of laborers and

Digging Cholla Roots

The roots of several species can be used for medicine, but the main cholla harvested for root medicine in the Sonoran desert is *Cylindropuntia fulgida*, chainfruit cholla, which grows abundantly in open plains and sandy bajadas, making for easy gathering. It is not necessary to dig up the entire plant to harvest some root; there are better, more sustainable options.

The first option is to go for a walk in an open plain where tall, top-heavy cholla (over 4–5 feet) can be found, right after a big storm with big gusts of wind. If the ground has been saturated and a strong wind comes by, cholla are readily toppled. The roots exposed to the air will soon dry out and die as the plant shifts its energy to the roots still in the ground. Simply trim back the exposed roots, at the base of the plant, or root crown, and work the ends of these roots out of the ground (they're likely running within 3 inches of the soil surface). Just one storm-toppled cholla can provide an ample harvest for a single family for one year.

The second option, best done when the soil has been moistened several inches down, also involves locating a cholla within a relatively open plain with little to no large boulders in the vicinity, or other large plants close by. With a mattock, begin striking the soil with the flat end of the pick 4-7 feet from the base of the plant or whatever distance is feasible given the circumstances. Tilt the handle, scooping up the soil in front of the flat end that just entered the soil; this maneuver is meant to check for distal rhizomes within a few inches of the soil surface. Continue entering the soil with the pick every few inches until a rhizome is encountered. They are about 1 inch thick, with a thin tan outer bark and a white inner flesh. They have a strong earthy aroma. Once encountered, pick/dig the root up out of the ground all the way back to within several inches of the base of the plant. Sever the root near the base of the plant. Take no more than 2-3 distal rhizomes per plant (Note: cholla are known to increase their root mass by over 35% within 72 hours of a large rain event.) If timed correctly, the plants will not suffer greatly and will continue to grow after your harvest.

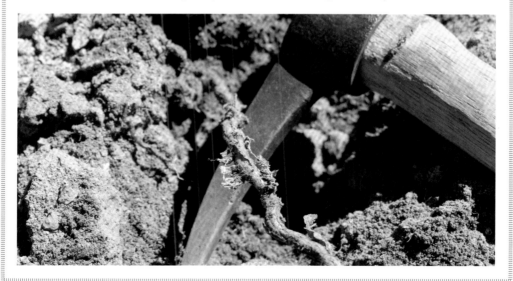

workers of the land, in our hot, dehydrating environment. The root has also been used for constipation and, conversely, diarrhea.

The dry flowers are taken as a tea to help repair tissue. They contain an abundance of flavonoids, each species varying somewhat in their content or variety of nutrients (perhaps relative to flower color). The tea is soothing and cooling to irritated and burned skin, and its antioxidant qualities help to heal digestive tract tissue.

The black sap, which forms misshapen lumps at joints along the stems and trunk, is a traditional food of the Seri and can be utilized as medicine both topically and internally. Powder the polysaccharide-rich sap to soothe irritated skin, or mix with water to make a drink that is soothing to the gastric mucosa, aiding in recovery from any type of inflammatory digestive condition, chemo-radiation, or injuries to the gut lining.

Future harvests

Follow the guidance provided in the sidebar on digging roots, and consider transplanting cholla stems that have fallen off the plant to appropriate areas, including the home landscape.

HERBAL PREPARATIONS

Flower Tea
Standard Infusion
Drink 4–8 ounces, as needed.

Root Tea
Standard Decoction
Drink 2–6 ounces, 2 times per day.

Powdered Sap Poultice
Apply topically, as needed.

Galium species
esculcona, bedstraw
PARTS USED aerial

Mild in flavor and unassuming in appearance, this delicate, clingy plant carries a medicine that acts slowly and deeply to stimulate the gradual release of waste products.

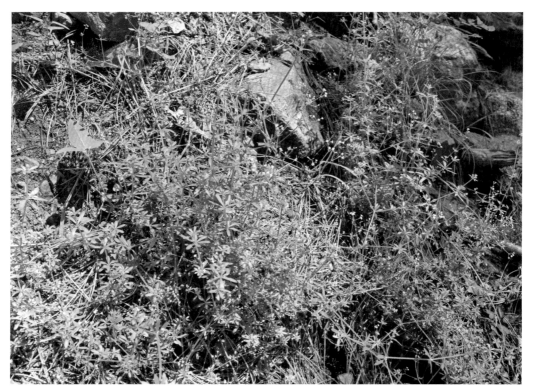

Galium aparine, growing in a ravine around 6,500 feet in a pine forest in Arizona.

How to identify

There are no less than 36 *Galium* species within our region, some annuals, some perennials. Despite this diversity, they are relatively similar in appearance. Leaves are covered in stiff hairs, and stems are markedly square, less than 12 inches high and in a tidy little mound, or luxuriantly long, growing over each other as thick mats, covering the ground and vining over other plants. The leaves occur in whorls of 4–8 along the stem (somewhat similar in form to its madder family relative, buttonbush). The 4-petaled flowers are white in our region, with the exception of *G. wrightii*, whose flowers are often red to pink, occasionally

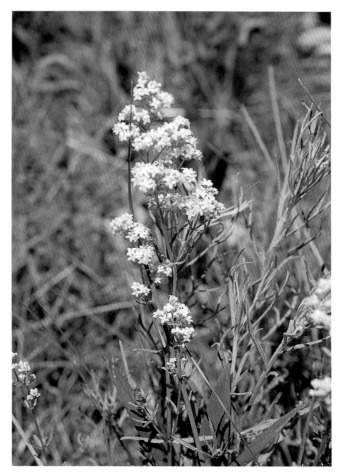

Galium boreale can be found at 6,000–10,000 feet in the western half of our region.

it can also be found under a mature tree canopy of cottonwood, willow, juniper, oak, pine, or occasionally mesquite. In the eastern third, it is nearly absent from the high plains but can be found just about anywhere else, including disturbed sites, oak woodlands, and the South Texas Plains and Hill Country. Cleavers flowers from midspring to early autumn but is relatively easy to identify even when not in flower. Where abundant, gather the whole plant by pulling up handfuls, or trim with scissors or pruners. Tincture or juice the fresh plant, or dry for tea.

Medicinal uses

This unassuming herb is, in fact, a potent remedy that deserves notice. Personally, I have often overlooked cleavers because its subtle power works slowly, but it can have a profound effect on shifting stagnation within the internal organs.

Cleavers was a classic remedy of Eclectic physicians, indicated for the kidneys and urinary tract, specifically for urinary gravel and painful urination in febrile or inflammatory states. The tea is a nice diuretic when urine is scanty. Herbalist David Winston employs it for inflammation of the vas deferens.

Cleavers can be combined with elder flowers, taken internally, and applied as a wash to cool and relax the child (or adult) for viral infections.

Aromatic species, such as *Galium triflorum*, fragrant bedstraw, may be used as tea

yellow. The tiny rounded fruits are usually covered in short but visible, stiff white hairs, which may be hooked or straight. Nearly all species have small flowers (1–2mm wide) openly spaced in spreading cymose panicles; the flowers of *G. boreale*, northern bedstraw, are a bit larger and in tighter, conical terminal panicles.

Where, when, and how to wildcraft

In the western two-thirds of our region, cleavers prefers canyons, streambeds, and other moist places, from 2,000–10,000 feet;

or tincture to open up the lungs and clear phlegm. Cleavers is also a useful remedy for internal hemorrhaging resulting from cough or acute injury. Applied topically, it relieves poison ivy rash and other hot, irritated skin conditions and makes a great hair tonic.

Folk herbalist Doña Olga Ruíz Cañez uses *Galium hystricocarpum*, esculcona, as a tea to help young girls adjust to the onset of menses. She says it doesn't stimulate the hormones but relaxes the nervous system and allays pain associated with menstruation.

Future harvests

Gather modestly from large stands, and leave at least 80% of the plants to go to seed. Spread to appropriate areas by casting seed in late autumn.

HERBAL PREPARATIONS

Herb Tea
Cold or Standard Infusion
Drink 4–8 ounces, as needed; apply topically to poison ivy, wounds, or rashes, or use as a hair tonic.

Fresh Juice
Run the fresh plant through a juicer and take ½–1 teaspoon, up to 4 times per day; preserve with 25% alcohol.

Whole Plant Tincture
1 part fresh plant, by weight
2 parts menstruum (50% alcohol, 50% spring water), by volume
Take 1–3 teaspoons, up to 5 times per day.

Acalypha species

yerba del cancer

PARTS USED aerial

An incredible tissue stimulant that's useful in all poorly healing skin conditions.
The tea taken internally provides soothing relief to acid reflux while stimulating healing.

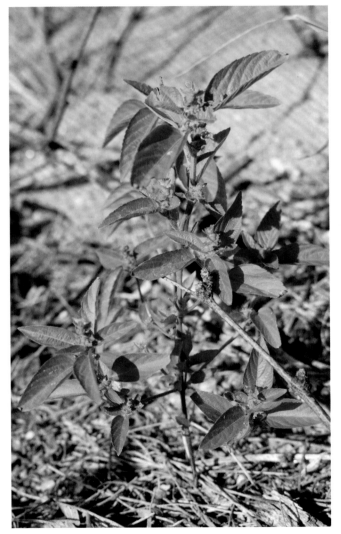

Acalypha neomexicana, an annual copperleaf, is found in abundance in the southwestern corner of our region.

How to identify

Copperleaf is a perennial or annual (depending on the species) and usually no taller than 2 feet. The various species (roughly 10 in our region) can be used interchangeably. The alternate leaves are serrated, often egg-shaped and downward drooping, and come to a point. The inflorescences of this spurge family plant are complex; they can appear as terminal spikes (*Acalypha phleoides*, *A. ostryfolia*, *A. monostachya*) or emerge from the leaf axils (*A. californica*, *A. neomexicana*). The bright red filaments of the petal-less flowers are distinctive. The bracts beneath the female flowers may be as large as leaves and also have toothed margins. The fruits are 3-celled, and the plant turns crimson or coppery red in autumn, distinguishing it from nearly all the surrounding vegetation.

Where, when, and how to wildcraft

Copperleaf is scattered throughout our region but is particularly abundant across

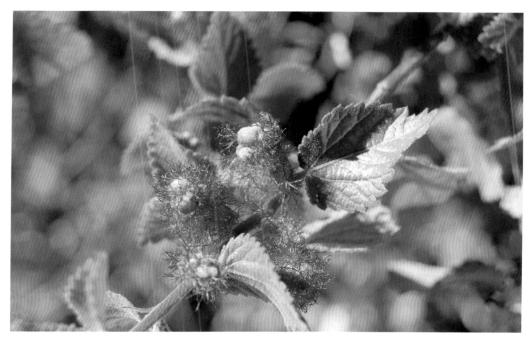
Note the sharply serrated leaves of *Acalypha californica* and the brilliant red filaments on the male flowers.

the southern tier. Look to floodplains and moist areas in desert grasslands, such as washes, as well as oak woodlands, prairies, and the South Texas Plains and Hill Country. In southern California and southern and central Texas, copperleaf can be gathered in mid- to late spring. Elsewhere (e.g., the Sonoran desert and higher elevations), seek it a month or two after summer rains have commenced. Gather several stems from perennial plants. Annual plants, when abundant, can be pulled straight from the ground; or, with 1–2 months still left in the season, cut them back to within several inches of ground level, and they may resprout and repeat bloom before the season ends.

Medicinal uses

Over a century ago, copperleaf was used as a diuretic and as an expectorant to relieve humid asthma; however, more recent generations of herbalists have given it little attention beyond its topical applications. It is a noted antimicrobial with a potent capacity to stimulate tissue repair, making it highly useful in slow-to-heal wounds and sores, such as diabetic ulcers. Prepare as an oil infusion and create a salve, or apply as a wash.

These vulnerary and tissue-healing actions serve excellently when a tea is drunk for acid reflux, or GERD. As an antimicrobial, it may combat an imbalance of digestive flora while also initiating a healing response from the gastric mucosa, thus bringing relief in short time. I've seen the tea work marvelously for this purpose. Another option is to chop the fresh leaf and infuse in honey, and without straining the macerated herb, apply directly to sores and take internally to heal the gut lining. Copperleaf can be combined with hopbush as a skin wash or lotion to reduce hyperpigmentation. Consider using copperleaf tea as a mouthwash with canker sores, gingivitis,

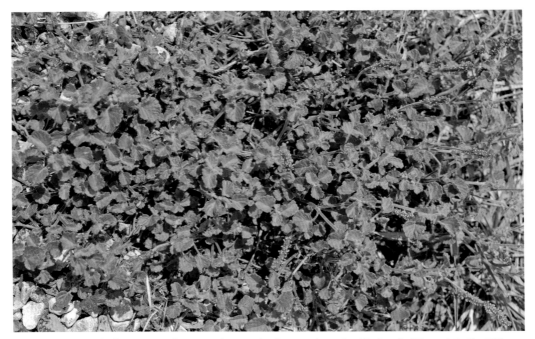

The prostrate *Acalypha monostachya*, round copperleaf, grows from the Big Bend of Texas into the Hill Country and South Plains.

or active infections in the mouth. Apply the fresh leaves to stop bleeding.

Its affinity for the lungs is demonstrated in its ability to relieve cough and reduce the discomfort and inflammation in stubborn cases of bronchitis.

Reviews of other *Acalypha* species have shown potent antidiabetic, hepatoprotective, anti-inflammatory, anthelmintic, and neuro-protective effects. This is certainly a plant we need to explore more thoroughly here in the Southwest.

Future harvests

Follow the guidelines given for gathering, and introduce the seed to disturbed areas in early spring or late autumn.

Caution

Do not ingest during pregnancy.

HERBAL PREPARATIONS

Leaf and Flower Tea
Standard Infusion
Drink 4–8 ounces, 1–3 times per day.

Oil Infusion
1 part dry leaf, stem, flower, by weight
5 parts extra virgin olive oil, by volume
*Prepare as alcohol intermediate oil infusion
(see page 38).*

Leaf Poultice
Apply topically to sores, infected wounds, or to stop bleeding.

Populus species
álamo
PARTS USED bark, leaf, bud

A pungent aromatic herb and a wonderful expectorant, effectively dispersing lingering dampness in the lungs. Cottonwood is also a great musculoskeletal pain remedy.

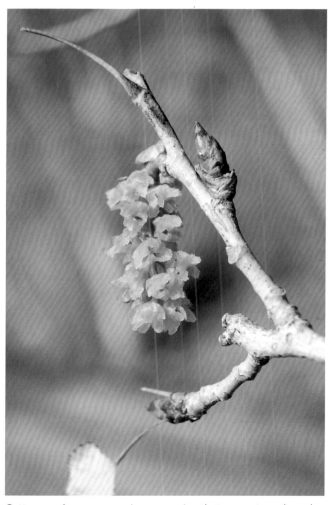

Cottonwoods are monoecious, meaning that separate male and female catkins are found on the same tree. Shown here are the female flowers opening in the early spring.

How to identify

Cottonwood, in all its forms, possesses a relatively light-colored and smooth bark, particularly when young. Its shiny, alternate leaves with rounded teeth vary in shape, depending on the species: *Populus angustifolia* (long, lance-shaped), *P. fremontii* (broadly triangular-ovate with a longer apex than *P. deltoides*). The high-contrast leaves of *P. alba*, the introduced white poplar, are dark green above, white-hairy below. All can hybridize, creating intermediate forms. Cottonwood leaves shimmer in the wind, glinting in a way similar to aspen (*P. tremuloides*). A quintessential marker of autumn in the Southwest, its burning yellow leaves light up the desert waterways as we descend into winter. Its long, thin branches are known to easily fall off in the strong winds brought by winter storms, thus falling to the ground beneath the trees. The bark grays and furrows with age, and in very old trees reaching 3–6 feet in diameter, one may

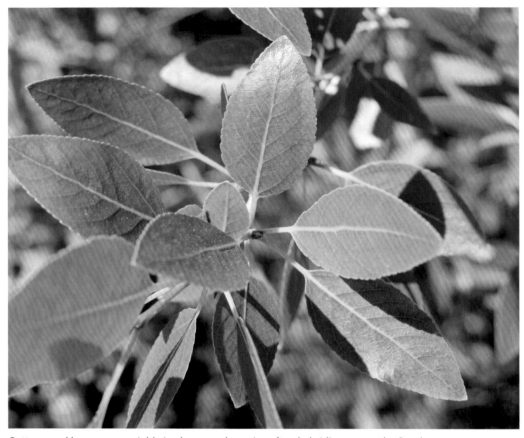

Cottonwood leaves are variable in shape, and species often hybridize across the Southwest.

find a brown ooze with a strong scent excreted near the base of the trunks.

Where, when, and how to wildcraft

Find cottonwoods in various locales of the Southwest but primarily in canyons, flood-plains, and alongside rivers. Like their close relatives willows, they are true phreato-phytes: plants that indicate the presence of surface or near-surface groundwater. Their medicine is available throughout the year. Upon entering a grove in early to mid-spring, the spicy balsamic scent of cottonwood is in the air. Gather both the leaf and flower buds of our cottonwoods from late winter to early spring; I prefer to gather just as they begin

to open, but I have gathered highly potent medicine from cottonwood leaves after they have fully opened from the bud but are still very sticky and resinous: the colder the winter, the thicker the resin, the stronger the medicine. The best source for this medicine is a very young tree, close to the ground, or young trees that have been severely bent or even partially buried by rushing floodwaters. Simply pinch the stem and strip the young, shiny, light green resinous leaves with your finger, and watch the dark green, bitter resin accumulate on your fingertips. The bark can also be stripped from young branches that still have smooth bark. See "Gathering Tree Medicine" (page 25).

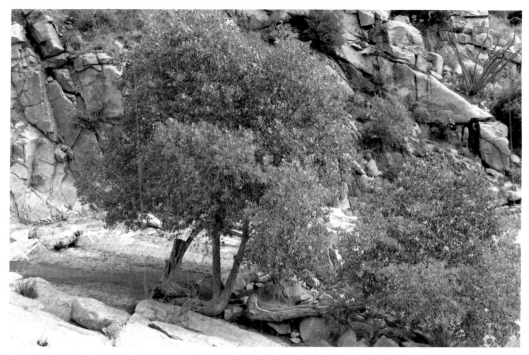

Populus fremontii grows close to water but is relatively drought-adapted, with the ability to reach down for water and pull it up to the ground's surface.

Medicinal uses

Cottonwood preparations are wonderful for relieving pain. Apply a fresh leaf poultice, wash, fomentation, oil infusion, or salve to acute musculoskeletal injuries, including broken bones. The same therapy can be applied to wounds, cuts, stings, and bites. A bark tea can also be applied to all the aforementioned.

The tincture of the fresh leaf bud or young, resinous leaves is an excellent warming expectorant to relieve dampness in the lungs and is useful to relax cough. This may speed healing from acute or chronic infections of the lungs, or certainly help prevent them. Taken internally, the tincture relaxes the musculature, aiding in pain relief from acute injuries. Pain relief can be experienced in the gut as well, along with softening and relaxing, which eases muscle pain as well as nervous tension along the digestive tract.

Future harvests

The young leaves of young trees are the most resinous and therefore the strongest medicine; happily, such leaves are more abundant than the leaves of mature trees and can sustain heavy gathering.

HERBAL PREPARATIONS

Leaf Bud Tincture
1 part fresh budding leaves, by weight
2 parts menstruum (95% alcohol),
   by volume
Apply topically to affected areas; take 15–60 drops, up to 4 times per day.

Oil Infusion
Dry leaves/leaf buds and prepare as alcohol intermediate oil infusion (see page 38).

cow parsnip

Heracleum maximum (H. lanatum)
yerba del oso
PARTS USED leaf, root, seed

Strongly pungent and warming to the lungs, cow parsnip clears damp heat congestion from the body by its counterirritant effects. It's a wonderful remedy for recent nerve damage.

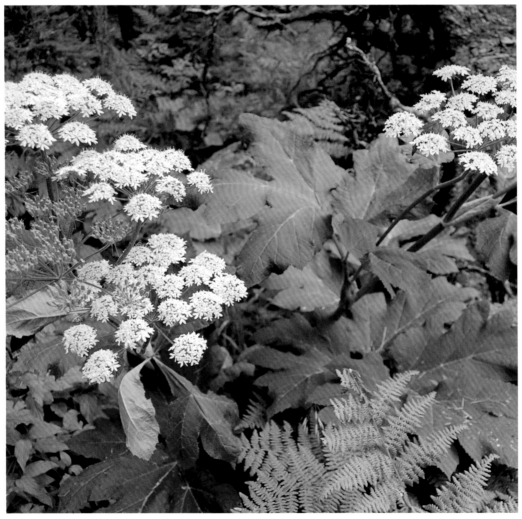

Cow parsnip, growing in a high-elevation conifer forest in Arizona in late summer, with both flowers and young seeds present on the plant.

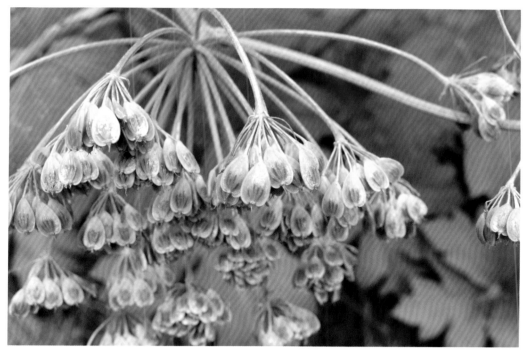
The flattened seeds of cow parsnip have thin wings along the margin and are aromatic.

How to identify

The large, toothed and sharply lobed leaves of this perennial herb arise from pale rootstock, on grooved, hollow stems that are sheathed before unfolding. The compound leaves are large (measuring about 2 feet square) and coarse, a bit rough to the touch, and slightly woolly beneath. Singly or in groups, compound rounded clusters of white flowers with unequal rays open above the leaves on leafless stalks. The semi-heart-shaped, yellowish green, sharply aromatic seedpods are compressed laterally, with thin ribs on the sides, and marked with 3–4 darker lines; they turn beige upon maturity. The similarly aromatic roots are white with a thin, light brown covering.

Where, when, and how to wildcraft

Cow parsnip inhabits seeps, creeks, and wet meadows at high elevations in the western half of our region, from the northwestern corner to some of the Sky Islands in south-eastern Arizona. Find it growing amid fir, spruce, rowan, and aspen. Leaves (1–2 per plant) can be gathered whenever present. Gather the seedheads in mid- to late summer by cutting off the entire cluster. Once the plant has gone to seed and its leaves turn yellow, gather the young roots for tea, syrup, or tincture. Fresh root poultices can be gathered whenever one can dig in the ground.

Medicinal uses

This widely used medicinal plant has a warm and dry energy and a strongly pungent flavor. It has an affinity for the lungs, nerve tissue, gut, and musculoskeletal system. As a topical counterirritant, it can be used to clear heat, blood stagnation, and pain from an area.

Nearly all parts of the plant have been applied as warm poultices to relieve painful swollen joints, sore limbs, back pain, and boils. The fresh root applied topically is counterirritant and works well to restore blood flow to the tissue (nerve, muscle, connective) following recent nerve and musculoskeletal injuries, including paralysis. Consider using the powdered root in salves. The seed tincture can be used similarly to help relieve pain and restore sensation to nerve injuries, or for facial paralysis, such as Bell's palsy, or trigeminal neuralgia. It may also allay various pains of the mouth. Consider taking it internally as well, for all these issues.

The root tea or seed tincture will relax intestinal cramping and act as a carminative to alleviate indigestion. It will diminish menstrual cramping and help start a delayed menses. It opens the lungs, helping to dry out damp conditions and relaxing bronchial spasms. Add the fresh or dry root to cough syrups.

Based upon some of the applications of the Eclectics, we may consider using the fresh root preparations for septicemia (combine with echinacea and oshá), glandular swellings, injuries to the spine (combine with anemone), painful menstruation accompanied by feelings of cold, or nervous indigestion. Fresh root preparations are considerably stronger.

Future harvests

Wild populations of cow parsnip are relatively protected in our national forests; nevertheless, gather modestly and spread seed where appropriate.

 Caution

Avoid during pregnancy. Unlike plants that grow further north, our cow parsnip is *not* known to provoke skin sensitivities upon contact.

HERBAL PREPARATIONS

Root Tea
Standard Infusion
Drink 1–3 ounces, up to 3 times per day.

Root/Seed Tincture
1 part fresh root (or seed), by weight
2 parts menstruum (95% alcohol),
  by volume
or
1 part dry root (or seed), by weight
5 parts menstruum (65% alcohol,
  35% spring water), by volume
*Take 20–60 drops (if seed tincture,
10–30 drops), up to 3 times per day.*

Geranium species
PARTS USED whole plant

Cranesbill is a classic astringent herb with a wide variety of topical and internal applications to dry excessive excretions and tone and tighten tissues.

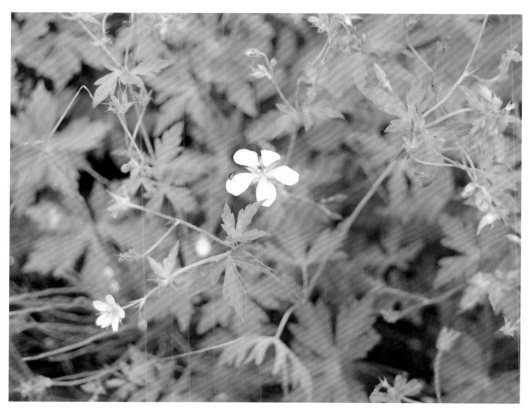

Geranium richardsonii has white to pale pink flowers; both it and *G. caespitosum* occupy high-elevation conifer forests in the western half of our region.

How to identify
Cranesbill is an herbaceous perennial with palmately lobed or divided, simple or compound leaves. The larger leaves occur at the base of the plant; stem leaves are smaller and opposite. Leaves often have deeply grooved upper surface venation. The white to pink to purple flowers have 5 petals, 5 stigmas, and 10 stamens. The carpels of the fruit become upright and elongated as they mature, reminiscent of a crane's bill, or beak; they eventually split lengthwise, ejecting seeds.

Where, when, and how to wildcraft
Cranesbill occurs throughout our region but is relatively sparse in the high desert

and high plains. Look to moist areas of oak woodlands, conifer forests, or desert canyons and arroyos. Those occurring furthest south and at lower elevations can be found in the early spring; high-elevation plants are found mid-spring through early autumn. Gather the foliage when needed, or gather the whole plant from abundant stands. Dry for tea.

Medicinal uses

Cranesbill is a classic astringent herb, not too dazzling. A tea of the whole plant is indicated for chronic diarrhea and dysentery and is especially useful in the subacute phases of inflammatory bowel diseases with a constant urge to evacuate. Use the tea or tincture for any and all types of excessive mucus discharge, such as leukorrhea, mouth sores, or recurrent strep throat. It can also be taken for blood in the urine, gleet, or abnormally heavy menstrual flow. Add to formulas where there's chronic dampness in the lungs and breathing is humid. Any ulcerations of the mucous membranes can be helped by consuming cranesbill preparations (combine with yerba mansa).

Topically, it's styptic (stops bleeding) and helps to heal ulcerous wounds or burns. Gargle the tea to alleviate sore throat, or apply a fomentation to sore eyes. The powdered herb is applied to a baby's navel to speed healing. For thrush, it's given orally as a rinse. It's been chewed for toothache and applied topically as a wash for aching joints. Snuff the powdered leaf for nosebleeds. It helps to dry the tissues in any excessively wet condition, as a poultice, powder, wash, or tincture.

Future harvests

Gather respectfully, only from large stands, and introduce to your home landscape, if appropriate.

HERBAL PREPARATIONS

Herb Tea
Standard Decoction
Drink 1–4 ounces, up to 4 times per day.

Tincture
1 part dry plant, by weight
5 parts menstruum (50% alcohol,
    40% spring water, 10% glycerin),
    by volume
Take 30 drops to 5ml, up to 4 times per day.

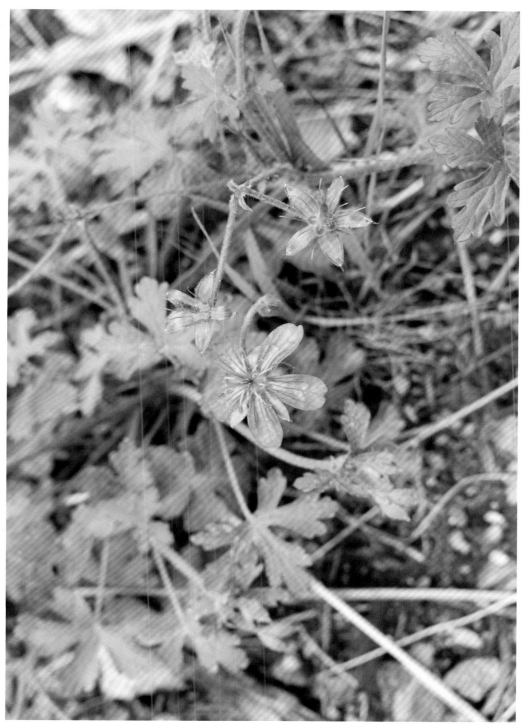

Geranium caespitosum, pineywoods geranium, has light pink to purple flowers.

creosote bush

Larrea tridentata

chaparral, gobernadora, hediondilla, guámis

PARTS USED leaf, stem, flower, gall

After rains, the desert air is filled with the pungent aroma of creosote bush—an herb that resolves any form of irritating, itchy, or inflammatory skin condition, such as burns, bites, stings, and fungal infections.

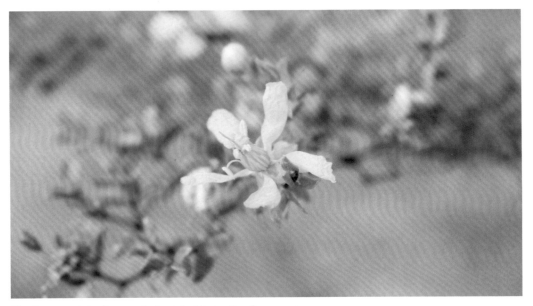

The flower petals of creosote bush twist shortly after opening.

How to identify

Creosote bush is a thin, scraggly woody shrub, usually 5–8 feet tall, occasionally to 20 feet. Plants respond quickly to rains, producing abundant green growth at the base and branch tips. Mature branches have swollen joints at each node and often zigzag or curve haphazardly, with the whole shrub generally growing in an upright V forma-tion. It may also take the shape of a mound, with the branches growing out and toward the ground. Yellow, 5-petaled flowers follow shortly after new leaf growth. The 2-parted resinous leaflets, opposite, rounded, and with a smooth margin, resemble a Pac-Man with an open mouth. As the dry season wears on, leaves turn amber-brown and fall off the plant. Seed capsules covered in silky white hairs soon cover the bush, giving it an air of seniority among other desert dwellers. A fitting countenance for one of the oldest recorded living plants in our North American deserts. In the spring and summer, look for bright green rounded growths (galls) with pointed scales on the branches; these will brown by winter.

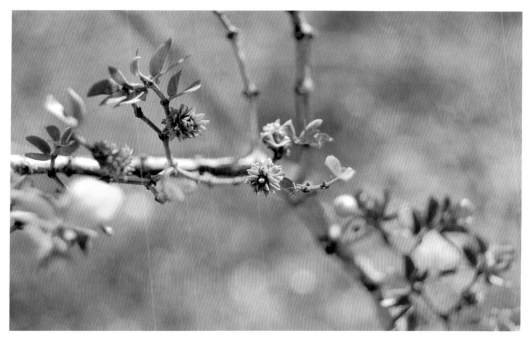

Tiny galls form on the branches of creosote bush in response to wasps. These galls are dried and smoked to alleviate asthma.

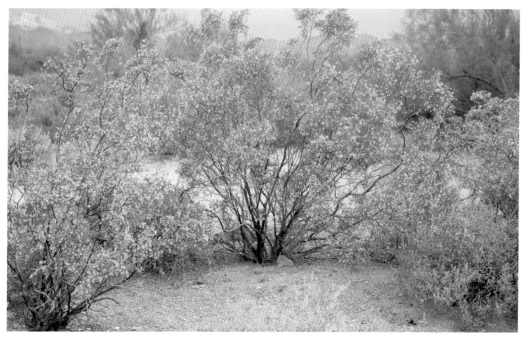

Creosote bush is known to occur in clonal stands but also easily reproduces from seed to create vast stands across desert floodplains throughout the Southwest below 5,000 feet.

Where, when, and how to wildcraft

Although creosote bush often grows abundantly as the exclusive shrub throughout a valley, it is also found intermixed with saguaro, brittlebush, ocotillo, and other plants. Its range extends from southern California to western Texas and the South Texas Plains in the open terrain of our desert grasslands and cactus forests. Harvest the fresh growth during periods of moisture, or after heavy rains, conditions which are most likely to occur in winter/spring toward the western edge of its range, in spring/summer/fall at the eastern, and at any time in the Sonoran desert. Simply pinch just below the fresh green growth and pull toward you; the leaves and tender stems will fall into your hand before you place them in your gathering bag. Be sure to look toward the base of the plant to find tall, fresh growth. The galls can be pinched off the stem by summer's end, while still green.

Medicinal uses

Creosote bush is one of the most widely and commonly used plants among the indigenous peoples of the desert Southwest. Its numerous external and internal applications have been relied upon for centuries. Apply the wash, oil infusion, salve, poultice, leaf powder, or tincture to a variety of wounds,

Safety Concerns with Creosote Bush

Creosote bush is not the panacea it was once purported to be, but is it safe to use it internally? The simple answer is a resounding yes. As with any herb, test small samples on the skin when using creosote bush for the first time to see if there's a reaction; this is uncommon but can occur. If creosote bush is taken in excess, over a period of months, concomitant with pharmaceuticals that significantly stress the liver (e.g., NSAIDs) or excessive alcohol intake (6 or more drinks per day), it is not too surprising that an individual may suffer an acute

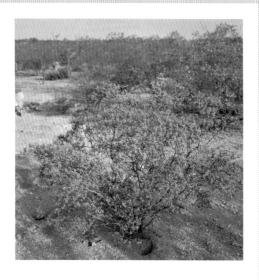

crisis. Be aware of its actions and closely monitor your body's responses on a daily basis. Any potential ill effects from the use of generally safe herbs can be quickly moderated: simply stop taking the herb. An individual who responds with a dramatically ill effect from the short-term use of an herb will have likely entered the situation with pre-existing health concerns. These can often be moderated through proper professional guidance as well as self-awareness practices.

In short, although creosote bush is a potent medicine, it can be used safely, both externally and internally, without fear of injury. When utilized for the applications mentioned in this profile, one can be assured of safety.

burns, cuts, abrasions, scrapes, bruises, damp inflammations, skin infections, fungal infections, mosquito bites, venomous bites, stings, or other blemishes or injuries to the skin.

Dry conditions beg for the oil or salve, whereas damp, hot conditions respond best to the wash, leaf powder, tincture, or poultice. Combine the powdered leaf with honey and apply to herpes sores (types 1 and 2). For acute cellulitis, cover the area with the fresh plant poultice, tincture, or powdered leaf (combine with self-heal), and cover again with a hot, moist towel. Continue until the pain is abated. A douche, or suppository, can be applied for HPV infections.

Creosote bush oil infusion is a truly remarkable remedy for burns of all sorts. Soak the feet for fungal infections, or for heat rashes. Perform a whole body soak once every 2–4 weeks for chronic inflammatory musculoskeletal pain or to simply induce deep relaxation. Make a decoction and, with a towel over the head, do a steam inhalation over the pot to abort the sudden onset of a head cold, to relieve sinus congestion, or to simply enjoy a deeply therapeutic experience. Place the fresh branches in athletes' shoes at night to reduce fungal overgrowth and odor, or simply dust feet with the finely powdered leaves.

Internally, the tea can be gargled for a sore throat or any ulcerations or lacerations within the mouth and throat; it is an excellent adjuvant to chemo or radiation therapy which affects this area. Among the O'odham peoples of the Sonoran desert, the tea of the leaves and stems is revered for its ability to treat a sore throat, cough, cold, chest congestion, sinus congestion, or other maladies brought on by cold, wet winter weather.

Women can utilize the tea or tincture to reduce feelings of discomfort around menses, especially when there is heat and dampness present. Also, take the tincture, or tea, internally for acute cellulitis infections, scorpion stings, brown recluse or black widow bites, atopic conditions, chronic joint inflammation, or upon ingesting a toxic substance. The use of the tincture before meals is helpful when fat digestion is poor. Consider its use in fatty liver disease but avoid protracted use (more than 2 weeks) where chronic fatigue is present.

Future harvests

Fortunately, this plant faces no imminent threats, but do plant one in your yard if it doesn't already grow there. You won't regret it.

HERBAL PREPARATIONS

Topical Wash
Strong Decoction
Apply to the affected area consistently until resolved.

Oil Infusion
1:5
Prepare as fresh plant oil infusion (see page 39).

Leaf and Stem Tincture
1 part dry herb, by weight
5 parts menstruum (75% alcohol, 25% spring water), by volume
or
1 part fresh herb, by weight
2 parts menstruum (95% alcohol), by volume
Take 15–60 drops, up to 3 times per day; apply to the affected area consistently until resolved.

Steam Inhalation
Strong Decoction
Inhale the steam deeply for 3–5 minutes while covering the head with a towel, 4 times consecutively; repeat this cycle several times a day during acute congestion or viral infection.

Pseudognaphalium canescens
manzanilla del rio, rabbit tobacco, gordo lobo
PARTS USED aerial

Resinous to the touch with a lemony scent, cudweed helps with colds, flu, and other respiratory illnesses. This anti-inflammatory herb can be used to relieve pain and spasm, topically and internally.

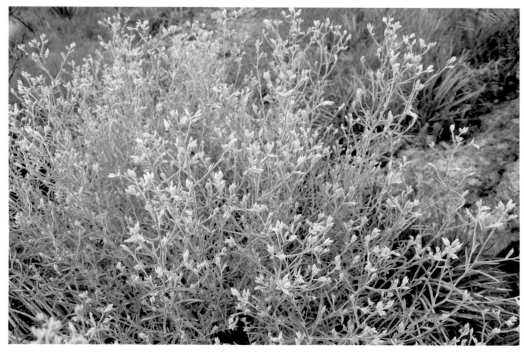

Cudweed has a multi-branched habit and rounded to almost square form.

How to identify
Cudweed is an annual or perennial reaching about 2 feet in height, pale gray-green, with a frosty white coating of soft, fine hairs covering the plant. Its flat, gray-green leaves are sessile, mostly linear in shape, and come to a fine point. Loose panicles of pearly white flowers emerge from the leaf axils on short branches throughout the plant, opening to reveal yellow corollas at the center. The ends of the seeds are covered in fine, feathery hairs. The plant appears grayish white in the winter.

Where, when, and how to wildcraft
This genial herb occurs throughout our region but is absent from the high plains. It can be used interchangeably with *Gnaphalium* species, particularly those with the lemony scent. *Pseudognaphalium californicum, P. macounii, P. viscosum,* winged cudweed, and

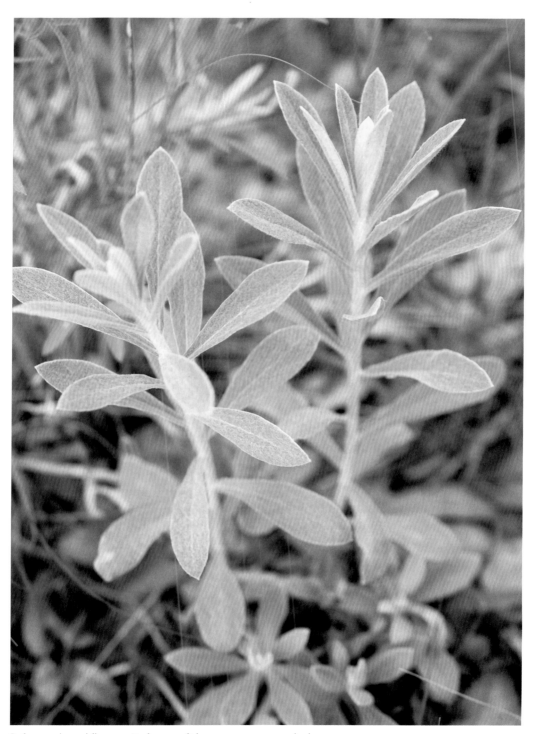

Before cudweed flowers, its fuzzy soft leaves appear more lush.

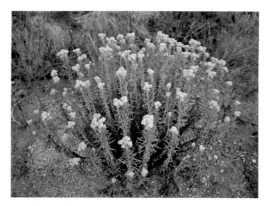

Pseudognaphalium leucocephalum, known in the Sonoran desert region as talampacate, can be locally abundant. Its foliage is resinous and lemon-scented.

Cold and Flu Formula

Combine the following dry herbs, by weight, and prepare as a standard infusion; drink 1–2 cups daily to help prevent colds and flu; drink 1 hot cup every 1–2 hours during acute infection.

- 2 parts cudweed
- 2 parts wild mint
- 2 parts elder flower
- 2 parts yerba mansa leaf
- 1 part yerba santa leaf
- 1 part wild oregano leaf

P. obtusifolium, rabbit tobacco, are also useful medicines. Gather the herb from late summer into late autumn, either just before flowering or after flowering has occurred. Bundle the herb and hang to dry in the shade, or place loosely in paper bags in a warm dry place out of direct sunlight.

Medicinal uses

A popular folk herb, cudweed is a highly useful remedy. As a tea, it helps reduce inflammation of the mucous membranes of the respiratory tract and lungs, enhancing immunity and reducing the severity of the illness. Beside being tasty, it aids in the recovery process. Consider adding to formulas for cough, asthma, and chronic lung inflammation. The tea relieves nausea, stomachache, and gastritis, while also calming the nervous system, making it a nice evening tea.

This relaxant effect can also be experienced via topical use of the herb, as a poultice or fomentation. It is relieving to muscle spasms, joint pain, and localized musculoskeletal pain. The infusion has also traditionally been used as an eyewash to relieve sore, irritated eyes.

Future harvests

Gather only from abundant stands, and leave the majority of flowering stems to go to seed.

HERBAL PREPARATIONS

Leaf Tea
Standard Infusion
Drink 4–8 ounces, as needed; apply topically as a fomentation, as needed.

Poultice
Mash up the fresh plant and apply directly to the body, as needed.

Rumex crispus

lengua de vaca, caña ágria, yellow dock, sour dock

PARTS USED leaf, root

Enlivens digestion while improving the health of the skin, liver, blood, muscle, and bone. A highly nutritious herb with different uses for the leaf and root.

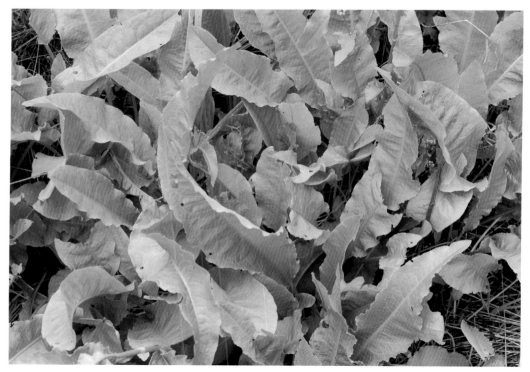

Curly dock produces large, abundant basal leaves in spring.

How to identify

Large, lance-shaped bright green basal leaves (reminiscent of a cow's tongue) arise in spring from a short-lived perennial rootstock; these 12- to 24-inch-long leaves are borne on long petioles and have curly or undulating margins, and they die back quickly once the plant goes to flower, turning rusty brown to brick-red as the plant ages. This buckwheat family plant produces inconspicuous yellow-green flowers in crowded, narrow, terminal inflorescences; the abundant seeds, or achenes, are rimmed by conspicuous 3-winged valves (which also turn rust brown). The flesh of the carrot-like or branched root is yellow, orange, or reddish orange; the root bark is a dark reddish brown-russet. Basal leaves re-emerge in late summer/early autumn in areas of sufficient moisture before turning rust-brown and falling off

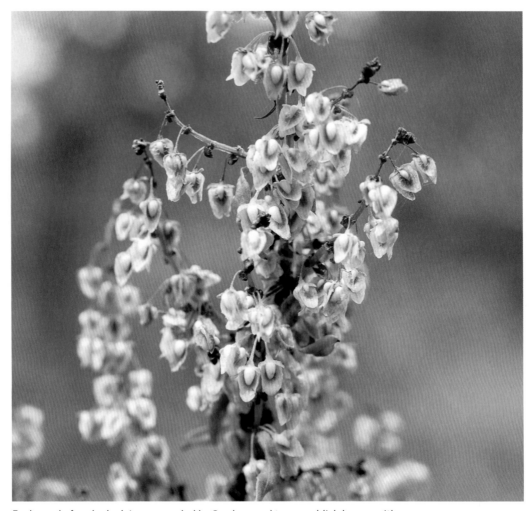

Each seed of curly dock is surrounded by 3 valves and turns reddish brown with age.

the darkened flower stalk, which persists through winter. The uses given here apply to most *Rumex* species found in the Southwest.

Where, when, and how to wildcraft

This introduced exotic from Europe is found throughout the Southwest, most often in disturbed ground, including pastures, roadsides, streambeds, or desert arroyos. It's particularly abundant in pastures in the high desert, high plains, and mid-elevation canyons. The leaves should be gathered prior to flowering (early spring to early summer) and during the second growth stage, after seeding, when available. Dig the roots in early spring (for best medicine) or late autumn.

Medicinal uses

Curly dock leaves are an excellent demulcent applied topically, or taken internally as a tea. Add them to tea blends to help preserve moisture in a dry climate. Both the leaves and root are particularly nutritious. A compound syrup made with molasses and the

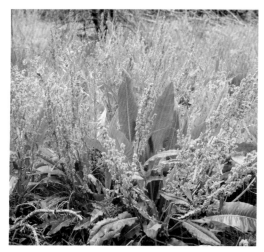

Rumex orthoneurus, Chiricahua dock, is a plant of the Mogollon Rim and of the Sky Islands in southeastern Arizona and southwestern New Mexico.

roots has been given to pregnant women to improve anemia. The root tea, applied both topically and internally, is terrific at clearing damp, stagnant conditions, particularly of the skin, lymph, and digestive system—think rashes, itching, chronic lymphatic swellings, or feelings of fullness and heaviness in the belly. Although strongly tonic, it has a mild relaxing effect on the nervous system, making it particularly useful in skin and digestive symptoms brought on by nervous system tension and agitation. The tea or tincture taken at bedtime is a reliable laxative for many, especially if lower back pain or tension is present as well. Conversely, it can also be used for diarrhea. Take a bath in the strong decoction whenever covered in insect bites, scratches, or any hot, itchy condition. This is a good application for an acetum of the leaf, which can also be taken internally for respiratory inflammation and restricted breathing. The powdered root helps fix loose teeth to the gums.

Future harvests

Many landowners and range management officials would be all too happy to see someone gathering this naturalized exotic and putting it to use.

HERBAL PREPARATIONS

Root Tea
Standard Decoction
Drink 4–8 ounces, up to 3 times per day.

Leaf Tea
Standard Infusion
Drink 4–8 ounces, up to 3 times per day.

Root Tincture
1 part fresh root, by weight
2 parts menstruum (95% alcohol),
  by volume
or
1 part dry root, by weight
5 parts menstruum (50% alcohol,
  50% spring water), by volume
Take 1–3ml, up to 3 times per day.

Leaf Acetum
1 part fresh leaf, by weight
2 parts menstruum (apple cider vinegar),
  by volume
Apply topically to affected areas, as needed; take 5–30 drops, up to 3 times per day.

dandelion

Taraxacum officinale
diente de león
PARTS USED whole plant

Cooling and soothing to the liver and kidneys, the leaves, flowers, and root are all highly nutritive. There are so many healing ways to ingest and cover oneself with dandelion remedies.

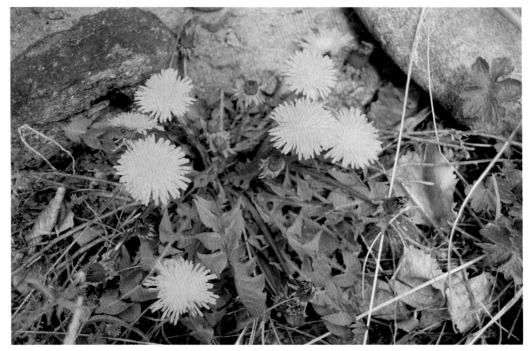

One can often find flower buds, open flowers, and closed flowers on one dandelion plant.

How to identify

Who doesn't know dandelion? The numerous, deeply and variably lobed and toothed, lance-shaped leaves of 3–7 inches, pointed like an arrowhead, arise from a taproot in the spring. Shortly thereafter, they're followed by a single terminal inflorescence arising on a hollow stalk that exudes a milky latex when broken. Dozens of bright yellow ray flowers are subtended by 2 rows of green, lance-shaped phyllaries, one of which adheres to the ray flowers while the other curves downward, away from the flower head. Attached to each gray-brown pointed seed is a feathery pappus, which floats away by the force of a toddler's breath.

Where, when, and how to wildcraft

A lover of disturbed ground, dandelion is found throughout our region. It favors damp soils or shady locations in our hotter, drier climes. It is largely absent from our lower elevations in the western portion of our region (and the South Texas Plains), save for well-watered lawns and parks (not particularly favored gathering locations due to irrigation with reclaimed water and spraying with herbicides), but may be found abundantly in clearings, and streambanks throughout high-elevation conifer forests. Gather the leaves before flowering, from early winter to late spring, depending on the location and elevation. The flowers are gathered upon opening when bright and fresh. The roots are gathered in the autumn after the plant has gone to seed.

Medicinal uses

Bridging the gap between healing food and medicine, dandelion has found its way from field to kitchen for centuries, all over the world. The bitterness of dandelion is indicative of its function in the body—it activates the secretion of digestive juices. This improved secretion helps to resolve simple constipation and improves poor appetite and sluggish digestion. Its delicate yet mildly stimulating effect on the liver gives us a medicine to apply to acute skin eruptions, and relieve stomachache, menstrual cramps, or hepatitis. For urinary gravel or stones, drink several cups of the root decoction, daily. Topical applications of the root can relieve chronic or acute inflammatory skin conditions as well. Roots harvested in the autumn, being sweeter, are more restorative to the liver, and, therefore, may be a useful aid for diabetics.

Future harvests

It will be there.

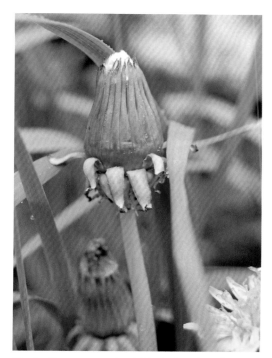

The feathery pappus is visible in this closed dandelion flower.

HERBAL PREPARATIONS

Root Tea
Strong Decoction
Drink 2-4 ounces, as needed.

Leaf Tea
Standard Infusion
Drink 4-8 ounces, as needed.

Root Tincture
1 part fresh root, by weight
2 parts menstruum (95% alcohol),
 by volume
or
1 part dry root, by weight
5 parts menstruum (50% alcohol,
 50% spring water), by volume
Take 1–5ml, up to 3 times per day.

Gossypium thurberi
algodoncillo
PARTS USED stem, root, root bark

One of our most important remedies for nourishing and supporting the female reproductive system.

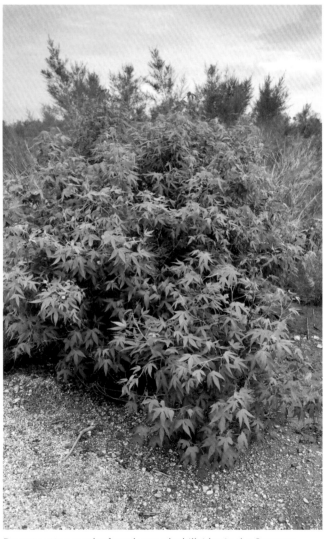

Desert cotton can be found on rocky hillsides in the Sonoran desert as well as floodplains of desert washes.

How to identify

This perennial shrub is generally 4–8 feet in height, at maturity. Its bark is smooth and gray to light brown. The palmate leaves with 3–5 pointed lobes appear in mid- to late spring on 1–3 inch petioles. The 5 white to pale yellow petals, appearing in late summer into autumn, often possess a pink spot at their base, and quickly turn magenta and pink as they age. A green fruit follows the flower, which matures to a reddish brown when it splits open to reveal a 3-celled capsule, each capsule opened in the middle revealing rows of brown rounded seeds on either side of the opening. The seeds and the inside of the capsule may have tufts of white hairs. The leaves turn an ochre or sienna red by late autumn.

Where, when, and how to wildcraft

Desert cotton is exclusively found at low to middle elevation rocky hillsides and floodplains of desert washes in the desert grasslands ecosystem from central to southeast Arizona.

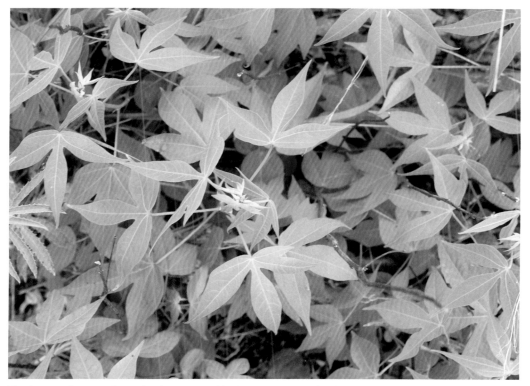

The leaves of young plants (and new growth) often start out with 3 lobes then expand into 5 lobes as they mature.

The root and stem bark should be gathered around the first full moon in March for optimal potency. Use just the root bark of thick (3 inches or more) older roots, and the whole root from younger plants. See "Digging Roots" on page 26 for further instruction. The seeds can be gathered from late autumn into winter.

Medicinal uses

Desert cotton is a specific medicine for the female reproductive system and the quint-essential female reproductive hormones (estrogen, et al.). The root and root bark tincture is used to resolve inflammation within the female reproductive system, which may otherwise lead to fibroids, painful menses, infertility, cysts, endometriosis, or cancers of these organs. It is commonly used to start the flow of a slow menses as well as initiate contractions during a slow to start labor. It relieves deficiency within the organ system delivering nourishment and enhancing the flow of vital energy to these organs, as opposed to being an irritant or a stimulant as many other herbs classified as emmenagogues may be.

The syrup of the root, or root bark, is a nutritive remedy for the uterus. It delivers warmth through increased blood flow, enhancing nutrition to develop a resilient and functional uterine lining. Take it daily during the weeks following menses. The seeds can be used similarly as a nourishing agent for the uterus. Males wishing to shift toward a more estrogenic hormonal profile

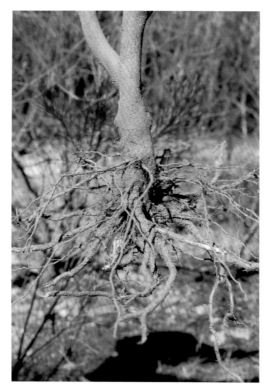

The entire root can be used for medicine when 1 inch or less in diameter (sometimes even larger). Strip the root bark of larger root crowns as well as the lowest few inches of trunk bark.

(reducing testosterone and libido) should consume the seeds regularly; otherwise, refrain from using this plant internally.

The stem bark tincture is a bit less nourishing in its action and more stimulating. It can be used to shift stagnant energy within the uterus within an otherwise nourished and full reproductive system. It combines well in formulation.

Although this plant's physiological effects are clearly indicated for the female reproductive system, its nature carries something that both sexes can tap into.

It may serve to balance the corresponding genders within oneself, transcending the external form to experience both sexes as equal manifestations of creative energy. This effect may be experienced through time spent with the plant, a flower essence preparation, or using drop dosages of the tincture.

Future harvests

This plant is often spread by floodwater. Scarified seeds can be planted in the fall in well-drained soil and transplanted to suitable areas shortly after germinating.

Caution

Avoid during pregnancy. The industrially processed seed oil has been known to induce sterility in males.

HERBAL PREPARATIONS

Seed Meal
Grind and take ½–2 tablespoons per day as a food supplement to nourish the female reproductive system.

Root Syrup
Take 1–2 tablespoons, up to 2 times per day. Use fresh root and/or root bark to prepare the syrup following the instructions on page 38.

Root Tincture
1 part fresh root and/or root bark, by weight
2 parts menstruum (95% alcohol),
  by volume
Take 10–60 drops, up to 4 times per day.

Stem Bark Tincture
1 part fresh stem bark, by weight
2 parts menstruum (95% alcohol),
  by volume
Take 15–40 drops, up to 3 times per day.

desert lavender

Hyptis (Condea) emoryi, H. albida
sálvia, xeescl
PARTS USED leaf, stem, flower

Cooling to inflammation throughout the body and relaxing to the nervous system, desert lavender offers an important medicine to the modern human.

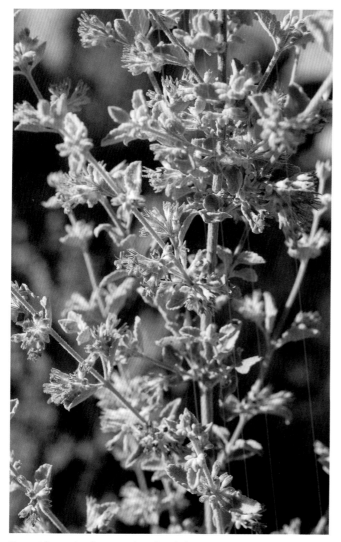

Desert lavender flowers abundantly in response to seasonal moisture.

How to identify

Our native desert lavender is an aromatic, drought- and frost-deciduous desert shrub, generally 4–7 feet tall, to 15 feet in optimal conditions. Its simple opposite leaves have crenate margins and are wrinkled and fuzzy, giving them a light greenish gray appearance. The light gray to beige opposite stems, arising from multiple thin trunks, are often leafless throughout the year. In response to moisture, leaves quickly emerge, and whorls of small, fuzzy lavender-blue flowers occur at the leaf axils and as terminal spikes. The lightly scented flowers have fuzzy, light gray calyces that may be tinged purple at the tips.

Where, when, and how to wildcraft

Desert lavender grows in the southwestern quadrant of our region, generally below 2,000 feet, sometimes as high as 4,000 feet, tucked into large boulders or at cliff faces, which wick off the day's accumulated heat into the night. Plants leaf

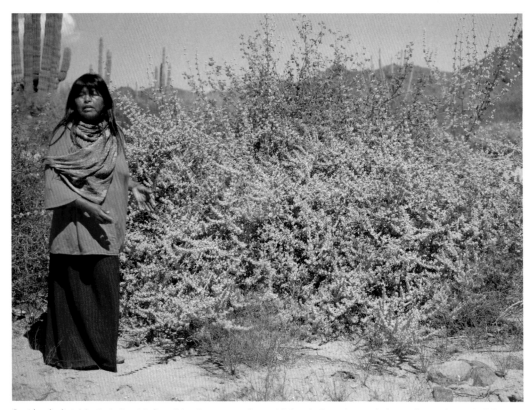

Seri herbalist Maria Luisa Molino Martinez, standing with her beloved *xeescl*, desert lavender, in full flower.

out and flower year-round in response to moisture. Look to the base of mature plants for fresh, luxuriant growth. Simply pinch the stem at the base of new growth and pull out, running the thumb and index finger along the stem. Young stems may break off as well; use the entire portion.

Medicinal uses

A gentle plant with a wide array of applications, desert lavender is a traditional remedy for internal hemorrhaging, coughs, colds, flu, sore throat, and toothache. Folk herbalist Doña Olga Ruíz Cañez uses it for a variety of female reproductive system issues, including leukorrhea, vaginal hemorrhage, inflammation, abnormal bleeding (metrorrhagia), and as a healing postpartum sitz bath. This same bath can be used for bleeding hemorrhoids. Related *Hyptis* species are also used for improving blood circulation.

Like other plants in the mint family (chia, sage, wild oregano), desert lavender calms inflammation throughout the body, applied both topically and internally. Topically, the herb is an effective poultice, tea, oil, or salve for cuts, wounds, burns, and general skin irritations.

Desert lavender has a particular affinity for the lungs. The tea or tincture is helpful in situations of chronic lung inflammation (combine with tree of heaven), asthma, allergies, or chest congestion. The cool tea is wonderfully tonic to the digestion, allaying a stomachache and reducing gastric inflammation. Drunk hot, the tea is diaphoretic, sedative, and astringent to the mucous membranes. The tincture (polyphenols present) also helps to relax and restore the liver.

Amongst the Seri, or Comcáac, in northwestern Sonora, Mexico, desert lavender is the most important herb applied for spiritual purposes such as cleansing a person or place when burning the bundled, dry herb, or for preparing the way and a person's mind for their journey ahead. It is also used as a protective covering for huts created for the purpose of going on an inward spiritual journey in the desert.

Future harvests

Gather no more than a quarter of what you find within a large stand. Consider planting in your home landscape to supply some of your medicine.

HERBAL PREPARATIONS

Herb Tea
Standard Infusion
Drink 2–8 ounces, up to 4 times per day.

Tincture
1 part fresh herb, by weight
2 parts menstruum (95% alcohol),
   by volume
or
1 part dry herb, by weight
5 parts menstruum (50% alcohol,
   50% spring water), by volume
Take 5–30 drops, as needed; take ½–1 teaspoon, 3 times per day, for acute viral infections or lung inflammation.

Oil Infusion
Dry leaves and flowers and prepare as alcohol intermediate oil infusion (see page 38).

desert willow

Chilopsis linearis
mimbre, bow willow
PARTS USED bark, leaf, stem, flower

This warming and drying remedy slowly resolves systemic fungal infections and is a great topical wound-healing agent. The plant's strong and motherly energy provides support even when we feel there is nowhere else to turn.

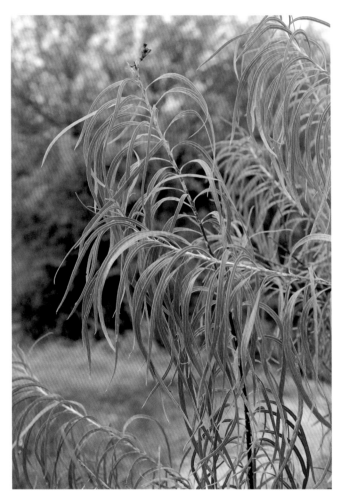

Gather young branches (stems and leaves) in spring and early summer. Gather branches that don't end in flower clusters to allow flowers to mature into seed.

How to identify
This deciduous tree is commonly found as a cluster of several trunks in close proximity within sandy desert washes; it reaches 15–35 feet tall at maturity. Bark is gray and smooth when young, becoming darker and furrowed as it ages. Young stems are fully brown to mottled yellowish green toward the tip. Leaves are long (up to 10 inches), thin, and aromatic, with little to no petiole; they are alternate, opposite, or whorled, and entire, perhaps slightly curved or straight as they hang down, similar to a willow's in appearance. The fuzzy, white bulb-like flower buds appear in clusters at the branch tips, opening into fragrant 2-lipped near-white to purple blossoms with streaks of yellow at the throat. Petal margins are wavy with rounded teeth. The long, thin seedpods open lengthwise upon maturity, releasing numerous flattened seeds with feathery ends, and remain on the plant for many months thereafter.

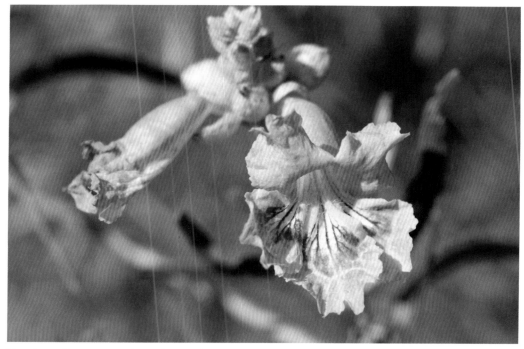

The showy flowers range from almost white to pink to purple, with yellow stripes down the throat and darker purple splotches across the lower lip.

Where, when, and how to wildcraft

Desert willow can be found scattered among the desert washes and high terraces adjacent to floodplains throughout our region below 5,000 feet, particularly along the southern portion, from southern Nevada and southern California eastward to Dallas and parts of southern Oklahoma; it is absent from the high desert and uncommon in the high plains. Gather the new leaf and stem growth from spring until the first frost arrives, and the flowers directly from the tree or as they fall to the ground, late spring through mid-summer. Gather bark in winter; see "Gathering Tree Medicine" (page 25).

Medicinal uses

Although there is a dearth of ethnobotanical information on desert willow as a medicine, and zero scientific data, numerous herbalists in the Southwest have explored its virtues for several decades now. This plant's antifungal properties and ability to improve conditions of candida overgrowth were first brought to the attention of the herbalist community by Michael Moore. I've used desert willow tincture, alone and in formula, to address valley fever (often characterized by sudden onset of cough and fatigue) with excellent results; Charles Kane (2011) recommends combining it with oshá for the same purpose. Michael Cottingham uses desert willow along with yerba mansa for toxic mold infections, particularly those centered on the lungs. A decoction of the flowers is a traditional remedy for cough.

Peter Bigfoot of Reevis Mountain School in Arizona discovered its use as a topical analgesic vulnerary through primary experience. Use as a powder to dust on wounds,

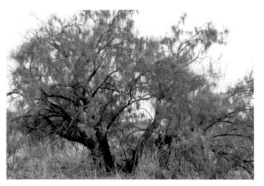

Desert willow is commonly found as a cluster of trunks emerging in close proximity within sandy desert washes. It may also be found as a single trunk tree, or with several singular trunks emerging from the ground in proximity to each other.

make an oil infusion from the leaf, or apply the tea as a wash against ringworm, athlete's foot, or dandruff.

Although its flavor profile will vary depending on the preparation, it tends to be bitter, with a pungent acridity that is experienced as a slight burning sensation at the back of the throat. This hints at its ability to break up congestion and relieve dampness, and to promote fluid movement through the tissues once again—it's a lymphatic. The effects of the flowers tend to center on the region above the diaphragm. Similar to ocotillo flowers, these are used as an emotional heart remedy. The nature of the plant is motherly, embracing us at times when we feel we could "break apart" from the weight we carry on our shoulders. Simply spend some quiet time alone beneath this tree, soften your heart, welcome her into your internal space, and allow the beauty to unfold within and before you.

Future harvests

Prune carefully and modestly to promote growth and maintain vitality. Consider bringing this tree into your home landscape.

HERBAL PREPARATIONS

Flower Sun Tea
Fill a jar half full with fresh flowers then fill with clean water and set in the sun, covered, for 2–4 hours. Strain and enjoy.

Leaf/Stem Tea
Strong Decoction or Cold Infusion
Drink 3–6 ounces, up to 4 times per day.

Leaf/Stem/Bark Tincture
1 part fresh plant, by weight
2 parts menstruum (60–80% alcohol,
   30–10% spring water, 10% glycerin),
   by volume; range of alcohol and water
   depends on moisture content of plant
or
1 part dry plant, by weight
5 parts menstruum (50% alcohol,
   40% spring water, 10% glycerin),
   by volume
Take 10–45 drops, up to 4 times per day; for severe candida infections, take ½–1 teaspoon, 3 times per day.

Echinacea angustifolia
PARTS USED leaf, flower, root

*Echinacea is our primary immune system enhancer for acute viral
and bacterial infections, both systemically and topically. Use it for cold,
flu, strep throat, or staph infections.*

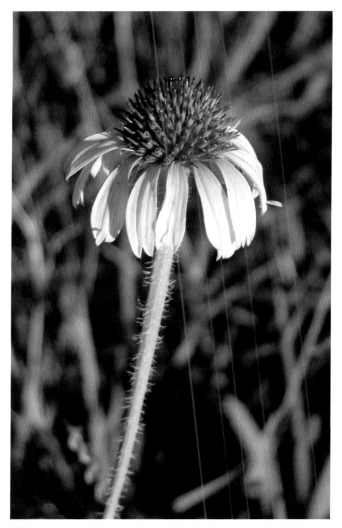

Echinacea angustifolia growing wild in short-grass prairie. Echinaceas have composite inflorescences, with dangling pink to purple ray flowers.

How to identify

Leaves are borne on a purple-tinged, bristly stem that arises from a fibrous taproot; they are alternate, coarsely haired, oblong to lance-shaped, with 3–5 nerves running the length of the dark green blade. Long, slender, and floppy pink to purple ray flowers with longitudinal ridges surround a darkened hump of disc flowers on a terminal inflorescence 2–4 inches wide. When you taste the fresh plant, it should cause a tremendous tingling in your mouth.

Where, when, and how to wildcraft

Echinacea occurs in sandy soils throughout the center of our region, from the grasslands of Kansas southward into the Texas Hill Country. It continues westward through the prairies into southeastern Colorado and northeastern New Mexico. Look to dry upland prairies with rocky soils. Dig entire plants after flowering using a mattock and shovel to pry them out; digging down 8 inches to remove the top of

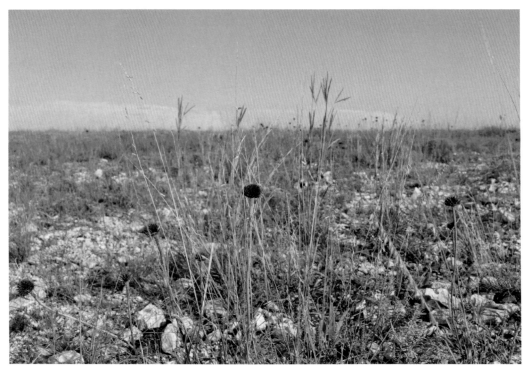

A small stand of *Echinacea angustifolia*, with just the dark disc flowers remaining by autumn, growing on a limestone ridge in the high plains.

the root while leaving root pieces behind is a sustainable practice.

Medicinal uses

First and foremost, echinacea is an immune stimulant and an immune modulator. The validity as well as the intricacies of this statement are still debated, yet the plant was a staple medicine of the indigenous peoples of the plains, has been loved by Europeans since the mid-19th century, and remains in wide use today. The root is the preferred medicine.

The tea or tincture is a useful remedy for tonsillitis, strep throat, cold, flu, staph infections (combine with red root), or other viral or bacterial illnesses. Use frequently (hourly) in acute infections. Some prefer to use it prophylactically as well during cold and flu season.

Traditionally used for snakebite, both topically and internally, it's known to inhibit hyaluronidase, thus reducing the spread of the venom; I carry echinacea tincture in my backcountry first-aid kit, in case a venomous snake strikes when the nearest hospital is hours away. Gargle a tea for strep throat, or apply as a wash or poultice for conjunctivitis, infected sores, septic wounds, burns, venomous bites and stings, enlarged glands, or swollen, painful joints (hyaluronidase inhibition potentially at play).

Future harvests

Echinacea has withstood 120 years of continuous wildharvesting for commerce. Studies by Kelly Kindscher of the University of Kansas show that 50% of wild echinacea

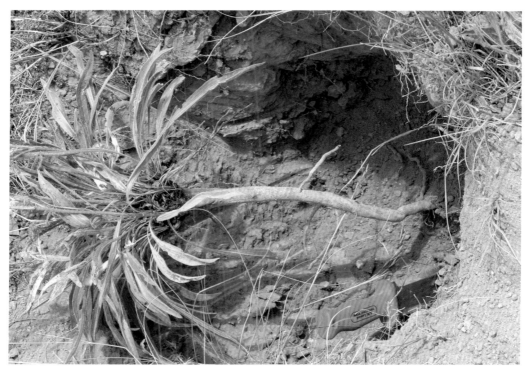

The long, thin root of this echinacea is likely decades old and may extend as much as 8 feet into the earth. It would be termed a "big carrot" by echinacea wildcrafters.

stands resprout after digging, so don't worry about leaving bits of root behind.

⚠ Caution

May cause increased pain or inflammation when used for arthritis or its immune-stimulating qualities. Simply discontinue use, and the symptoms will abate.

HERBAL PREPARATIONS

Root Tea
Cold Infusion
Apply topically, as needed; drink 2–6 ounces, up to 5 times per day.

Root Tincture
1 part fresh root, by weight
2 parts menstruum (95% alcohol), by volume
or
1 part dry root, by weight
5 parts menstruum (70% alcohol, 30% spring water), by volume
Take 30–90 drops, as needed; in acute infections, take every 30–60 minutes.

Sambucus species
tápiro, sauco, elderberry
PARTS USED leaf, stem, flower, fruit

Exemplifying grace and quick to rejuvenate, elder is the perfect remedy for young children. It is a valuable cold and flu remedy, and an essential herb for bone healing.

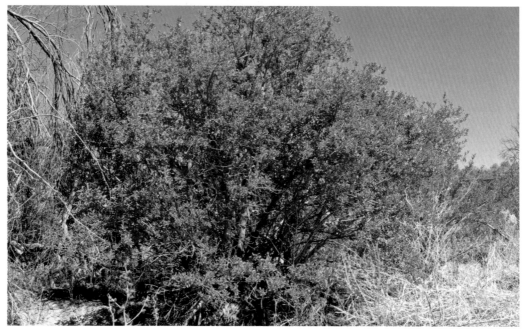

Sambucus mexicana (*S. nigra* ssp. *canadensis*), Mexican elder, is common in southern California, riparian areas of the upper Sonoran grassland in Arizona, and south into Sonora, Mexico.

How to identify

Elder is a large shrub or small deciduous tree with opposite, pinnately compound leaves in a series of 3–9 finely serrated leaflets. The smooth, shiny, pointed leaves are on long, thin, grooved stems that may turn reddish brown or magenta as the berries ripen. Flat-topped clusters of tiny, fragrant, creamy white flowers with 5-lobed corollas, also borne on long stems, are followed by green berries that turn light blue to blue-black when ripe, with a white bloom covering the outer skin. In southern California, berries may be light green to white when ripe. The bark and mature stems are reddish brown to white or ashen gray, with thin ridges running vertically. *Sambucus* nomenclature has recently undergone revision and remains a bit confused.

Where, when, and how to wildcraft

Elder inhabits areas with access to ground-water, from the lower desert riparian areas

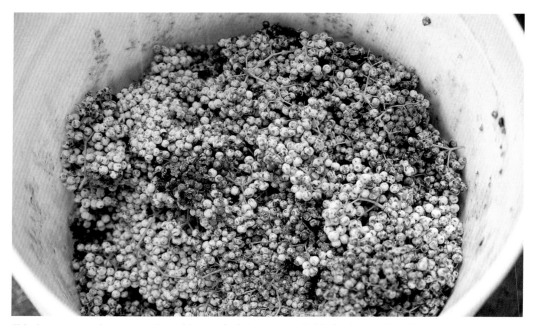

Elderberries are often covered in a bloom of white yeast, suitable for fermenting the sugars present in the fruit.

to the high-elevation conifer forests; it is found most abundantly in the western third of our region. However, *Sambucus mexicana* can also be found scattered along the eastern edge of our region beginning just south of San Antonio and moving northward in Oklahoma and west into the panhandles of Texas and Oklahoma. The flowers are gathered from late spring to early summer, and the berries ripen from early summer (low desert riparian stands) to late summer (at higher elevations). The leaves can be gathered whenever present, usually from early spring to late autumn. Simply pinch the clusters of fully ripened berries (or flowers) with your fingertips (or cut with pruners) and place in a bucket, bag, or gathering basket. Be sure to process the berries quickly, as they ferment readily (not altogether a bad thing, especially if intended). Gather the green stems with attached leaves and process promptly for fresh leaf tincture as they, too, spoil quickly.

Medicinal uses

Elder flowers are a first-rate remedy for the common illnesses of childhood. Always have some dry elder flowers on hand for infants and toddlers for whenever a hot, irritated, feverish condition presents itself. Apply the cool tea as a wash to an infant's body, feed by teaspoon, apply to the nursing mother's nipples, or have the nursing mother drink the tea herself to relax the child, through the release of excessive heat from the body.

Elder is a phenomenal immune enhancer in the presence of respiratory viral illnesses, serving as both a prophylactic and for acute symptom relief. It's been shown that elderberry preparations reduce the ability of the flu virus to attach to the cell, thus disabling them from replicating within the cell. Take internally as the berry tincture, the berry syrup, or a hot infusion of the flowers (combine with wild mint, oshá tincture, or yerba mansa). Elderberry wine, jelly, or other berry

Fresh Elderberry Syrup

Begin by filling a large stainless steel pot about two-thirds full with clusters of fresh elderberries. Pour in several inches of clean water and heat to simmering. Once warm, begin mashing the berries with a potato masher to help release their juice into the liquid. Continue mashing and simmering until the stems become pale and all the berries have been smashed. Pour the liquid through a strainer and return to the pot. Gently simmer with the lid off for 1–2 hours. Consider adding additional spices (clove, ginger) or herbs (oshá, spikenard) to your syrup at this stage. The liquid should be quite tart and rich with elderberry flavor. Adding honey at ½–2 parts to the volume of elderberry "juice" will create a short- to long-term shelf-stable product, with or without pressure sealing. The more honey, the longer the syrup should be expected to remain stable. Store in the fridge for even greater longevity. The elderberry pectin content is occasionally high enough that a jelly spontaneously forms when following this recipe.

Use elderberry syrup in 1 tablespoon doses to prevent colds and flu, or take hourly during the initial stages of acute respiratory viral infections to reduce the severity and duration of the infection.

preparations may also work to improve the immune response.

Elder flower skin tonics were in vogue during the Victorian era, and the fermented blossom tea has been a traditional drink throughout northern Europe for centuries. Infuse the flowers in oil and add to salves to improve skin healing.

Stephen Buhner recommends a fresh leaf tincture to heal broken bones as well as improve osteoporosis. The use of elder leaves in ointments or salves to treat bruises, sores, and various injuries is a traditional circumboreal application.

Future harvests

Elder is often abundant where found; however, its habitat is restricted by drought and dropping water tables in the lower desert. Consider introducing it to your home landscape, within a graywater or rainwater harvesting system.

 Caution

Consumption of fresh elderberries (and their seeds) may cause nausea.

HERBAL PREPARATIONS

Flower/Berry Tea
Standard Infusion
Drink 2–4 ounces, up to 3 times per day.

Berry Tincture
1 part fresh berry, by weight
2 parts menstruum (brandy), by volume
Take 30–90 drops, as needed.

Leaf Tincture
1 part fresh leaf, by weight
2 parts menstruum (95% alcohol), by
　volume
or
1 part dry leaf, by weight
5 parts menstruum (50% alcohol, 50%
　spring water), by volume
Take 25 drops to 3ml, up to 5 times per day.

Artemisia ludoviciana
simonillo, western mugwort
PARTS USED aerial

This gentle, relaxing aromatic bitter goes "straight to the liver," addressing a wide array of health concerns, from musculoskeletal and nervous tension to digestive ailments and irregular menses.

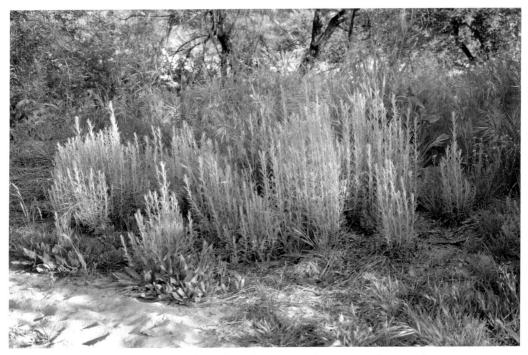

Estafiate is one of the most common plants throughout our region—it's nearly everywhere.

How to identify

A highly variable species, this aromatic plant morphs into several colors, forms, and sizes, depending on its locale. In oak or piñon-juniper woodlands, it may be no more than knee-high and appear only as numerous individual stems; in the desert grasslands and canyons of the Sonoran desert, it grows in tall clumps, ascending to 5 feet on occasion, which by summer's end appear to billow out from rocky cliff faces. The soft, short, white hairs atop the sessile green to gray-green leaves and stems—along with its sweet aromatics—help distinguish this rhizomatous perennial from so many other similar-looking plants. The mostly ascending stems develop distinctive longitudinal ridges as they approach maturity. The tiny disc flowers, borne on compact panicles originating at leaf axils as well as at the stem tips, are

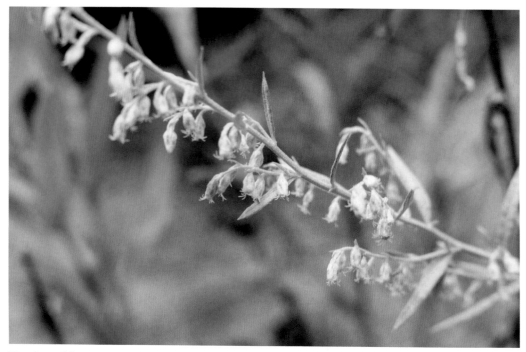

The discoid flowers of estafiate are held in drooping panicles all along the stem; leaf morphology is highly variable.

not showy in the least, but may show some yellow from the pollen or a slight redness upon the bracts. As the seasons move on, leaves at the base of the stem will dry yet remain clinging, even into the following spring. These leaves, when crushed, do not completely disintegrate into dust but are largely held together by the fluffy white hairs that cover the entire leaf when fresh. This is a clear and distinctive feature of estafiate.

Where, when, and how to wildcraft

Estafiate is one of the Southwest's most common plants. Look to moist, north-facing canyon walls at lower elevations in the west of our region, to open roadsides or disturbed areas from south Texas through the Hill Country, and up into the high plains of Oklahoma, Colorado, and New Mexico. In the middle elevations and mountains of the West, find estafiate growing beneath cottonwoods, junipers, pines, or oaks, or out in the open on rocky outcrops at 9,000 feet adjacent to Douglas fir, Gambel's oak, or pine. The preferred time for gathering is pre-flowering once the plant has reached 1–2 feet in height. As the plant flowers in late summer, the leaves will gradually become smaller. Cut or break the stems near ground level to use fresh as a poultice, tea, tincture, or oil, or dry for tea or tincture. Once dry, strip the leaves to remove from the stem, if desired, but be sure to retain the medicinally potent stems.

Medicinal uses

To borrow a homeopathic term, estafiate is a polycrest, an herb with many uses and minimal toxicity (i.e., it may be used frequently over long periods of time). It is the primary digestive folk remedy of our region, relieving inflammation along the GI tract, allaying gas and cramping, enhancing digestive secretions, and improving appetite. It's a wonderful aromatic bitter nervine with musculoskeletal relaxant effects. Additionally, use the tea or tincture internally for acute respiratory viruses, hay fever, musculoskeletal injuries, gall bladder "attacks," liver tension or inflammation, or slow bile secretion, urinary tract pain and inflammation, painful menses with or without bloating, headache, nervous tension, or anxiety. Coupled with wild mint, it is a wonderful remedy for post-food-allergen consumption. Crushed leaves are placed up the nose for headaches or nosebleeds—a fast and effective remedy.

Although not as potent as other *Artemisia* species in this regard, estafiate does possess anthelmintic properties that are useful to combat common pinworms or other intestinal parasites (combine with algerita, goatbush, tree of heaven, or walnut hulls).

The fresh plant poultice, fomentation, oil infusion, or salve can provide soothing relief to strained, overworked, or excessively tense musculature. Apply to the IT band to relieve runner's knee—internal use of the tea or tincture is also useful.

Collect the old dry leaves from the base of the stem to use in moxibustion. Place a fresh ginger slice, ¼ inch thick, over a meridian point, with some herb atop it; light the herb and allow it to burn out, driving warmth into the point.

Future harvests

Replant rhizome cuttings with stems attached to expand the stand. Be sure to establish some estafiate around your home so it's always available to you.

HERBAL PREPARATIONS

Herb Tea
Standard Infusion (or add a small amount to formulas)
Drink 2–4 ounces, up to 4 times per day.

Tincture
1 part fresh herb, by weight
2 parts menstruum (95% alcohol), by volume
or
1 part dry herb, by weight
5 parts menstruum (50% alcohol, 50% spring water), by volume
Take 10–60 drops, up to 5 times per day.

Oil Infusion
1 part fresh herb, by weight
6 parts extra virgin olive oil, by volume
Apply to the affected area consistently until resolved.

evening primrose

Oenothera biennis, O. elata
PARTS USED whole plant

Nutritious seeds support the immune and female reproductive systems. Strongly acrid leaves and root help break up stagnation, relieve indigestion, or stimulate a slow-to-start menses.

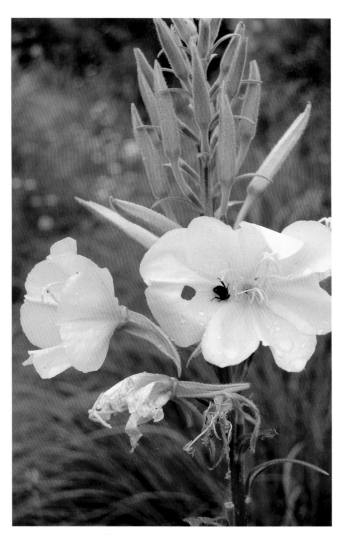

Evening primrose's flowers are distinguished by a 4-parted stigma that reaches beyond the stamens; seedpods are long and thin, with ridges running end to end; stems turn red as plants reach maturity.

How to identify

This erect biennial to short-lived perennial is 3–8 feet tall. It begins as a basal rosette of pointed, lance-shaped leaves with wavy margins and a milky white midrib. Usually in the second year, the plant sends up an erect green and red, unbranched flower stalk with clasping leaves. Single yellow flowers with 4 heart-shaped petals open near the top of the plant; the elongated ovary is inferior (i.e., below the base of the hypanthium). Flowers turn pink to reddish orange the day after they open, giving way to the elongated seedpod, which splits open lengthwise into 4 parts, each capsule filled with 2 rows of tightly compressed, brown seeds.

Where, when, and how to wildcraft

Fond of disturbed ground, evening primrose prefers roadsides, rocky slopes, canyon bottoms, woodlands, and moist meadows throughout the western two-thirds of our region, up to 9,000 feet. The basal leaves and taproots can be gathered year-round but are best harvested in early spring. The flowering stems can be gathered, along with young plants, from mid-summer to early autumn. Seeds are available mid- to late autumn.

Medicinal uses

This acrid-tasting plant has an affinity for the digestive tract and female reproductive system, and to some extent the upper respiratory tract.

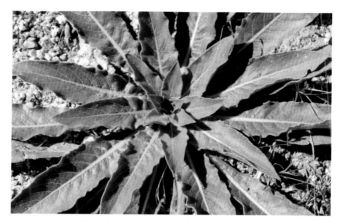

At the center of each basal rosette, the overlapping leaves form a starry whorl.

It breaks up stagnation, clears dampness, and tones tissues and organs that have become too relaxed and deficient in function, perhaps leading to a stagnancy type of inflammation.

A tincture of the whole plant can be used for depression related to indigestion. Look for a swollen tongue with scalloped edges and enlarged organs indicated by swelling or tenderness of the abdomen. It can also stimulate a menses delayed by torpor in the pelvic region (combine with ocotillo). Labored breathing associated with heavy, full digestive conditions may also respond well to the tea or tincture. Try a small dose of the tincture (5–10 drops) if wakefulness occurs midway through sleep. Add the root to cough syrups or as a tea for colds. It's also indicated for dysentery.

Leaves are applied topically as a poultice, oil infusion, or salve to ulcers, sores, poorly healing tissue, or any rheumatic swellings. The seeds are nutritious and particularly rich in gamma linolenic acid (GLA), a beneficial omega-6 fatty acid; consuming them can help alleviate a variety of conditions (PMS, menopausal symptoms, eczema, allergies) resulting from a deficiency of GLA.

Future harvests

Gather only from areas of abundance. Consider casting seeds in appropriate areas.

⚠ Caution

Excessive use of GLA supplements may increase the risk of blood clotting; it is not known whether this could pertain to consuming an abundance of the seeds.

HERBAL PREPARATIONS

Leaf and Flower Tea
Standard Infusion
Drink 2–4 ounces, as needed.

Root Tea
Standard Decoction
Drink 2–4 ounces, up to 3 times per day.

Leaf, Flower, and Root Tincture
1 part fresh leaf, flower, and root, by weight
2 parts menstruum (95% alcohol),
  by volume
or
1 part dry leaf, flower, and root, by weight
5 parts menstruum (50% alcohol,
  50% spring water), by volume
Take 30–75 drops, up to 4 times per day.

fanpetals

Sida species
yerba del pollo, wireweed
PARTS USED whole plant

This universal remedy helps to regenerate red blood cells and protects the liver and nervous system. Apply topically for ulcers, sores, wounds, and itchy skin, or take internally for a variety of inflammatory conditions.

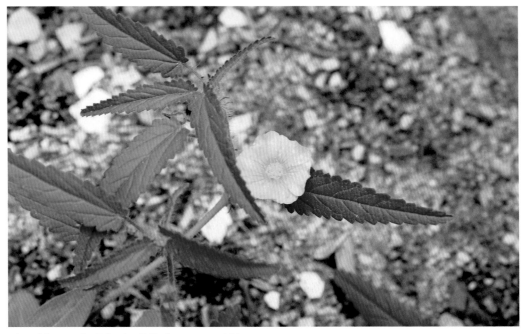

Like all fanpetals, *Sida abutifolia* flowers at midday.

How to identify

All 11 species of *Sida* that occur within our region look quite similar, differing mostly in growth habit. Some are prostrate with stems that crawl along the ground (*S. abutifolia*, *S. neomexicana*), emerging from a central taproot; others are more upright (*S. spinosa*). Some may be upright under shady, moist conditions but become prostrate in bare, dry ground (*S. rhombifolia*). The thin, round stems may be smooth or covered in short, stiff hairs. The leaves may be thin and lance-shaped, rhomboid, ovate coming to a fine tip, or elliptic, and are generally toothed. The white, yellow, orange, or red flowers (primarily, yellow-orange) of this mallow family plant are 5-petaled, with a dense cluster of stamens in the middle (think hibiscus); they arise singularly from the leaf axils and open midday. Each petal is offset with a rounded lobe, which gives the impression of motion (hence the common name). The round seedpod is a

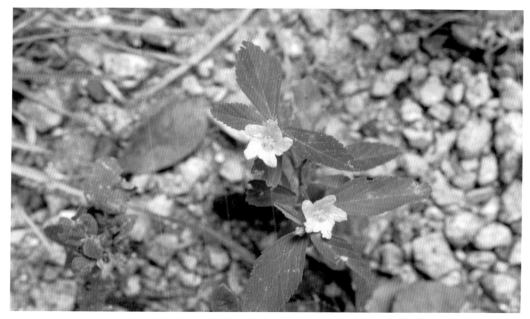

Sida rhombifolia's specific epithet tells you it has rhomboid leaves.

schizocarp, meaning that it splits into separate parts when mature.

Where, when, and how to wildcraft

Fanpetals occurs along the southern tier of our region, from the desert grasslands of southern Arizona eastward to the South Texas Plains, then up through Dallas and into central Oklahoma. It is found in a variety of disturbed habitats, with more or less moisture, depending on the species. The plant often goes unseen for its prostrate habit. Although *Sida abutifolia*, *S. acuta*, *S. rhombifolia*, and *S. spinosa* have the most well-known tradition of use and are the most studied, our other species are safe to explore and are likely to have similar attributes. Gather the leafy stems, in flower, or the whole plant when particularly abundant. Tincturing the whole plant when in seed, with a bit of acid (10–15% vinegar), may optimize extraction of the adaptogenic qualities of the plant.

Medicinal uses

A plant rich in phytochemicals, with a rich history of folk usage (outside of the United States). In Mexico, for example, it is well known for treating upper respiratory illnesses, as well as being employed against "evil eye," loss of soul (*susto*), and to cleanse patients spiritually and emotionally. It is also nutritious and high in protein; some cultures use it as a potherb. There are many ways to take our medicine!

The tea has been used for joint pain and as a general pain reliever, and to relieve stomachache, diarrhea, and constipation, stimulate appetite, reduce blood pressure, and calm the nervous system.

Several important research discoveries inspired by traditional folk usage of *Sida* species have helped bring this plant to the awareness of a greater audience (Buhner 2012). This adaptogenic herb is hepatoprotective and neuroprotective. It's particularly effective against *Plasmodium falciparum*, the infectious

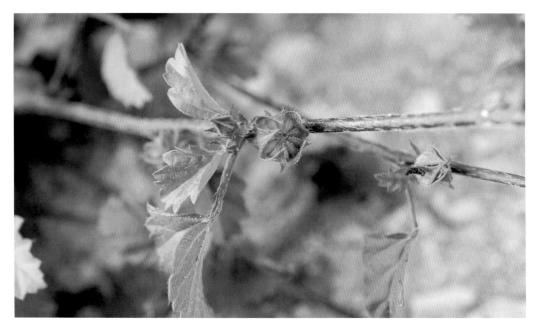

Maturing schizocarp and appressed hairy stems of *Sida rhombifolia*.

agent in malaria, confirming its traditional use for malarial fevers. Additionally, it protects, strengthens, and regenerates the red blood cells, making it highly useful in babesia infections (a common coinfection with Lyme disease) as well as anemia. It is also effective against mycobacteria, and it reduces inflammation within the nerve tissue. An effective emollient, it can also be topically applied to both bacterial and fungal infections.

Respiratory viruses, as well as asthma, are treated effectively with fanpetals. Its cooling, anti-inflammatory qualities have been employed to relieve arthritis, gastritis, gingivitis, and liver inflammation. It's been used for hepatitis and excess bile conditions.

Future harvests

I have developed stands of fanpetals by tilling the soil and letting it be for several years, an invitation for this perennial plant to seed itself.

 Caution

Avoid during pregnancy: it was traditionally used as an abortifacient.

HERBAL PREPARATIONS

Herb Tea
Standard Infusion (plus a teaspoon of vinegar or lime/lemon juice)
Drink 4–8 ounces, as needed; apply topically, as needed.

Whole Plant Tincture
1 part fresh plant, by weight
2 parts menstruum (85% alcohol, 15% apple cider vinegar), by volume
Take 30–60 drops, up to 5 times per day; apply topically as a liniment to sore joints, muscle pain, and injuries.

figwort

Scrophularia species
PARTS USED aerial

A remedy for dampness and all its manifestations, figwort slowly clears lymphatic stagnation and accumulation of fluids throughout the body. The oil or poultice is a classic remedy for ulcerations.

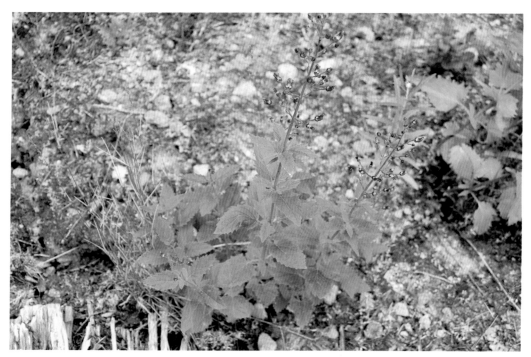

Scrophularia californica, California figwort, is found at high elevations in Arizona and in the mountains of southern California.

How to identify

With its 4-angled stem (8-sided with age) and opposite leaves (which may occur in whorls of 3 or 4), this tall herbaceous perennial may be mistaken for a mint family plant; however, it has no aroma. The deep green, lance-shaped leaves have toothed margins and a truncated base. Loose clusters of tiny flowers (2–4mm wide), which at first appear as if they're still opening, occur at the top of the plant; in all species, the upper lip is light to dark red, the lower, smaller lip a yellowish to solid green (dark red in *Scrophularia californica*). Further aiding in identification, *Scrophularia* species possess a nonfertile, scalelike stigma adhering to the wall of the corolla.

Where, when, and how to wildcraft

Figwort is predominantly found within the western half of our region in high-elevation

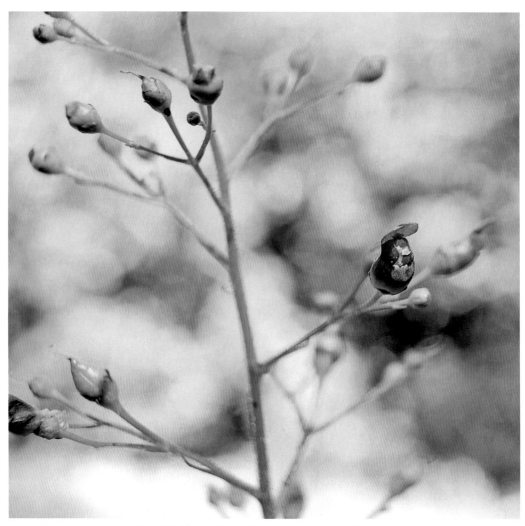

Like all figworts, the upper lip of California figwort's flowers sticks out like a hood or canopy. Unlike the rest of our species, which have bicolor flowers, its flowers are solid red.

conifer forests as well as the plains of central to western Oklahoma. *Scrophularia lanceolata*, lanceleaf figwort, is also found in the lower Rocky Mountains of southern Colorado, northern New Mexico, and southern Utah. *Scrophularia parviflora*, pineland figwort, prefers rich soils in conifer forests and moist canyons at 5,000–8,000 feet. Gather the aerial portions (or the whole plant, including root, in very large stands).

Medicinal uses

Use figwort in formulations whenever dampness is significant and skin or lymph detoxification is indicated. Use to move stagnant lymph in chronic infections, with slow-to-heal ulcerations or red congested swellings, such as plugged mammary glands, testicular pain, or ringworm infections. Figwort is considered soothing to the female reproductive system. The fresh plant poultice and the leaf oil infusion can also be applied topically in these cases.

Use figwort internally for joint inflammation and chronic viral infections (EBV, CMV, HIV) and topically for fungal infections, eczema, rashes, burns, or hemorrhoids (Moore 2003). Use in formulation with red root, curly dock, and queen's root. Use the oil infusion, tea, or fresh plant poultice for skin sores, sore nipples, hives, or other skin eruptions.

Saikosaponin, a triterpenoid found in our native *Scrophularia* species, has been studied extensively. In vitro studies have shown it to be effective against a wide array of cancers, hepatoprotective when used concurrently with acetaminophen, and effective against viruses. Evidence also indicates it may be a weak phytoestrogen.

Future harvests
Gather with respect and gratitude from large stands.

HERBAL PREPARATIONS

Herb Tea
Standard Infusion
Drink 2–4 ounces, up to 3 times per day; apply topically, as needed.

Whole Plant Tincture
1 part fresh plant, by weight
2 parts menstruum (75% alcohol,
   25% spring water), by volume
Take 10–40 drops, up to 4 times per day; apply topically, as needed.

Oil Infusion
1:5
Prepare leaves as a fresh plant oil infusion (see page 39).

Erodium cicutarium, E. texanum
alfilerillo, storksbill
PARTS USED whole plant

A commonly overlooked herb with cooling, astringent, and anti-inflammatory effects on the gut, skin, and urinary tract. It is also mildly stimulating to liver function.

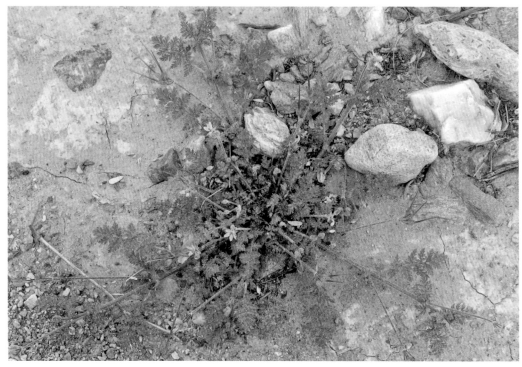

Filaree in midspring with both flowers and seeds; note its prostrate habit, stems growing close to the ground.

How to identify
When there is ample moisture, plants may grow to be 8 inches tall, but this naturalized annual herb is otherwise prostrate, spreading out across the ground in arachnoid fashion. Its finely and deeply divided, featherlike leaves are on short petioles arising from the taproot. In the flowering stage, the plant produces runners that may extend several feet from the taproot, branching out with opposite leaves at the swollen nodes. Stems become red with age. The flowers, borne on long stalks, grow in clusters of 2–8 and are pale pink to purple with 5 petals and 5 sepals. Fruits are long and pointed, reminiscent of a stork or heron's bill, with an interesting mechanism for seed dispersal: upon maturing, they split open

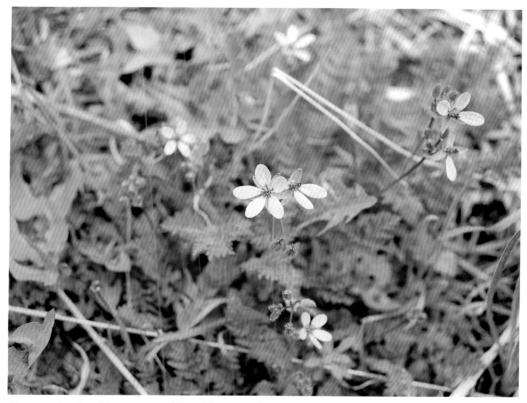

Filaree is closely related to cranesbill and has a similar flower structure. Flowers are generally bright pink.

into 5 segments, each of which twists into a screw shape, preparing them to penetrate a wide variety of surfaces and tissues and be dispersed throughout the landscape.

Where, when, and how to wildcraft

Look to roadsides, disturbed ground, and overgrazed areas. Filaree occurs as a winter annual from southern California eastward to central Texas and Oklahoma; in dry, exposed places up to 8,000 feet it may be found growing into the autumn season. Texas storksbill, *Erodium texanum*, is a plant of the winter and spring throughout this same range (as well as summer and autumn in Texas and Oklahoma); its simple, 3-lobed leaves can be used similarly to filaree. Gather the whole plant, in flower. Dry for tea.

Medicinal uses

Filaree is a useful plant that is too often overlooked and underestimated. It is a mild astringent and cooling herb with an affinity for the skin, gut, and liver. The tea will aid in detoxification when there is sluggishness present in the liver, such that it may provoke the outbreak of a rash when the liver is really overworked or if too much is taken, initially. Start with 2 ounces of tea, in the evening. This therapy is well timed during the spring season, when the liver energy is naturally activated and engaged. It is also great to add to tea blends for this purpose.

Its astringent and antiseptic properties can be applied as a gargle for sore throat, or topically for cuts, infected wounds, animal bites, sores, or rashes. Apply a fomentation

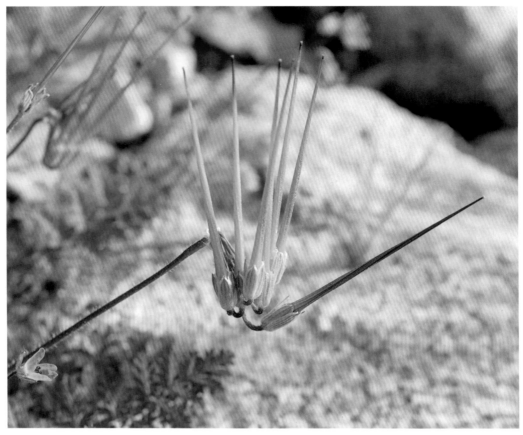

The seedpods are often hard to see when first forming, but their shape is very distinctive. Upon maturing, they split open and, within moments, twist into a tight screw.

over the eyes to relieve conjunctivitis. The tea is drunk for diarrhea (similar to cranesbill in action) or to relieve stomachache. Traditionally, the plant is eaten by nursing mothers to increase milk production.

Joint inflammation may be relieved by the tea's anti-inflammatory action. Its diuretic effect may also help to alleviate rheumatic joint pain. Charles Kane (2011) recommends filaree as a urinary tract anti-inflammatory and to reduce heavy menses.

Future harvests

Filaree was brought to this continent from Europe and Africa on the hooves of sheep, so the story goes. It is common and abundant throughout our region. Gather for medicine to your heart's content.

HERBAL PREPARATIONS

Herb Tea
Standard Infusion
Drink 2–8 ounces, up to 3 times per day; apply topically, as needed.

fireweed

Chamerion (Epilobium) angustifolium
willow herb
PARTS USED whole plant

*Cooling and detoxifying, this potent anti-inflammatory herb can relieve pain
and discomfort throughout the body used both topically and internally.*

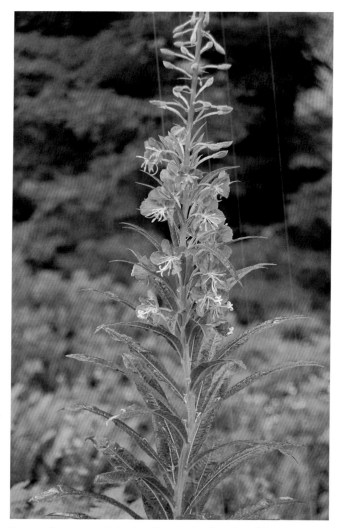

Fireweed occurs in high-elevation conifer forests within our
region. This colony-forming plant is often clearly visible, even
from a distance, from flowering through to seeding.

How to identify

This erect, non-woody perennial plant forms large colonies via underground rhizomes. The whitish midvein on the leaves of the young plant help identify it prior to flowering (it can appear quite similar to *Pedicularis racemosa* at this stage). The central flower stalk is crowded with lance-shaped, alternate leaves possessing smooth margins (rarely, with teeth). The inflorescence is a terminal spike rising above the leaves. There are 4 pink to lilac, rounded to obovate petals with thin, darker reddish purple sepals in the back. The top of the plant turns fire red in autumn, contrasting with the bright white hairs on the seeds, which are exposed as the long, thin pods split open.

Where, when, and how to wildcraft

Fireweed is found scattered throughout the higher elevations of the western two-thirds of our region. It occupies clearings in conifer forests. True to its name, one will find fireweed growing in abundance in the years, or wet seasons, following forest fires. The leaves and flowers can be gathered throughout the summer into early autumn. Cut back the entire stem and dry in the shade. Once dry, strip the leaves and flowers for tea. Gather the roots in spring as the plants appear, or in the fall after they have gone to seed.

Medicinal uses

This close relative of evening primrose clears inflammation in the digestive tract and is a reliable remedy for dysentery, with or without fever present. Its anti-inflammatory effects are experienced both internally and externally for a variety of pain relief. Use for painful rheumatic joints, bruises and strains, irritating skin conditions, gastritis, stomachache, intestinal discomfort (drink daily for irritable bowel), or with intestinal hemorrhaging. It can also relieve a sore throat. Apply a warm poultice to boils or use as a drawing poultice for an infected wound or to remove foreign matter. The whole plant can be used topically and internally to resolve candida and other yeast overgrowth. The root decoction was traditionally used to resolve chronic lung congestion or bacterial infections of the lungs.

The leaf tea is a traditional remedy for kidney and urinary problems. It's also been traditionally used for "male urinary problems."

The tea or tincture can be a valuable remedy for prostatitis and benign prostatic hypertrophy. A 1996 study revealed that this herb has the ability to inhibit aromatase.

Future harvests

This plant has its own niche in our mountain habitats. Gather respectfully, and only gather the roots from large stands, and it should continue to produce medicine for us while fulfilling its role.

HERBAL PREPARATIONS

Leaf and Flower Tea
Standard Infusion
Drink 4–8 ounces, as needed.

Leaf and Flower Tincture
1 part fresh leaf and flower, by weight
2 parts menstruum (95% alcohol),
  by volume
Take 30–60 drops, up to 4 times per day; apply topically as a liniment to sore joints, muscle pain, and injuries.

Leaf and Flower Oil Infusion
1 part dry leaf and flower, by weight
5 parts extra virgin olive oil, by volume
Prepare as alcohol intermediate oil infusion (see page 38).

Conopholis and *Orobanche* species
bear corn, cancer root, broomrape
PARTS USED aerial

Low-growing parasitic herbs that heal burns and wounds, as well as induce a deep relaxation of the musculoskeletal and nervous systems.

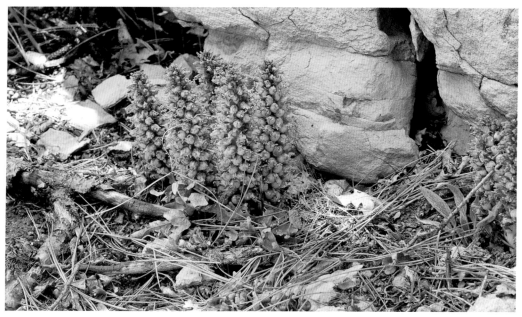

Conopholis alpina var. *mexicana*, bear corn, growing in canyon shade off the roots of Gambel's oak, *Quercus gambelii*.

How to identify

Conopholis and *Orobanche* are closely associated, botanically and medicinally. Both are genera of holoparasitic plants that contain no chlorophyll and gain their nutrients from the roots of photosynthesizing plants—note: the compounds of the host plants may affect their medicinal qualities. Plants are 8 inches tall at most, generally much less, growing out of bare ground or from within surrounding vegetation in our wetter Southwest habitats. *Orobanche* flowers have a curved corolla tube with upper and lower lobes in white, yellow, pink, lilac, or purple to almost gray. The naturalized *O. ramosa*, branched broomrape, grows on a relatively tall and slender beige and brown stem. The corollas of *Conopholis* are beige-yellow (as is the entire plant) and also tubular and bilabiate, with both stamens and pistil included.

Where, when, and how to wildcraft

We find *Conopholis* in the moist, shady woodlands of mid- to higher elevations in the

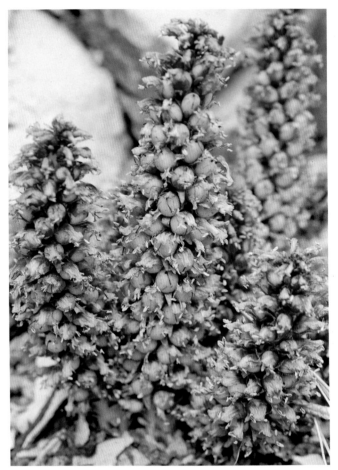

Conopholis fruits are round and contain hundreds of tiny seeds upon maturity.

aerial parts of each genus are gathered as they emerge and the flowers open, from mid-spring in the lower deserts to mid-summer at higher elevations. Simply slice off the aerial portions with a sharp long, thin blade, reaching down below the leaf layer. In dry, sandy areas, you may dig down a couple of inches to expose the underground stem to gather an optimal amount. Leave the roots intact.

Medicinal uses

These parasitic plants possess some very potent medicine. Many of the over 200 *Orobanche* species that occur worldwide are used as both food and medicine. Traditionally, they have been used topically to treat burns, wounds, sores, and hemorrhoids; powder the dry plant to apply topically. They are used internally for pneumonia and other pulmonary conditions, viral illnesses, and cancer. Diné healer Emerson Gorman uses *O. fasciculata* internally to heal broken bones.

Recent scientific trials have revealed neuroprotective properties associated with the constituent acteoside, found in many *Orobanche* species. Acteoside has been shown to reduce the aggregation of amyloid plaque. *Orobanche* is potently antioxidant, and several species have been studied for their anti-tumor potential based, initially, on folk or modern clinical usage. *Orobanche aegyptiaca*, which is naturalized in California, is given as a decoction for breast and ovarian cancer in the West Bank–Palestine. Studies

western half of our region. It's most often associated with oaks but can also be found growing near walnut, pine, and cypress. Approximately 11 *Orobanche* species occur in our region, but the genus is largely absent from the high plains; plants are found primarily in relatively drier environments, and flower in warm, dry periods following cool, rainy seasons. *Orobanche ramosa* contains potent antioxidants and is considered invasive in eastern and central Texas; inhabitants of these areas would do well to tincture the whole plant for its valuable medicine. The

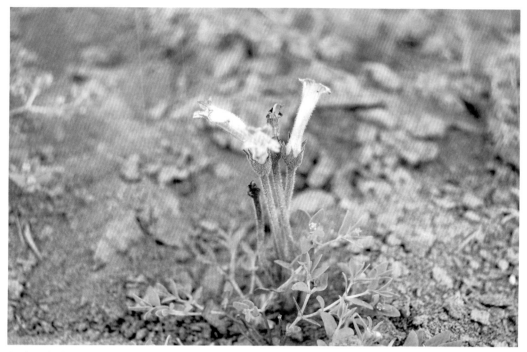

Orobanche fasciculata occurs in dry soil at 4,000–8,000 feet, within our region. In this photo, it is likely growing as a parasite on the roots of *Artemisia tridentata*, sagebrush.

have revealed that *Orobanche* inhibits tumor metastasis and induces apoptosis in the cancerous cells.

Interestingly, cancer root is a common name for *Conopholis* (which was previously classified as *Orobanche*). My experience with bear corn has shown that it is a powerful relaxant nervine that induces a deep, restful sleep, particularly when eaten fresh; an excellent remedy—if at all possible to administer—for someone who is overworked and cannot stop working. It is a muscle relaxant that acts deeply on the body. Michael Moore considers bear corn an astringent sudorific with relaxant properties. The Tarahumara of northern Mexico use bear corn during the birthing process to calm the mother, as well as to limit bleeding and promote lochial discharge. Bear corn is best eaten fresh, or made into a tea.

Future harvests

Gather only from large stands and leave the roots of native plants in the ground for future flowering. Harvest and transport seeds to new locations to expand the population.

HERBAL PREPARATIONS

Herb Tea
Standard Infusion
Drink 2–4 ounces, up to 3 times per day; apply topically, as needed.

Tincture
1 part recently dry herb, by weight
5 parts menstruum (40% alcohol,
 60% spring water), by volume
Take 30–60 drops, up to 3 times per day, in water.

globemallow

Sphaeralcea species
mal de ojo
PARTS USED leaf, flower, root

Topical application of this cooling, soothing member of the mallow family heals sores and relieves inflammation. It's an all-around digestive remedy that's also useful with colds and flu.

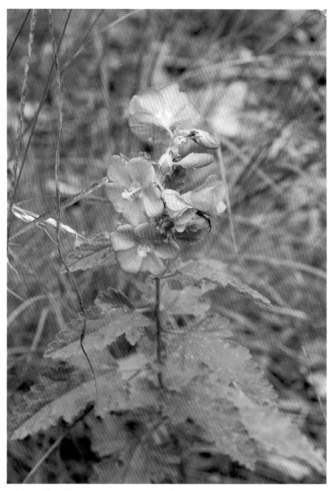

Although *Sphaeralcea* is closely related to *Hibiscus*, globemallows are normally covered in tiny white hairs; hibiscus are not. Salmon-flowered globemallows (here, the type of *S. fendleri*) are most common throughout our region.

How to identify

Several species of these erect perennials are found in our region, with little variability among them, aside from flower color, overall size (1–5 feet in height), and degree of hairi-ness. The alternate leaves are commonly toothed and 3-lobed (with a longer middle lobe), usu-ally crinkled and covered with fine white hairs (these often covering every part of the plant but the petals), giving them a grayish, almost white appear-ance. The variably red, orange, salmon, peach, lavender, or lilac flowers have 5 petals, each petal with a notch at the end, with the quintessential mallow family cluster of anthers in the center. The 5 triangular sepals extend beyond the schizocarp fruit (like the "cheese wheels" of mallow), which dries to a light tan.

Where, when, and how to wildcraft

Globemallow exists in a wide variety of habitats throughout our region but is only sparsely present from the Hill Country

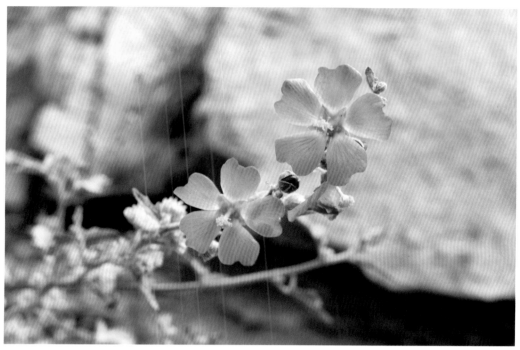

The lavender flowers of *Sphaeralcea fendleri* var. *venusta* are found at middle elevations in the western half of our region.

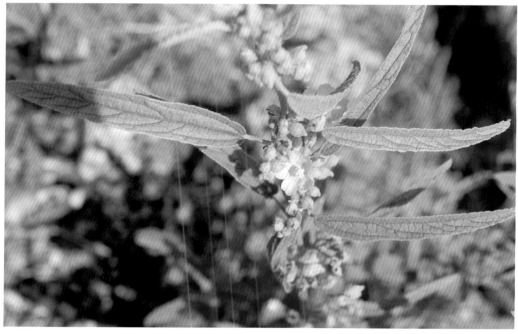

The pink flowers and long, narrow leaves of *Sphaeralcea angustifolia*, growing in the Texas Hill Country.

northward to Dallas. From nearly sea level to over 8,000 feet, look to dry ground in lower desert washes and bajadas, desert grasslands, disturbed ground in urban areas, oak woodlands, high desert, high plains, and clearings in conifer forests. Plants may flower year-round when moisture is available and temperatures remain above freezing. Gather the flowering branches and dry in the shade. When abundant, the root can be gathered and prepared for a fresh poultice or dried for tea.

Medicinal uses

A ubiquitous plant across the Southwest deserts, globemallow helps to soothe hot, dry, and irritated conditions of the skin, gut, and urinary tract. It is closely related to mallow in its medicinal applications. Combine in tea blends to help relieve inflamed lung conditions, such as are typical of acute viral illnesses.

A traditional remedy for snakebite, boils, wounds, sores, rheumatic joints, and sore eyes, the root is particularly demulcent. The fresh, mashed root is poulticed onto recent rattlesnake bites. Seri herbalists in northwestern Mexico prepare an eyewash with the root and include it in formulas for cancer. The tea is traditionally drunk as a laxative (as well as for diarrhea) and to soothe a stomachache, stop internal bleeding, calm agitation, and help heal broken bones. Clinical trials have confirmed its folk usage as a topically applied remedy that relieves the pain of arthritis. It is still a well-known hair rinse in the Southwest.

Future harvests

If globemallow is uncommon in your area, consider dispersing seeds over disturbed ground in late autumn.

Caution

Be sure to thoroughly strain any tea: the tiny hairs on this plant can be irritating when ingested.

HERBAL PREPARATIONS

Herb Tea
Standard Infusion
Drink 4–8 ounces, as needed; apply topically, as needed.

Root Tea
Standard Decoction
Drink 2–6 ounces, as needed.

Poultice
Mash up the fresh plant (or moisten dry leaf powder) and apply directly to the body; repeat, as needed.

---

goatbush

Castela species
amargosa, chaparro amargosa, crucifixion thorn
PARTS USED stem, fruit

A queen of bitters, goatbush is a first-rate digestive aid and remedy for amoebic dysentery. It's the perfect remedy to carry when traveling to distant lands where Montezuma's Revenge is a possibility.

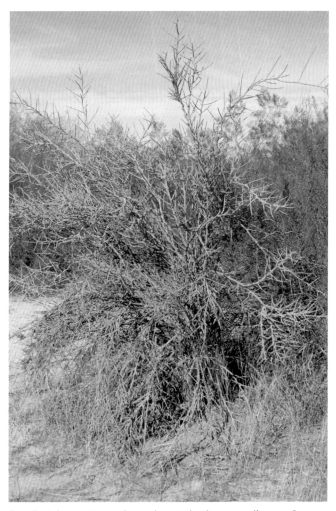

Our *Castela* species are large desert shrubs or small trees. Seen here is chaparro amargosa, *C. emoryi*, which is found throughout the lower Sonoran desert.

How to identify

Castela erecta ssp. *texana*, our common goatbush, has gray bark on short, pointed stems growing at nearly right angles and reaches 5–7 feet in height. Its small alternate leaves (present when sufficient moisture is available) are simple, glossy green, and entire; they appear semi-succulent and are very bitter. Its small 4-petaled flowers are red with a yellow center; mature fruits are bright red. *Castela emoryi* reaches upward of 15 feet in height with age and rarely possesses leaves beyond germination. Its flowers have 5–8 yellow to green petals, tinged with pink, and triangular sepals. The rigid yellow to lime-green branches are often intricately interwoven and entangled. Dark brown to black, dense seed clusters may persist on the plant for years.

Where, when, and how to wildcraft

Castela erecta ssp. *texana* is a plant of the South Texas Plains, the lower Gulf Coast, and up

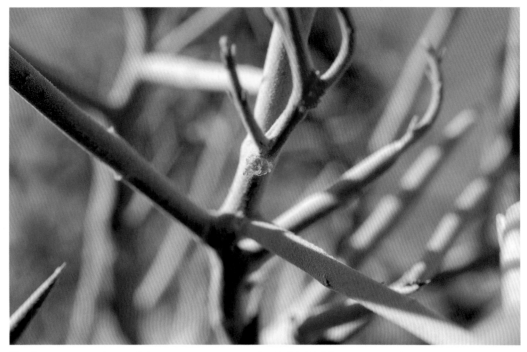

The thorny young stems of chaparro amargosa are frosted to bluish green; as spring warms up, an amber-colored mucilage is excreted from their joints.

along the Rio Grande into the Big Bend area of Texas, often in sand dunes. It is also found along the northeastern edge of the Edwards Plateau. *Castela emoryi*, a plant of the lower Sonoran desert, occupies floodplains from the Phoenix basin to Yuma and up to Barstow, California. Both plants can be gathered year-round, and both can put on tremendous growth in a short time in response to substantial rains. Select the newest growth, which is relatively soft and flexible; stems are otherwise very difficult to chop. Grind the dry stem pieces in a powerful blender and macerate for 2–4 months to extract the medicine thoroughly. It can otherwise be decocted. Berries ripen in late summer.

Medicinal uses

Goatbush has a long history of use as a medicinal plant in south Texas (where it is known as amargosa). The very bitter alcoholic extracts have been applied for dysentery, fever, eczema, or jaundice, to relieve intestinal ailments, as a diuretic, as a digestive aid, and to reduce biliousness. The tea or tincture is used as a mouthwash for periodontitis or for amoebic infections of tooth cavities.

Chaparro amargosa is used very similarly. There is less of an extant tradition of use for this plant, however, as it often exists in unpopulated areas. It too is nonetheless a fantastic remedy for intestinal parasitic infections, such as giardia and amoebic dysentery, and likewise a wonderful remedy to have on hand when traveling to an entirely new locale with different foods and unusual microbes in the air, soil, and water that could possibly disrupt the balance of one's gut flora. Take 15–30 drops per day in water as

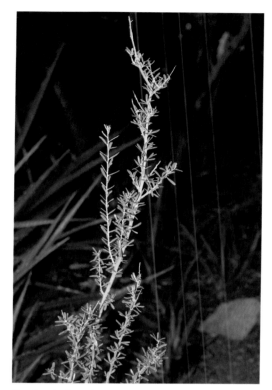

Goatbush, *Castela erecta* ssp. *texana*, also known as amargosa, grows along the Rio Grande and up across the South Texas Plains.

a prophylactic in these situations, especially when dealing with a sensitive digestive tract or when sampling suspect food and drink. The Yavapai smashed the flower buds of chaparro amargosa and applied to the face as a poultice to resolve acne.

Its affinity for the biliary apparatus is significant. I was once suffering from a severe case of nausea coupled with mild abdominal distension and rib pain with tension. It took no more than holding the tincture bottle of chaparro amargosa, and I felt a sudden upsurge of bile and the release of that pressure upon emesis—without even ingesting the tincture. Following emesis, I began to ingest it (at 30-drop doses), and the situation stabilized over the next 2–3 hours.

Future harvests

Gather only from large stands, pruning stems from the trees/shrubs as is appropriate for their current health status and growth rate. Gather and plant seeds in well-drained soil in early winter, after scarifying. Although *Castela emoryi* is on United Plant Savers' To-Watch list, I feel what is most important "to watch" is our rapid urban expansion across its habitat in the lower Sonoran desert.

HERBAL PREPARATIONS

Stem Tea
Standard Decoction
Drink 2–4 ounces, as needed; apply topically, as needed.

Stem Tincture
1 part dry stem, by weight
5 parts menstruum (50% alcohol,
  50% spring water), by volume
Take 20–60 drops, up to 5 times per day; use 5 drops as a bitter tonic.

goldenrod

Solidago species
PARTS USED aerial

A long-standing folk remedy, this astringent and aromatic herb helps to stimulate deficient kidney function, allay hay fever, and relieve arthritic joints.

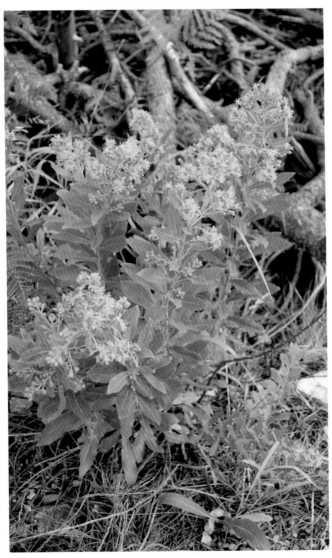

Solidago missouriensis, seen here growing in oak woodland in Arizona, is only one of many species that occur in our region.

How to identify

The leaves of this rhizomatous herbaceous perennial are mostly elongate with entire or toothed margins, sessile or petiolate, smooth or hairy, and some-times coarse to the touch with age. Brilliant yellow terminal clusters of radiate (ray and disc flowers) or discoid (disc flowers only) inflorescences appear by late summer. The form of the inflorescences is often most indicative of goldenrod: look for either an erect conical spike (among a patch or thicket of identical plants) or a series of drooping, semi-parabolic inflo-rescences all originating from one side of the stem.

Where, when, and how to wildcraft

Except for the most arid areas, various native *Solidago* species, more than 24 in number, are found throughout our region. As a general rule, look to moist cli-mates and microclimates, such as oak woodlands, grasslands, rivers and canyons, higher eleva-tions, or north-facing slopes of drier areas. South Texas (away from the coastline) is the least

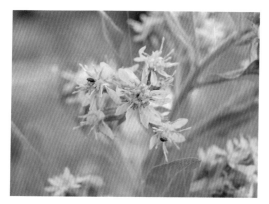

Goldenrod flowers are yellow and often arranged in conical or pyramidal terminal clusters. Most heads have ray flowers; some are purely discoid.

likely place within our region to find goldenrod. *Solidago velutina* is a common goldenrod in much of the western half of our region; it can be found in moist locations from lower-middle to higher elevations. *Solidago missouriensis*, Missouri goldenrod, is scattered throughout our region, appreciating a broad range of elevation (650–9,000 feet) and a variety of soils and habitats, from sandstone ledges to conifer forests. As with most aster family plants, goldenrod flowers quickly turn into a light fluff shortly after gathering. Avoid that by cutting back the stems just ahead of flowering. At lower elevations, begin looking in mid-spring to gather before flowering; at higher elevations, goldenrod begins flowering in late summer and continues into autumn.

Medicinal uses

Eclectic physicians employed the essential oil of goldenrod for a variety of diseases of the kidneys and bladder; and for centuries, teas, liniments, or poultices of the whole herb were familiar folk remedies in the Americas and Eurasia.

The tea of the herb, or root, makes a great anti-inflammatory for the kidneys; take after stones have been passed. Drink a half-cup of this astringent tea daily during allergy season to allay the symptoms of hay fever. Combine with estafiate, brittlebush, and yerba mansa. Consider using the tea in a neti pot for sinus congestion or infection. The hot tea is also taken for cough, cold, flu, retained menses, or joint pains, and as a diaphoretic to help break a fever when the patient is excessively cold.

Apply the tea or plant poultice to heal burns, boils, or infected wounds. The young leaves are a food and can be made into a tea to aid the digestion and promote appetite, particularly the more aromatic species.

Future harvests

Gather modestly from large, healthy stands. Consider bringing it into your home landscape, if appropriate.

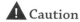 Caution

Avoid in acute cases of kidney stones or nephritis: it may be too stimulating. It's best to begin using goldenrod just past the acute phase.

HERBAL PREPARATIONS

Herb Tea
Standard Infusion
Apply topically to affected areas; drink 1–4 ounces, up to 5 times per day.

Tincture
1 part fresh flowering tops, by weight
2 parts menstruum (95% alcohol),
  by volume
or
1 part dry herb, by weight
5 parts menstruum (50% alcohol,
  50% spring water), by volume
Take 20–60 drops, up to 3 times per day.

---

golden smoke

Corydalis aurea, C. curvisiliqua, C. micrantha
fumewort
PARTS USED whole plant

Golden smoke is a wonderful pain remedy. Its bitter flavor indicates its ability to stimulate appetite and promote digestive secretions, as well as signaling its effects on the cardiovascular system as a blood mover.

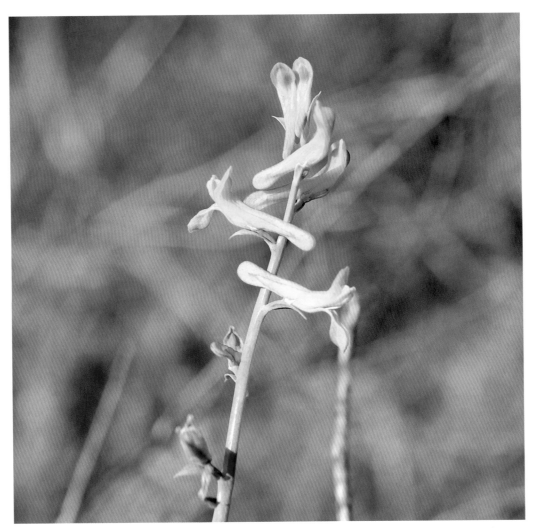

Corydalis aurea is the predominant species in the western half of our region. The flowers may rise above the foliage, or appear within the foliage.

How to identify

This annual poppy family plant grows to about 1 foot in height, producing dozens of stems and spreading out in a short mound. Leaves are smooth and blue-green, divided into leaflets of oval or diamond-shaped lobes. The yellow flowers are quite complex: the upper petal and lower petal are separate, and 2 fused petals are noticeable at the mouth of the corolla; the upper outer petal has a flat-tened or compressed rounded spur at its tail, and the lower outer petal possesses a rounded lip at the mouth of the flower. The end result is a horizontally balanced sculpture, elegantly poised at the end of a short ped-icel. The seedpods are upright and erect (curved in *Corydalis curvisiliqua*). The taproot is pale in color.

Where, when, and how to wildcraft

Golden smoke covers a wide range of habitats. Find it as a winter annual in the low desert of Arizona, a spring annual in southern New Mexico (*Corydalis aurea*), and a summer annual in the high-elevation conifer forests of the western half of our region (*C. aurea* or *C. curvisiliqua*). *Corydalis micrantha*, smallflower fumewort, can be found abundantly from the South Texas Plains northward along the eastern edge of our region, into the plains and prairies of Oklahoma, and westward into the high plains of the Texas panhandle. If you encounter a large stand, gather the whole plant in flower, grabbing from underneath

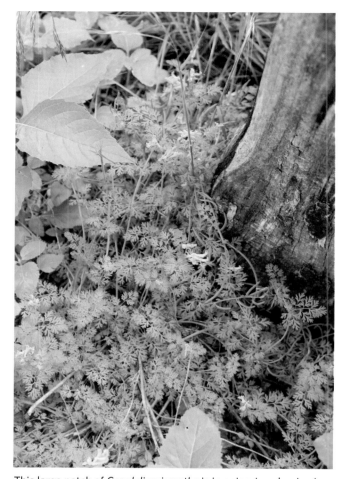

This large patch of *Corydalis micrantha* is in a riparian clearing in the northwest corner of the Edwards Plateau.

the leaves; golden smoke is often found growing in loose, sandy (regularly disturbed) soil, so it is easily pulled up by hand. In years of sparse production, trim only a portion of the stems and allow the rest to go to seed. Tincture the plant fresh.

Medicinal uses

Golden smoke is traditionally used as an alterative; it has an ability to tonify weakened tissues and improve their ability to transport wastes and take in nutrition—two important aspects of healing. It also promotes blood movement, thereby relieving pain and stagnation. Consider using it both topically and internally for ulcers and hemorrhoids.

The tincture will promote lymph movement, stimulate digestive secretions and improve appetite, relieve nerve pain, clear dampness from painful rheumatic joints, and increase the overall evacuation of wastes from the body. It's also useful as a post-partum tonic in cases of fever arising from infection.

In cases of an enlarged abdomen, combine with figwort, alder, and curly dock. It's best to use it in small to moderate doses, frequently; don't take heroic doses.

Most historic accounts of *Corydalis* are in fact referring to *Dicentra*, a closely related genus with overlapping uses. About two-thirds of the over 400 *Corydalis* species are native to China, where yanhusuo (as the herb is commonly known there) has been studied extensively and used for fever, hepatitis, edema, gastritis, cholecystitis, and hypertension. This matches well with some indigenous uses of golden smoke in North America. *Corydalis* species are currently being employed for neuropathic pain and preventing drug addiction relapse. It has a cool energy which can help us move into a quiet, self-reflective space beneath the pain.

Future harvests

Gather from areas of abundance only. Cast the seed over disturbed ground in appropriate areas.

Caution

Do not ingest during pregnancy. Consult a health practitioner if you have liver disease or are taking any pharmaceuticals (particularly blood thinners or neurologics).

HERBAL PREPARATIONS

Whole Plant Tincture
1 part fresh plant, by weight
2 parts menstruum (95% alcohol),
   by volume
or
1 part recently dry plant, by weight
5 parts menstruum (50% alcohol,
   50% spring water), by volume
Take 10–40 drops, up to 4 times per day.

Grindelia species
PARTS USED leaf, flower

An aromatic bitter with a complex flavor, gumweed is warming and drying with an affinity for the lungs and the urinary tract. Applied topically, it also stimulates healing from injuries or infections of the skin.

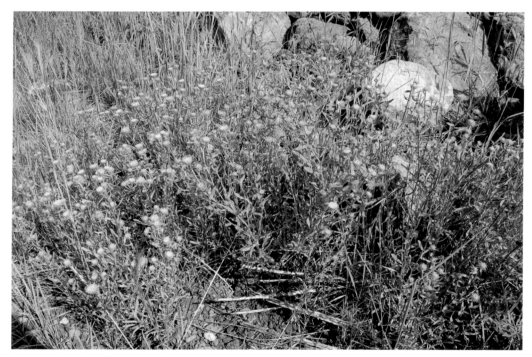

Gumweed prefers disturbed and exposed areas, such as roadsides and the edges of meadows. It can be difficult to spot unless growing alone or already in flower.

How to identify
Gumweed is often forming stands due to its rhizomatous habit, although some species are annuals and taprooted as well. The alternate leaves are mostly smooth and a bit glossy, sometimes gland-dotted, often resinous and serrated; they clasp a rounded, yellow-green or reddish stem. Inflorescences may be radiate or discoid; the flower buds, with pointed and often recurved phyllaries, develop a milky white resin—a good indication of their medicinal value.

Where, when, and how to wildcraft
The roughly 24 species of gumweed that occur in the Southwest regularly inhabit roadsides, clearings, and disturbed areas. Heavily grazed rangeland is a good place to look. In the western part of our region, it occurs mostly at higher elevations; in the

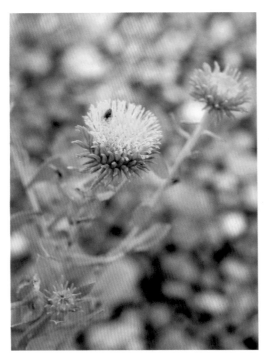

Grindelia squarrosa inflorescences are often discoid (ray flowers absent). Look for unopened buds (far right of photo) as the preferred plant part to gather.

eastern portion it occurs throughout, from western Oklahoma to just south of San Antonio. Gather the barely opened flower buds, usually in late summer/early autumn. You may notice a milky white resin coating the top of the bud; this is the preferred medicine. Simply pop buds off by hand, or clip with pruners or scissors. The whole flowering stem can also be harvested, with the entirety used for medicine, stem and all. *Grindelia arizonica*, *G. nuda*, and *G. squarrosa* are all good medicines and found within our region.

Medicinal uses

Gumweed's aromatic compounds are useful for the lungs as a disinfectant from viral and bacterial infections, serving as a functional expectorant. Its acridity helps to slowly break up and disperse cold, congested mucus deep in the lungs. Also, consider gumweed for chronic lung inflammation, dry cough, or labored breathing associated with asthma. The tincture is also somewhat relaxing and has a diuretic effect; it stimulates the appetite and relieves gastric discomfort due to cold or congestion.

Its warming resins are excreted through the urinary tract, serving to disinfect and increase blood flow to the epithelial tissue in the presence of infection. Use the fresh plant poultice or fresh plant tincture to soothe poison ivy rash or to stimulate tissue healing in wounds, scrapes, or skin infections.

Future harvests

Consider casting gumweed seeds into your local disturbed soils, then sit back and wait.

hackberry

Celtis species
cúmero, cumbro, sugarberry
PARTS USED bark, leaf, stem

The leaf tea is delicious and nutritious, aiding in digestion and relaxing the musculature of the body.

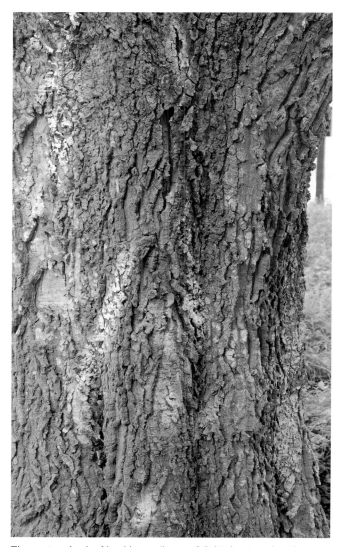

The mature bark of hackberry (here, of *Celtis laevigata*) with stout ridges running vertically along the trunk in the Texas Hill Country.

How to identify

This stout deciduous tree develops a wide, rounded crown with age and grows up to 30 feet in height. The smooth, light gray bark develops corky-warty, pointed vertical ridges with age. The rough, sandpapery leaves with smooth margins (serrate in *Celtis occidentalis*) are heart-shaped, asymmetrical at the base and lengthening out to a point; their underside has raised veins that branch out in a netlike pattern. The inconspicuous flowers are either male or female, on the same tree. The fruit is classified as a drupe, with a hard stone seed taking up much of the volume, and covered by a thin, orange sugary tissue. Its outer covering is thin, dry (fleshy in *C. pallida*), and matures to a dark reddish orange to purple. The tree takes on a grayish purple tone in the winter when leafless.

Where, when, and how to wildcraft

There's a good chance you'll find hackberry in nearly any area of our region. It prefers moist soil, so look to drainages, rivers, canyons, flood-plains, and roadsides. It is ubiquitous along the eastern edge of our region, to such an extent that many people consider it a weed. The bark and stems can be gathered year-round, and the leaves are best gathered before or after fruiting. Look for luxuriant new growth (a much more common occurrence on the eastern edge of our region) and prune back young branches to gather the leaves and stems. Harvest smooth bark from slightly older branches that are in need of pruning.

Medicinal uses

Despite the dearth of medicinal information on hackberry, it shows promise as a useful medicinal agent. Bark preparations were considered cooling and pain relieving by 19th-century physicians. A tea of the bark was traditionally used to alleviate sore throat and indigestion, while also addressing vene-real disease and serving as an emmenagogue. A leaf infusion is sweet and pleasant with a mild, relaxing effect. It also acts as a mild astringent and demulcent to the gut lining.

I consider both the leaf and bark tea to be nutritious. A decoction of the bark is slightly more astringent than the leaf preparation but perhaps more nutritious. Add the tea to a mushroom soup with wild greens as a convalescent aid. Although it is in the same plant family as *Cannabis* and hops, hackberry is not a narcotic.

Future harvests

If you're in the western half of our region, consider bringing this tree into your home landscape; along the eastern edge, this "weed" is doing fine on its own.

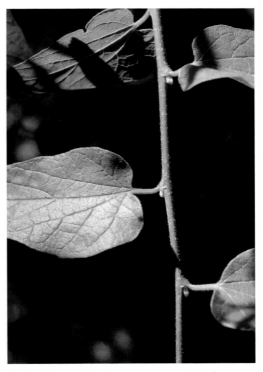

The leaf base of hackberry is asymmetrical.

HERBAL PREPARATIONS

Leaf Tea
Standard Infusion
Drink 4–8 ounces, as desired.

Bark Tea
Standard Infusion
Drink 2–4 ounces, up to 3 times per day, or combine in formulation.

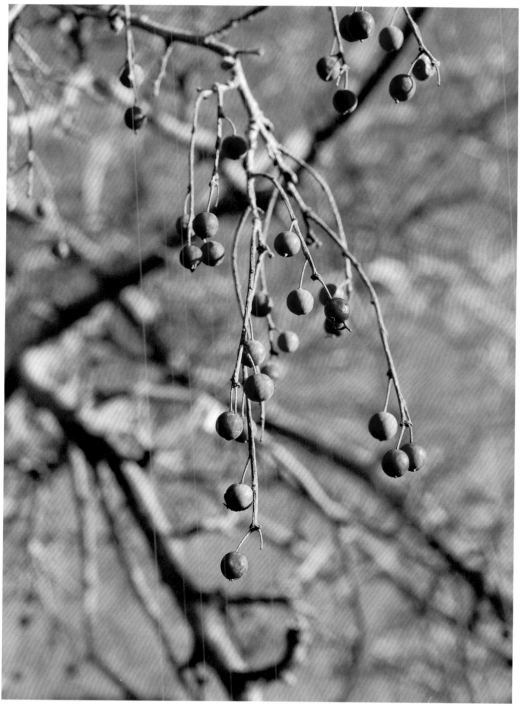

The green fruits last all summer, ripening in mid- to late autumn and persisting on the tree through to spring (here, on *Celtis reticulata*) if not consumed by birds or humans.

hawthorn

Crataegus species
tejocote
PARTS USED leaf, stem, flower, fruit

Hawthorn is our premier cardiac remedy. Balancing in its effects on the heart, both the tea and tincture are taken daily for their nourishing and restorative effects.

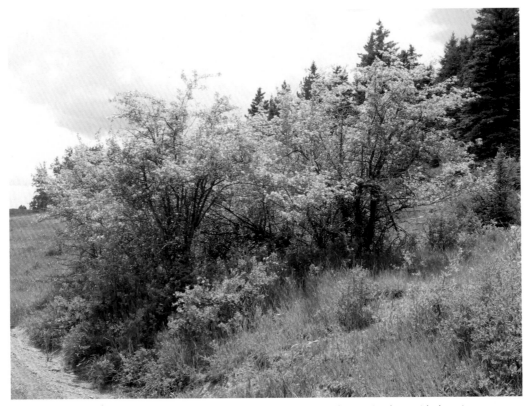

Hawthorn occurs in a variety of relatively moist habitats in the Southwest. Look to mid-elevation canyons, pine-oak woodlands in the northwestern quadrant, and humid forests along the Balcones Escarpment.

How to identify

Hawthorn is a large shrub or small tree found along waterways in our driest areas, or as a forest understory plant where moisture is more abundant. Most species can be identified by the stout to thin thorns studded along their branches from trunk to tip, although some do lack thorns entirely. The simple alternate leaves are toothed and often lobed; leaves on flowering branches often differ from those on vegetative branches. The 5-petaled flowers appear in clusters and are mostly white, occasionally tinged pink. Bark varies from dark to light gray to

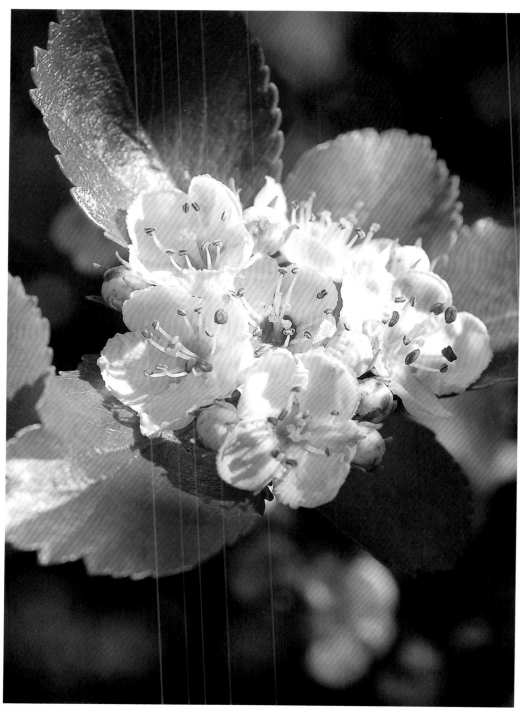

Hawthorn flowers bear a strong resemblance to its rose family relatives, such as apple, plum, and serviceberry.

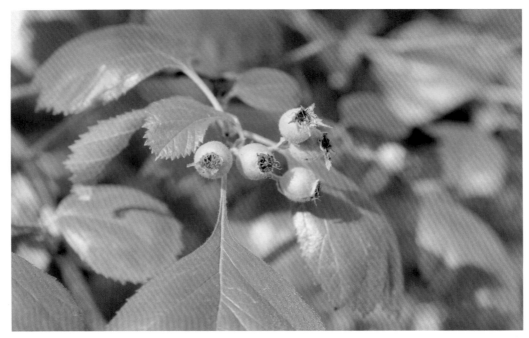

Crataegus mollis is a frequent understory shrub from Dallas to Corpus Christi. Its leaves make a delightful tea, and its berries are food and medicine in one.

reddish brown; it is smooth to start with, often becoming scaly, or peeled, with age. Each fruit, or haw, possesses a "crown" of persistent petals (often long and thin) at the apex of the fruit; ripe berries are bright red.

Where, when, and how to wildcraft

Although hawthorn is found throughout North America, it is a somewhat rare and special find in the Southwest, with the vast majority of our dozen or so *Crataegus* species found only in Texas. Hawthorn naturally occurs in the mountains of the Big Bend, near San Antonio, and along the edge of the blackland prairie moving north toward Dallas; north and south of San Antonio, you'll find *C. mollis*, downy hawthorn, growing in riparian oak woodlands, along with mulberry, pecan, hackberry, and many other favorites. In the western half of our region, look to mid- to high-elevation moist ravines,

mostly along the Mogollon Rim or in southern Colorado. The showy white blossoms appear at the height of spring; fruits follow in mid-summer. The leaves and twigs can be gathered at any time. Gather the fruits before the first frost hits.

Medicinal uses

Our application of hawthorn as a cardiovascular remedy comes directly from traditional European usage. Eclectic physicians saw it as the primary remedy and preventative medicine for cardiovascular maladies. It was used for hypertension, angina pectoris, cardiac neuralgia, tachycardia, and pericarditis, with an understanding that it was an indispensable tool in helping to prolong life for patients with these and other cardiac conditions. Modern herbalists throughout the Western world follow suit today, employing hawthorn as tea, tincture, or fruit paste for supporting heart health. It opens the chest, gently clearing and mildly astringing dampness. It enhances circulation to the heart and helps to moderate cardiac excess and deficiency. It's often used for arrhythmia, palpitations, anxiety, and insomnia (combine with skullcap).

In China, the berry is a preferred medicine for relieving food stagnation in the digestive tract, as well as for nourishing and strengthening the heart. Use the berry in tea for slow transit times, indigestion, foul belching, or general digestive debility (combine with cinnamon and orange peel

for a tasty elixir). The berry is nutritious. Combine the flower and leaf tincture with the fresh or dry berry tincture to round out its gentle effects.

The tea of the leaf and stem is mildly astringent. Native Americans applied this (and bark tea) for diarrhea, stomachache, and topically as an eyewash or for skin inflammation and swellings.

Future harvests

Treat the trees with respect and consider introducing to your home landscape, if appropriate.

Cooling Summer Formula

Consider making a tea blend with the following herbs to help cool the tissues and relieve dampness, which accumulates during the long, humid days of summer in the Southwest. These herbs may help reduce stress on the cardiovascular system, which hot weather may provoke. They reduce inflammation of the mucous membranes and tone and astringe organs as they "swell" and become diminished in their function; as tissue is relaxed and cooled, the spirit is lifted. Combine the first 6 herbs in equal amounts, and the final 3 at ½ part, and prepare as a sun tea or standard infusion. It's okay to omit herbs you don't have.

- hawthorn leaf and flower
- elder flower
- ocotillo flower
- mulberries
- nettle leaf
- plantain leaf
- rose petals
- prickly pear flower
- desert willow flower

HERBAL PREPARATIONS

Flowering Branch Tea
Standard Infusion
Drink 4–8 ounces, up to 3 times per day; apply to the affected area consistently until resolved.

Berry Tea
Cold Infusion
Drink 2–4 ounces, up to 3 times per day.

Flowering Tops/Berry Tincture
1 part fresh herb, by weight
2 parts menstruum (95% alcohol), by volume
or
1 part fresh herb, by weight
5 parts menstruum (50% alcohol, 50% spring water [berries, 60%, 40%]), by volume
Take 10–30 drops, up to 4 times per day.

hopbush

Dodonaea viscosa
tarachíque, saucillo
PARTS USED leaf, stem

A smooth muscle relaxant with a strong effect on the liver and gall bladder,
hopbush moves blood throughout the body, relieving pain and promoting
relaxation when tension or spasm is present.

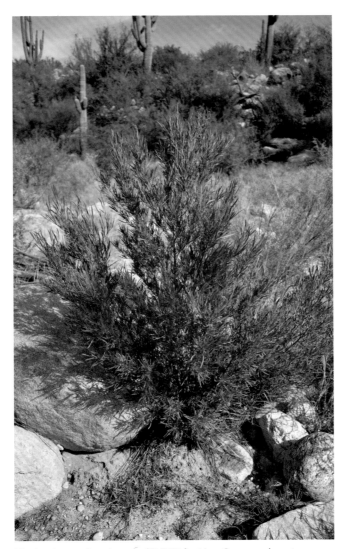

Hopbush, growing at around 3,000 feet in a Sonoran desert canyon.

How to identify

Hopbush is a perennial ever-green shrub but may lose its shiny, somewhat sticky alter-nate leaves following prolonged freezing temperatures. It is dioecious (male and female flowers on separate plants), occasionally polygamodioecious (bisexual flowers on either male or female plants). The long, lin-ear, simple leaves have a raised midvein on the underside; stems are yellowish green when very young, eventually reddish brown to gray. Tiny, incon-spicuous, pale yellow petal-less flowers occur in clusters near the branch tips. The fruit is a 3- to 4-winged capsule (samara), often tinged with pink or magenta before maturing to a beige-brown.

Where, when, and how to wildcraft

Fascinatingly, this plant is native to every continent except Europe and Antarctica. Within our region it is found exclusively in the Sonoran desert at 2,000–5,000 feet,

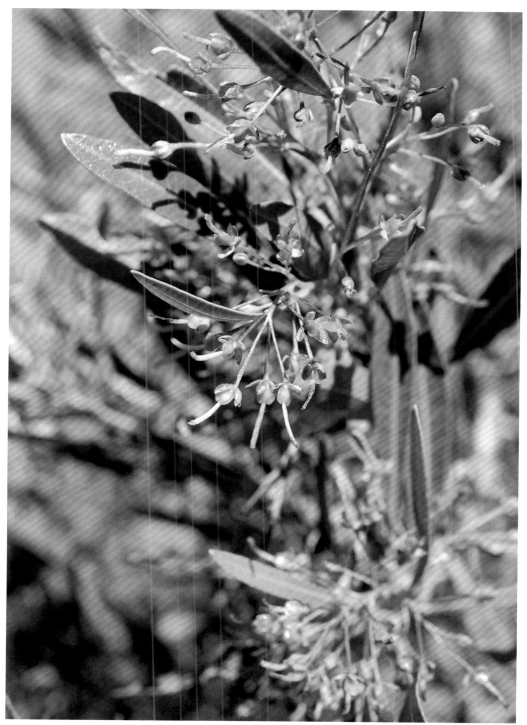

Plants often flower in late winter, with young fruit formation by mid-spring.

occupying the rocky banks of desert washes, or boulder-strewn bajadas and mountainsides of desert grasslands. Although it isn't as common in these areas as cholla, saguaro, or prickly pear, it is often abundant when found. Gather the young leaves after winter rains, before the plant flowers (the plant may flower in late autumn after rains, as well), or after the summer rains begin. Simply snip at the base of the young stem to use the entirety of the tender growth. Tincture fresh, or dry for tea or oil infusion.

Medicinal uses

The energy of this plant strongly correlates with the spring season. It exemplifies the Bile humour, mobilizing its release, delivering warmth throughout the body, promoting fluid movement, stimulating digestion, enhancing metabolism, and relieving restrictions in the liver and gall bladder and muscle spasm of the digestive tract. As a hepatoprotective herb, it also enables the liver detoxification pathways. Its slightly acrid flavor is indicative of its ability to relieve and disperse congestion.

It is calming to the nervous system, allaying tension and anxiety (start with 5 drops of tincture) as well as muscle pain and spasm. In Tasmania, where it natively occurs, it is used topically for sprains and bruises. Locally in Sonora, it is applied topically to cuts, wounds, and skin irritations as a poultice. It can also be prepared as an alcohol intermediate oil infusion for these applications. A wash made from the leaves may help reduce skin pigmentation.

Applied topically, its antifungal, antimicrobial, and anti-inflammatory properties can be experienced through the resolution of lingering fungal infections or antibiotic-resistant sores. It is also strongly active against *Streptococcus mutans* and has been shown to reduce biofilms, making it effective as a mouthwash to prevent dental caries. A strong infusion of hopbush leaves can be applied to recently abraded and irritated skin.

This species has been used against malaria and diabetes, prompting widespread interest and scrutiny of its therapeutic potential. Its antioxidant and anxiolytic properties, and its effectiveness against *Plasmodium*, are other important areas of study, currently.

Future harvests

Hopbush can live for decades. Gather the leaves prudently from healthy individuals within large stands, and it will continue to produce for many years to come. Consider introducing it to your home landscape, if appropriate.

HERBAL PREPARATIONS

Leaf Tea
Standard Infusion
Apply topically, as needed; drink 2–4 ounces, 1–3 times per day.

Leaf Tincture
1 part fresh leaf, by weight
2 parts menstruum (95% alcohol),
  by volume
or
1 part dry leaf, by weight
5 parts menstruum (50% alcohol,
  50% spring water), by volume
Take 5–30 drops, up to 3 times per day.

Oil Infusion
1:5
Dry leaves and prepare as alcohol intermediate oil infusion (see page 38).

Poultice
Mash up the fresh plant and apply directly to the body, as needed.

---

hop tree

Ptelea trifoliata
wafer ash
PARTS USED bark, leaf, seed

Use hop tree in cold, congested states with restricted circulation, such as poor digestion, chronic infection, asthma, or joint pain.

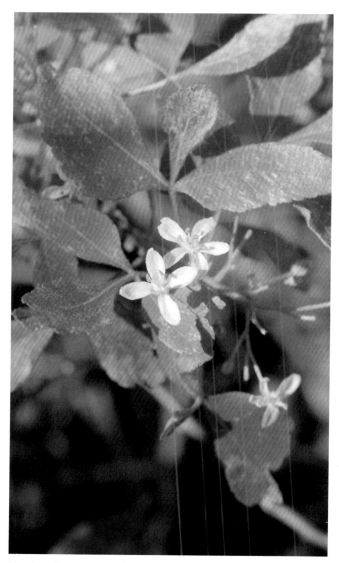

Hop tree flowers are either 4- or 5-petaled.

How to identify

This tree is often nearly invisible at a distance within its prime habitat, due to the abundance of green surrounding it and the overstory shadowing of the forest canopy. Its leaves are 3-lobed throughout the Southwest, but the leaflets of plants in the western half of our region are more rounded (ovate-obovate) and less pointy than those of eastern populations. The alternate leaves occur on long petioles that extend beyond the flowers and seedpods, often hiding them from sight. The smooth brownish gray bark is mottled with white. I once entered a canyon believing a mountain lion might be present, taking the aroma in the air for its urine—but no: it was the pungent spring scent of hop tree, wafting down the cool drainage.

Where, when, and how to wildcraft

Hop tree is found in the middle elevations of moist canyons from northwestern to southeastern Arizona and

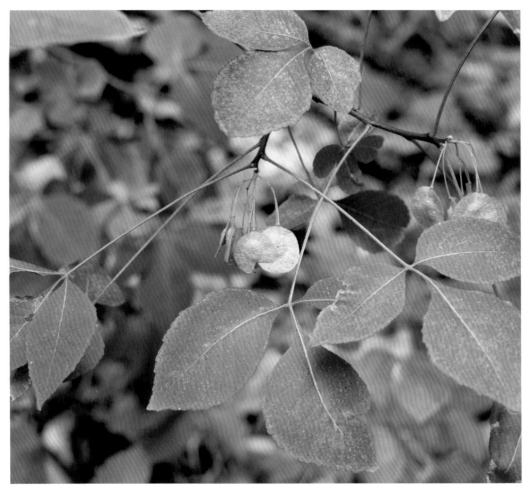

Hop tree is known as wafer ash in the Texas Hill Country. Crush the leaves to experience its distinctive smell.

mountainous areas of north-central to southern New Mexico. It occurs in great abundance in the Texas Hill Country, sparingly in the Big Bend of Texas, and relatively rarely in the moist canyons of the Texas and Oklahoma panhandles. Since hop tree grows as an understory plant, look to roadside forests (eastern half) and canyons (western half). Gather leaves and/or bark whenever the plant is not in flower or going to seed. In autumn, select the bark, as the leaves lose much of their aromatic appeal after the long summer. Simply prune the tree at the base of healthy stems, 1.5 inches or less in diameter; then strip the bark and chop the leaves for fresh plant tincture. Look to harvest branches that are lower on the trunk, which may be shed naturally by the tree in the coming years.

Medicinal uses

This is strong medicine. Much of hop tree's value derives from its bitter aromatics. Its nature is warming and drying with a strongly pungent flavor. Salivary secretions kick in almost immediately after tasting it, stimulating the appetite. This may lead to a laxative effect, when appropriate. The initial lubricating effect from the digestive stimulation may cause a rebound drying effect (this can be ameliorated through herbal formulation). The plant is a strong Bile-inducing herb, sending warmth throughout the body, enhancing mobility, and improving digestive secretions.

Consider using hop tree in combination with tickseed, red root, and other herbs for chronic infections where there's an accumulation of waste products, poor circulation, fatigue, and poor appetite. Physicians effectively employed hop tree for rheumatism, asthma, or constriction in the chest (combined with mullein) well into the 20th century.

Future harvests

No worries in the eastern part of our region, where hop tree is abundant, but in the western portion, it can be a thin, tall, delicate tree, so gather modestly or not at all. Consider introducing it to your home landscape, if appropriate.

HERBAL PREPARATIONS

Leaf/Seed Tea
Standard Infusion
Drink 2–4 ounces, up to 3 times per day.

Bark Tea
Standard Decoction
Drink 1–4 ounces, up to 3 times per day.

Bark/Leaf/Seed Tincture
1 part fresh herb, by weight
2 parts menstruum (95% alcohol),
  by volume
or
1 part dry herb, by weight
5 parts menstruum (65% alcohol,
  35% spring water), by volume
Take 10–30 drops, up to 4 times per day.

Equisetum species
cola de caballo, scouring rush
PARTS USED aerial

Horsetail, an ancient remnant of forests long gone, is an excellent aid in chronic inflammatory lung conditions. A tea of it is exceptionally nutritious, speeding the regeneration of tissues that are in the process of recuperating or rebuilding.

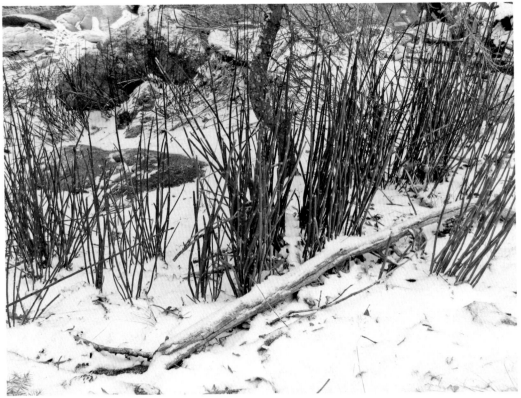

An identifying characteristic of *Equisetum* ×*ferrissii* (a hybrid of *E. hyemale* and *E. laevigatum*) is that the stems last through winter.

How to identify

Horsetail always grows near groundwater. The erect green stems, 1–6 feet tall, are made coarse by vertical ridges. Each stem is circumscribed by toothed, black-banded sheaths of various thicknesses; at these junctions, you can pull the pieces of the plant apart and put them back together again (hence another common name, puzzle plant). Bushy *Equisetum arvense* looks the most like a horse's tail, with its smaller side stems coming out in whorls from top to bottom of the stem, but

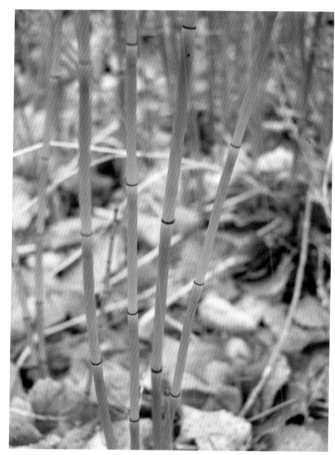

The black-banded sheaths occurring along the stem are thinner in *Equisetum laevigatum*.

to mid-spring to avoid excessive silica content, and avoid gathering when sporangia are present. Nicotine is found in appreciable quantities in various species of horsetail; to minimize this, only gather early in the season. Often, the stems can simply be pulled up out of their sheaths near ground level. If that proves too difficult, clip or prune back at the base of the stem.

Medicinal uses

This nutritious herb is particularly high in silica, supporting its use as a tea to rebuild injured connective tissue (tendons, ligaments, cartilage, mucous membranes, bones, epithelial tissue of the lungs). It is an excellent tonic to support the growth of luxuriant hair and nails. Enhance its grassy flavor or direct its influences to particular areas of the body by adding some orange peel, cinnamon, or beebalm to

these can occur on any injured or cut horsetail. Sporangia, or spore-producing segments, appear at the end of the stems in early summer; they're a bit like a spine-tipped football, shoved down into the sheath below (*E. laevigatum*, smooth horsetail, has no point).

Where, when, and how to wildcraft

Horsetail is found throughout our region in places of significant moisture, such as springs, creeks, streams, or high-elevation canyons and rivers. You will not find it in drier, more exposed areas—it likes moisture *and* shade. Gather the stems in early

your decoction. Numerous properties are attributed to horsetail; besides its ability to relieve joint pain, it is diuretic, vulnerary, anti-inflammatory (due to inhibition of lymphocyte activity), hemostatic, anxiolytic (potential cannabinoid receptor modulation), and antioxidant.

A decoction of horsetail may benefit urinary incontinence, ulcers, internal bleeding, chronic respiratory inflammation, osteoporosis, kidney stones, UTIs, prostate pain, edema, eczema, heavy menses, and nosebleeds. The tincture is potentially hepatoprotective. Apply the oil or salve topically to heal wounds (used traditionally to heal from an episiotomy).

Future harvests
Gather modestly from established stands without disrupting the rhizomes and it will continue to produce healthy stems.

 Caution
Avoid during pregnancy: horsetail may inhibit CYP1A2. Avoid while on antiretroviral pharmaceuticals and during regular cortico-steroid use. Gather only early-season horse-tail to avoid potentially toxic concentrations of silica or nicotine; avoid gathering horsetail downstream of agribusiness, as horsetail concentrates heavy metals (aluminum, arse-nic, lead) from the soil and water. Unheated, ground horsetail in capsules contains thi-aminase, which will lower the body's levels of vitamin B1, eventually causing beri-beri. Dermatitis may be experienced through use of high-nicotine horsetail.

HERBAL PREPARATIONS

Herb Tea
Standard Decoction
Let stand overnight to enhance micronutrient extraction. Drink 4–8 ounces, up to 3 times per day.

Tincture
1 part fresh herb, by weight
2 parts menstruum (75% alcohol, 25% spring water), by volume
or
1 part dry herb, by weight
5 parts menstruum (50% alcohol, 50% spring water), by volume
Take 1–4ml, up to 3 times per day.

Oil Infusion
1:5
Dry stems and prepare as alcohol intermediate oil infusion (see page 38).

horseweed

Conyza canadensis
yerba del caballo, mare's tail, Canadian fleabane
PARTS USED whole plant

A hot and dry counterirritant for topical use, including burns, joint pain, and acne. It's also ingested for its ability to stop internal bleeding and heal the gut lining from chronic inflammation or leaky gut.

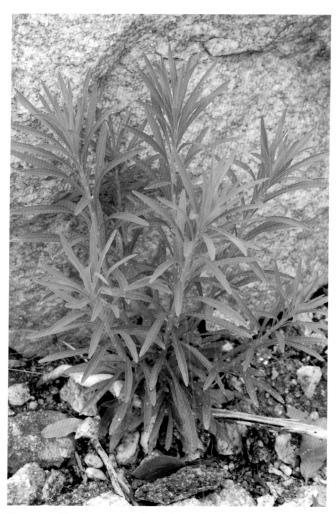

Horseweed is a common sight in desert washes and along roadsides.

How to identify

This naturalized annual from Europe is often difficult to make out in the early stages of its growth; however, with a little practice you can train your eye to identify it at any stage by searching for its key traits. The basal and stem leaves have tiny hairs sticking out from the leaf margins, and there is usually at least one small tooth on either side of the leaf, toward the tip. Young leaves often have a pink or red midrib. The leaves attach directly to the stem and come off all sides of it, often quite close together. They hang off the stem in a bit of a parabolic shape, giving it the appearance of a mare's tail (another common name). At maturity, the plant is 3–5 feet tall, 8 feet or more in optimal conditions. Clusters of tiny inflorescences of inconspicuous white ray flowers and yellow disc flowers appear at the branch tips and the leaf axils. The plant gradually turns light brown and dies by late autumn/early winter.

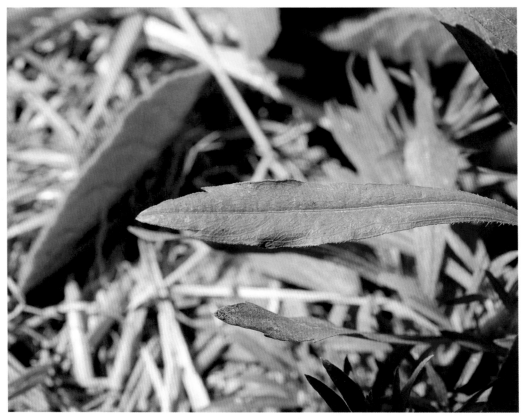

Two key features will aid in identifying horseweed prior to flowering: the pair of teeth near the apex of the leaf, and the tiny hairs along the leaf margin.

Where, when, and how to wildcraft

A colonizing plant if ever there was one, it can be found on nearly every continent on Earth. Needless to say, it's everywhere. Look for it in disturbed areas, starting in late autumn to early spring in our lowest and warmest areas, in mid-summer at the higher elevations. Gather the whole plant just prior to flowering for optimal leaf size. The whole plant is chopped and dried for tea or prepared as fresh or dry tincture.

Medicinal uses

The essential oil of horseweed ("oil of erigeron") was a highly rated hemostatic employed by the physiomedicalists and Eclectic physicians. The tea, tincture, or poultice can work similarly to stop bleeding, internally or externally. It is of great use in chronic inflammatory bowel disease (note: blood in the stool should always be evaluated by a physician); regular use of the tea is essential for relief as well as for restoring the gut lining (combine with plantain and mallow). Tea is perhaps our most effective and efficient use of this plant.

Horseweed is useful in all manner of kidney and bladder conditions for its diuretic action, in particular, conditions which show accumulation of fluid in the body, shortness of breath, and a slow or thick pulse. Its acrid quality helps relieve the damp conditions while stimulating the heart–kidney feedback loop, improving fluid movement throughout the body.

Apply the tea or poultice topically to stiff, achy joints, injuries, burns, bleeding hemorrhoids, boils, skin infections, or venomous bites and stings. The tea can also be used as a steam inhalation for sinus congestion, earache, or chest congestion (combine with brittlebush, internally).

Future harvests

I have seen these plants come in by the millions after floods and fires. If we have any sort of future on this planet, horseweed will be here, too.

HERBAL PREPARATIONS

Herb Tea
Standard Infusion
Drink 2–4 ounces, up to 4 times per day; apply topically, as needed.

Tincture
1 part fresh herb, by weight
2 parts menstruum (95% alcohol),
   by volume
or
1 part dry herb, by weight
5 parts menstruum (50% alcohol,
   50% spring water), by volume
Take ¼–1 teaspoon, up to 4 times per day.

inmortál

Asclepias asperula
contrayerba, antelope horns
PARTS USED dry root

This very bitter remedy stimulates the appetite and secretions throughout the body; it is a wonderful remedy for both acute and chronic lung afflictions.

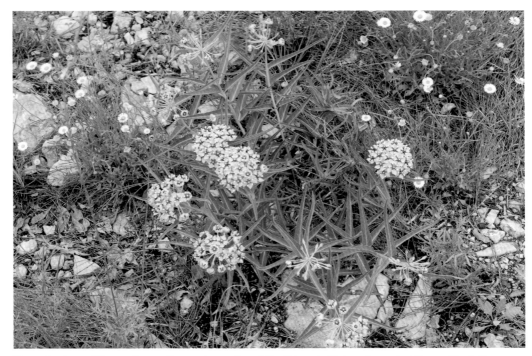

Flowering inmortál, growing on the western edge of the Edwards Plateau in central Texas. The inflorescence is shaped like a ball overall.

How to identify

Before flowering, this herbaceous perennial easily escapes notice; however, when the rounded umbels of greenish white and purple flowers pop out over the rangelands, from central Texas to eastern New Mexico, it is very easy to spot. A key feature of inmortál is the erect corolla lobes (these typically point downward in other *Asclepias* species). Before flowering, the rough, linear, irregularly alternate leaves with short petioles show a yellowish, sometimes pinkish, midrib and leaf margin. Stems are trailing; the main stem is usually yellowish (occasionally reddish pink). The seedpods, borne on long, curved pedicels, are quintessentially milkweed, with a teardrop shape that's pointed at the top. As the green, fleshy pods mature, they wrinkle and turn beige, finally opening along a lengthwise split to spew forth fluffy, winged seeds. The root is thick and often massive relative to the slender vegetation; its outer skin is dark brown, the inner pith milky white and juicy. All plant parts exude a milky white sap when broken.

Where, when, and how to wildcraft

With the exception of southern California and southeastern New Mexico, inmortál occurs throughout our region, but it is far more abundant in the eastern third. Look to grasslands, plains, rocky hillsides, old pastures, and roadsides. Refrain from gathering it within the western two-thirds of our region, where it is relatively scarce. Gather the root before the plant begins to flower, or conversely, in the autumn once the plant has gone to seed. Digging the roots of inmortál is legitimate physical labor, especially when the soil is rocky; for guidelines, see "Digging Roots" (page 26), to ensure you gather your optimal medicine and steward the health of the stand as well. Use only dry root for medicine.

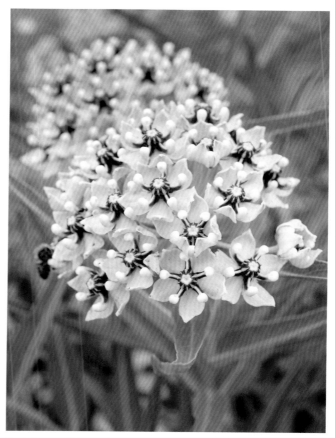

Each inmortál flower has 5 curved and ascending bowl-shaped lobes; the 5 "hoods" attached to the hypanthium give the appearance of antelope horns.

Medicinal uses

Beginning in the 19th century, as they began to learn about them from the indigenous healers, Eclectic physicians put our native *Asclepias* species to use; however, inmortál's medicinal uses were relatively unknown outside its Southwest home until Michael Moore helped spread the word. The uses listed here overlap with other *Asclepias* species used for medicine (not all are), but inmortál is considered stronger in its effects, and it's the most abundant species overall within our region (with the exception of *A. speciosa* at higher elevations in our northwestern quadrant).

Use the tincture to stimulate appetite and promote digestive secretions while simultaneously improving peripheral circulation and enlivening blood flow. Moore ranks it as one of our country's prime plant medicines and a great remedy for asthma, pleurisy, bronchitis, and lung infections. It stimulates secretions within the lungs, just as it does throughout the entire body (skin, kidneys, reproductive system). I've used it when dampness settles in the lungs causing episodic asthma (often worse at higher elevations during particularly humid weather); *Asclepias tuberosa* can be used similarly.

Moore also considers inmortál a safe cardiac tonic for the deficient, aged heart—traditionally administered as root powder taken in hot water. It's also used in a variety of ways to stimulate the female reproductive system, from delayed, painful menses to improving the efficiency of contractions during labor and postpartum lochial discharge.

In northern Sonora, the root is ground and mixed with hot water to relieve epileptic seizures (a common use of warming herbs in the region) and sexual debility.

Future harvests

Gather only from large stands (several dozen plants or more). Larger root pieces left in the soil tend to regenerate in subsequent years (hence "inmortál"). Bring the seeds to disturbed ground throughout middle elevations in the western half of our region.

Cardiovascular Formula

Combine the following tinctures to support cardiovascular health; take 60–120 drops, morning and evening.

- 2 parts chia tincture
- 2 parts hawthorn tincture
- 2 parts Bermudagrass tincture
- 1 part tree of heaven tincture
- 1 part inmortál tincture

HERBAL PREPARATIONS

Root Tea
Add ½ teaspoon dry root to hot water and drink up to 4 times per day.

Root Tincture
1 part dry root, by weight
5 parts menstruum (50% alcohol, 50% spring water), by volume
Take 5–30 drops, up to 3 times per day.

jojoba

Simmondsia chinensis
PARTS USED leaf, seed

*This Sonoran desert native has been used as medicine for centuries,
if not millennia. The oil from the nuts is a hair tonic, and the leaf tea is
used to relieve intestinal inflammation.*

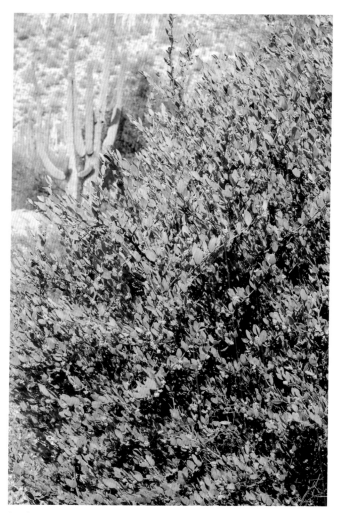

Jojoba, growing in the Sonoran desert alongside saguaro in the open sunshine.

How to identify

The opposite gray-green leaves of this evergreen perennial shrub (4–6 feet in height) are leathery, thick, and pointed; when exposed to full sun, they often point straight up to reduce sun exposure. Jojoba is dioecious (male and female flowers, which first appear in mid-winter, are borne on separate plants). The male flowers are inconspicuous and dangly; female flowers, even less conspicuous, have long green sepals that cover the top of the fruit like a fan-shaped sombrero. Female plants are easy to identify when covered in fruits, which may cling to the plant for months after maturing. Mature fruits are covered in a thin, wrinkly, light brown husk and contain a dark brown ovoid seed (nut) with a pointed end and smooth grooves running along its length. The nuts are a favored food of javelina, so their tracks, scat, and signs of activity are often found near jojoba populations.

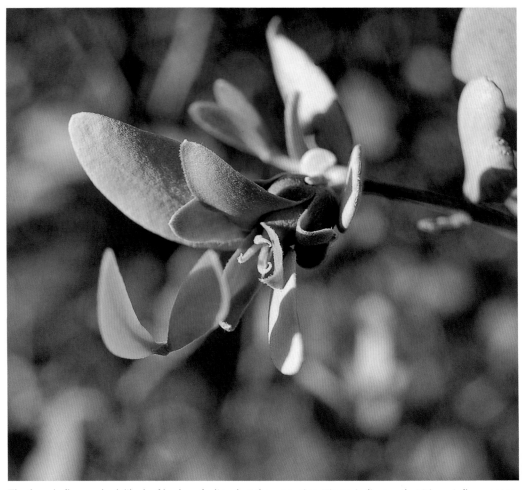

The female flowers look like leaf buds unfurling, but the emerging stigma indicates that it's an inflorescence.

Where, when, and how to wildcraft

Jojoba is found throughout the lower elevations of the Sonoran desert in Arizona and southern California, often in the company of cholla, ocotillo, or rhatany. Look to dry, rocky slopes, bajadas, and desert washes. After a significant rain, gather the fresh green leaves by pruning at the new growth. As with other desert shrubs, avoid gathering leaves when in flower (generally, late winter to mid-spring). Seeds ripen from late spring to early summer. Pick directly from the plant or look to the ground beneath it to gather freshly fallen nuts, still in their husk. Dry the leaves for tea; crush the seeds to make a cold infusion. Seeds can also be smashed and boiled to extract the oil, or wax, in a simple, non-industrial fashion.

Medicinal uses

To this day, homemade jojoba oil is used in northwestern Mexico as a hair dye and to help remedy balding; the paste is applied directly to the skin where new hair growth is desired. In Sonora, the ground nut was traditionally roasted with bovine bone marrow to extract its properties. Industrially prepared jojoba oil (more properly, wax) is an expensive yet popular ingredient in herbal skin care products, desirable for its chemical similarity to the skin's sebaceous secretions and the pleasant sensation it produces when applied to the skin; it is also known for its topical antimicrobial and anti-inflammatory effects.

The cold infusion of the nut is used to alleviate sore throat or a bad case of *empacho*, a condition marked by a stuck feeling in the middle of the gut, digestive torpor and discomfort, and (possibly) an inability to swallow. The Seri of northern Mexico make eyedrops from a cold infusion of the ground, raw nut to alleviate red, itchy eyes.

The leaf tea is an aid to inflammation of the digestive tract, particularly the large intestine. Add it to formulas with horseweed, evening primrose, and walnut leaf for irritable bowel disorder or similar inflammatory conditions of the large intestine. The tincture, applied topically, has an anti-inflammatory effect and is inhibiting to herpes viruses.

Future harvests

Gather with respect and gratitude, and consider introducing this plant to your home landscape, if appropriate.

 Caution

Consuming excessive amounts of the nuts, or drinking the nut tea, may cause intestinal griping, diarrhea, or constipation. The small amount of nut tea suggested here is not known to cause any ill effects.

HERBAL PREPARATIONS

Leaf Tea
Standard Decoction
Drink 4–8 ounces, 1–3 times per day.

Nut Tea
Cold Infusion
Grind the nut and prepare overnight; drink 1–4 ounces, 1–3 times per day.

Leaf Tincture
1 part dry leaf, by weight
5 parts menstruum (50% alcohol,
   50% spring water), by volume
Apply the tincture topically to resolve herpes sores or to relieve the pain of shingles.

Nut Oil
Grind and roast the nut with a bit of oil high in saturated fat (e.g., coconut oil); apply topically, as needed.

Juniperus species
cedar
PARTS USED leaf, berry

The warming oils of the berries are sweet and pungent in flavor, stimulate the appetite, and promote urination and sweating.

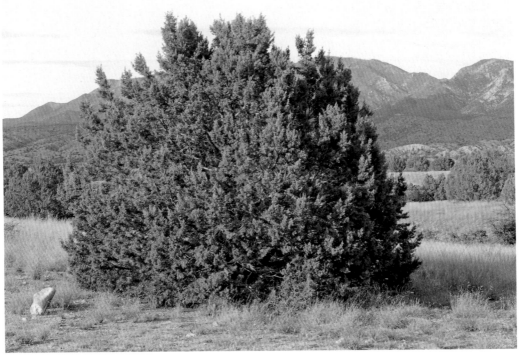

Juniperus monosperma is common at middle elevations and high desert habitats throughout the western two-thirds of our region.

How to identify

Many juniper species in the Southwest are quite similar in form and color; all are evergreen conifers with rounded, scalelike leaves. The short (2–4 feet tall) *Juniperus communis* grows at high elevations within our region and has thin, flat leaves that end in a sharp point. *Juniperus monosperma*, one-seed juniper, has a shrub-like appearance and shredding gray bark. *Juniperus deppeana*, alligator juniper, has an overall white tinge to its light green foliage and produces larger (2cm) berries than most species; its bark is characteristically checkered, akin to alligator skin. *Juniperus pinchotii* can be distinguished by its red berries. Shredding bark is a trait common to many junipers, as are the fruits, which appear green when young; fruits mature into

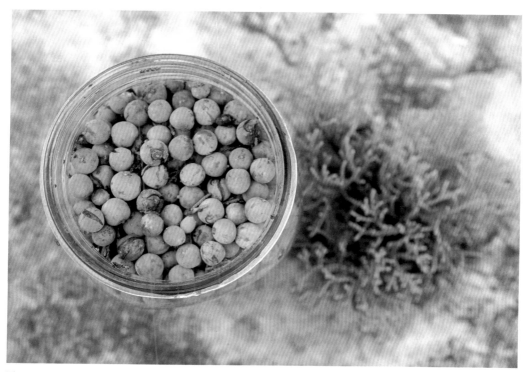

These ripened purple berries of *Juniperus ashei* contain 1-2 seeds. The white bloom easily rubs off the berry's surface.

red, blue, or purple cones, which often have a white yeast bloom coating the outer surface (this is easily rubbed off with a swipe of the finger). The tiny male cones usually appear at the tips of the leaves in autumn. Most junipers are dioecious, with berries only on female trees; *J. osteosperma*, Utah juniper, is largely monoecious, with both male and female cones borne on the same plant.

Where, when, and how to wildcraft

Junipers are found in nearly every habitat of the Southwest, with desert grasslands, high plains, high desert, Hill Country, and oak woodlands being the most common locales. *Juniperus monosperma* is abundant in Arizona, New Mexico, and southern Colorado, often overlapping with *J. osteosperma* and *J. scopulorum*, Rocky Mountain juniper,

which is found at slightly higher elevations as well. In the Texas Hill Country, *J. ashei*, Ashe's juniper, colonizes areas that are no longer grazed or maintained by fire as they were in ancient times, just as *J. pinchotii* does in western Texas and the panhandle. Juniper leaves are best gathered when the tree is not flowering, from spring to autumn. The berries are gathered when ripe, which may be anywhere from late autumn to mid-spring, depending on the location and species. It's always best to take hikes and observe your local populations throughout the year; weather variations from year to year can skew the seasons by weeks, if not months. Trim the leaves with pruners where they emerge from the woody branch; the ripe berries come off easily by hand. Both can be dried or used fresh.

Medicinal uses

Juniper berries are laxative and diuretic, stimulating the bladder and kidneys as well as digestive secretions. Specifically indicated for UTIs with mucus in the urine; combine with gumweed, yerba santa, or manzanita. The warming and drying energy has a beneficial effect on the lungs in cold, damp respiratory infections. The leaves can be used similarly but the flavor is more bitter and acrid.

Simply chewing on a berry is a basic yet effective way to employ juniper as a remedy. It's a worthwhile arthritis remedy in the cold, deficient, and aged. The berries can also be made into a tea or tincture. A heated decoction of the berries, leaves, or twigs acts as a moderate circulatory stimulant, treating rheumatic joints, sores, or boils when applied topically.

Future harvests

Gather sparingly, and never harvest all available berries: you will damage wild populations. Consider adding junipers to your home landscape, if appropriate.

HERBAL PREPARATIONS

Leaf/Berry Tea
Standard Infusion (Standard Decoction to apply topically)
Drink 2–4 ounces, up to 3 times per day; inhale steam from leaf tea.

Berry Tincture
1 part berries, by weight
5 parts menstruum (75% alcohol, 25% spring water), by volume
Apply topically to affected areas; take 20–40 drops, up to 4 times per day.

kidneywood

Eysenhardtia species
palo dulce, palo azúl, vara dulce
PARTS USED bark, leaf, stem, flower, seed, wood

Wonderfully aromatic, this pea family shrub makes a pleasant-tasting tea that helps to allay irritation in the urinary tract and to relieve the pain of rheumatism and similar complaints.

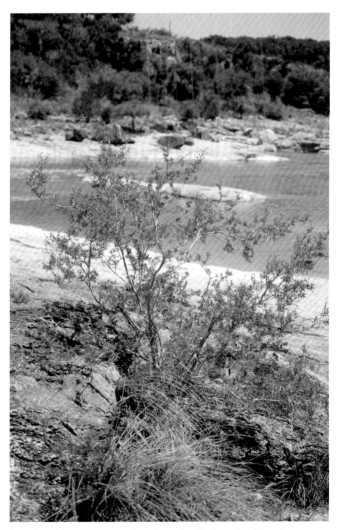

Eysenhardtia texana, growing along the Pedernales River in central Texas.

How to identify

This deciduous pea family shrub has odd, pinnately divided compound leaves; they are quite similar to mesquite, but upon closer inspection, one can see the tiny dark glands dotting the underside of their 2–5 dozen rounded leaflets. The long terminal racemes of beautiful white flowers, in *Eysenhardtia orthocarpa*, emerge from the center of leaf clusters with the arrival of moisture in the warmer months, distinguishing it quite readily from mesquite and other desert legumes. Flower clusters on *E. texana*, the larger of the two species, are more widespread across the whole shrub. When crushed, the leaves of both species emit a strong scent reminiscent of tangerine. Clusters of small, greenish yellow seedpods are another key characteristic. The bark is light gray and peels back slightly on the trunk.

Where, when, and how to wildcraft

Look for kidneywood along drainages in the understory,

or out in the open, on exposed rocky ledges. *Eysenhardtia orthocarpa* occurs in southern Arizona and the extreme southwestern corner of New Mexico; *E. texana* is found in the Texas Hill Country and southward, then west into the Big Bend. Where it is present, kidneywood is common, but there are large swaths of land in between where it is completely absent. Some part of kidneywood can be gathered year-round. Harvest the bark from healthy, abundant stands, particularly in the early spring or autumn; gather only from pruned young branches, ¾ inch thick or less. The leaves (alone, or with flowers or seeds) can be pruned from branch tips.

Medicinal uses

Along with *Pterocarpus indicus* (the national tree of the Philippines), kidneywood was a source for "lignum nephriticum," the reigning diuretic of the 16th through 18th centuries. Traditional uses of kidneywood in the Southwest and Mexico reflect this usage.

Cold infusions of the wood and bark are used to decrease kidney and urinary tract inflammation and resolve kidney or bladder stones and scanty urination. There's a tradition of using the bark tea for diabetes in northern Mexico; scientific trials attribute this to the flavonoids present in the bark. The tincture can be taken for rheumatic joints and general pain and inflammation, both topically and internally.

Future harvests

Gather carefully and sparingly from wild populations, following the guidelines in "Gathering Tree Medicine" (page 25).

⚠ Caution

Bark and leaf preparations lower blood sugar levels significantly, even for individuals with normal blood sugar.

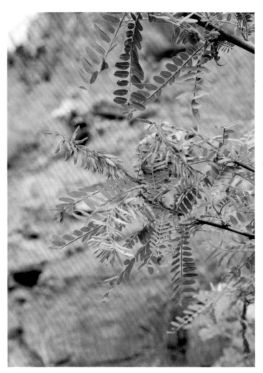

The densely crowded terminal seed clusters help distinguish *Eysenhardtia orthocarpa* from mesquite.

HERBAL PREPARATIONS

Bark/Herb Tea
Standard Decoction
Drink 4–8 ounces, up to 4 times per day.

Bark Tincture
1 part fresh bark, by weight
2 parts menstruum (95% alcohol),
  by volume
or
1 part dry bark, by weight
5 parts menstruum (50% alcohol,
  50% spring water), by volume
Take 15–30 drops, up to 4 times per day.

Lobelia cardinalis, L. anatina
cúralo todo, cardinal flower, tobacco plant
PARTS USED whole plant

This relaxing herb improves respiration and tones the parasympathetic nervous system, enhancing digestion as well as shifting us into "rest and recovery" mode.

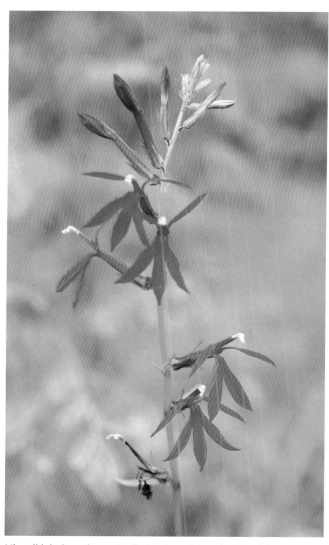

Like all lobelias, the typically bright red (rarely white) flowers of *Lobelia cardinalis* have 2 top lobes and 3 bottom lobes.

How to identify

As an herbaceous perennial, lobelia becomes visible in the summer, when it actively grows and flowers. The long grass-like leaves of *Lobelia cardinalis*, cardinal flower, with tiny teeth along the margins, cause it to blend in until its exceptionally brilliant red flowers appear at the top of the plant. It can occasionally grow to be over 7 feet tall when growing in groups or clumps, but *L. anatina*, Apache lobelia, grows to no more than 30 inches and has blue flowers. *Lobelia* species possess a 2-lipped corolla with 5 deeply cut lobes: 2 pointing up and 3 pointing down and to the side.

Where, when, and how to wildcraft

Lobelia likes consistently moist soil like seeps, wet meadows, and creeks. In the western half of our region, look to mid-elevation springs and riparian woodlands at the edge of streambeds. Lobelia may also be found in grassland ciénegas in the eastern half of our region. It is not a common plant in our region by any means, but it can occasionally be found in abundance. Plants generally flower at the end of summer, perhaps as early as mid-August. Gather the aerial parts once the plant has begun to seed. Although the roots are stronger medicine, avoid gathering the whole plant unless a larger (more than 50 plants) stand presents itself. The fresh plant is much preferred for tincture or acetum.

Medicinal uses

This phenomenal native North American herb facilitates healing for the human body in many ways, although taken in excess it is a strong emetic. Lobelia was the centerpiece of a healing system developed by New England farmer Samuel Thomson in the early 1800s, from herbal wisdom imparted by indigenous healers in his area. Eclectic physicians used it for angina pectoris, neuralgia of the heart, and other cardiac conditions. Small, frequent doses of 5–15 drops stimulate the parasympathetic nervous system, enabling the body to shift out of productivity mode. Digestive secretions are stimulated, creating a smooth movement within the GI tract, which in turn allows the gentle and fluid release of waste products throughout the body. The induction of this nervous system response is conducive to repairing tissues and revitalizing the mind-body connection.

Use lobelia for acute respiratory distress from asthma, acute viral illness, cough, or chronic fungal or bacterial infections. A wonderful antispasmodic for smooth muscle cramps (part of how it helps with asthma), it is particularly adept at relaxing small duct cramps (gall bladder, bladder). Taken internally, it relieves upper back, neck, and shoulder tension. Topically, it has the same effect on muscle tension as well as helping to heal sprains and bruises.

Herbalist Matthew Wood (1997) notes lobelia's ability to heighten the effects of other herbs and states some of the primary circumstances in which to apply it: impacted mucus, spasm, a feeling of oppression in the chest, profuse sweating and overheating, muscle ache and tension, and asthmatic paroxysms (sudden onset).

Apply the acetum topically to relieve poison ivy rash or other skin sensitivities. *Lobelia cardinalis* is also anthelmintic. Taken internally, the acetum can be stimulating to the senses when fatigue and torpor set in from hot weather or long, arduous activity.

Future harvests

Never gather indiscriminately. Lobelia habitats are sensitive areas, especially in the Southwest, so spend time observing and learning about its local habitat first. Consider cultivating it in your yard, if you can sustainably give it consistent water.

HERBAL PREPARATIONS

Whole Plant Tincture
1 part fresh plant, by weight
2 parts menstruum (75% alcohol,
   25% spring water or apple cider vinegar),
   by volume
Take 10–40 drops, up to 5 times per day.

Whole Plant Acetum
1 part fresh plant, by weight
2 parts menstruum (apple cider vinegar),
   by volume
Use topically, as needed; take 20–60 drops, up to 5 times per day.

Malva species
PARTS USED whole plant

A nutritious herb with cooling and soothing qualities, it's healing to the entire digestive tract and the genitourinary tract. It also helps to moisten the lungs and relieve inflammation.

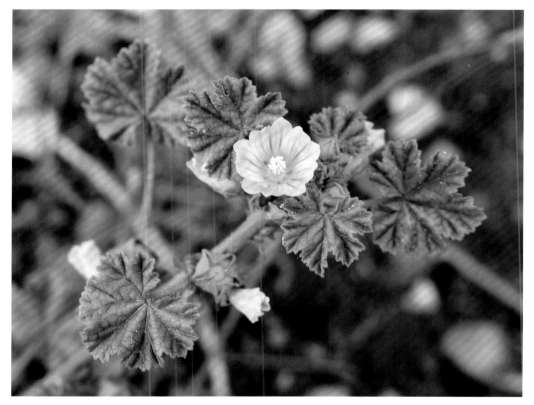

Malva neglecta flowers with parallel pink veins on each petal.

How to identify

Mallow is an annual herb with an erect or prostrate habit, depending on the species and habitat. Its rounded to kidney-shaped leaves are held on long petioles; margins are toothed, lobed, and/or undulate. Each of the leaf's main veins (usually 7) radiates out in a straight line, from the base to the margin.

The leaves can be somewhat (or not at all) hairy, depending on local growing conditions. The small, white to lavender, 5-petaled flowers are often hidden beneath the leaves; they grow from the leaf axils, singly or in clusters. Fruit is a disc-shaped schizocarp, divided numerous times within its outer coating, resembling a wheel of cheese. In

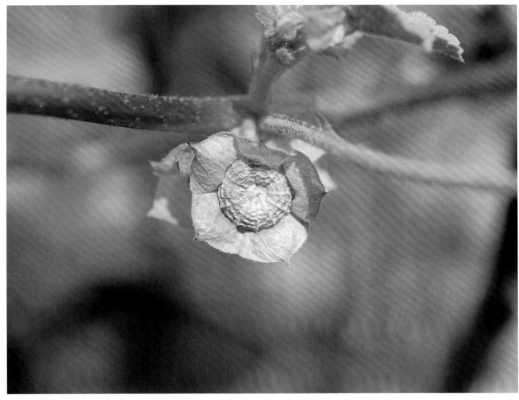

The dry seedpod of *Malva parviflora*. Notice the short pedicel.

ideal conditions and if left undisturbed, mallow can grow to 6 feet tall and wide. *Malvella leprosa*, alkali mallow, can be used similarly.

Where, when, and how to wildcraft

Look to recently disturbed ground throughout our region, including yards, gardens, vacant lots, pasture, horse corrals, streamsides, and mountain meadows. The lower the elevation, or hotter the climate, the more likely you'll find mallow in winter and spring. If you go up in elevation, or further north, mallow will be more of a spring and summer plant. Gather the whole plant from spring to mid-summer, depending on the location, as it begins to flower; the leaves are at their most robust at this time. If necessary, rinse off in clean water and simply trim the root from

the whole plant to dry separately. If the root is thicker than 1 inch, then split it lengthwise before drying. Spread out the aerial portions of the plant to dry; once dry, garble or strip the leaves and stems.

Medicinal uses

Mallow is a wonderfully soothing and cooling demulcent, applicable in a wide variety of mucous membrane and skin irritations. As a tea, it helps replenish moisture at the level of the mucous membranes, enhancing our resiliency to pathogens and augmenting our immunity (it is rich in polysaccharides). Combine this weedy herb in formulas for gut health, urinary tract irritability, cold and flu teas, or any dry, hot respiratory condition. Simply crush some fresh leaves in cool water and allow to infuse over a couple hours, make an overnight cold infusion with dry herb, or prepare as a standard infusion for quicker application. This makes a nice remedy to relieve sore throat, laryngitis, or hoarseness (add some wild oregano honey infusion for flavor and effect).

The root decoction is an excellent aid in relieving heat in the lower intestines. Administration of an enema of the root tea to children or infants with fever or respiratory viruses is a long-standing traditional remedy in the Southwest. It helps resolve loose stool from excess heat in the colon (combine with algerita or walnut leaf). Look for a yellow coating at the back of the tongue.

The tea of any part of the plant aids in relieving inflammation of the digestive tract and rehabilitating its entire lining. I often add mallow in small amounts to any tea preparation to help balance the dryness of our climate. It is a nutritious herb with a vulnerary, or wound-healing action, both within the body and on the surface. The leaf tea also makes an excellent hair rinse.

Future harvests

This naturalized plant is often abundant when present. Inquire at your local organic farms, as they may invite you to gather to your heart's content.

 Caution

Beware of the soil conditions where mallow is growing. It is best to avoid areas with any potential for agricultural run-off, reclaimed water, or regular animal traffic that may dirty the leaves. Use sparingly in damp conditions.

HERBAL PREPARATIONS

Herb Tea
Standard Infusion
Drink 4–8 ounces, as needed; apply topically, as needed.

Root Tea
Standard Decoction
Drink 2–6 ounces, as needed.

Poultice
Mash up the fresh plant and apply directly to the body, as needed.

manzanita

Arctostaphylos species
kinnikinnick, pingüica
PARTS USED leaf, fruit

*A prime remedy for the urinary tract, the leaf tea helps to relieve UTIs,
reduce kidney inflammation, and prevent bladder stone formation.*

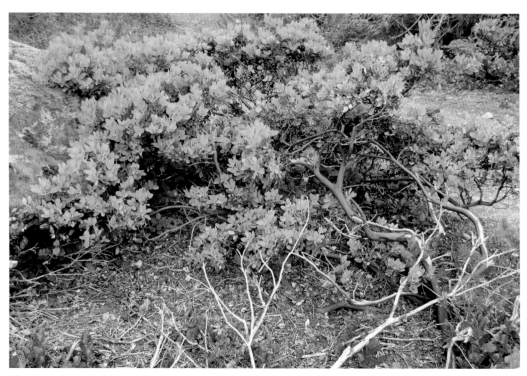

The smooth, reddish brown bark is an unmistakable identifying characteristic of manzanita.

How to identify

Its conspicuous smooth, reddish brown, often-peeling bark makes manzanita one of the most attractive shrubs in our region. We have 4 species in the Southwest, with *Arctostaphylos pringlei* and *A. pungens* particularly prominent. Although the growth habit of *A. uva-ursi* is low to the ground and spreading, its leaves and flowers are otherwise similar in appearance to our larger manzanitas, which have pointy, rigid evergreen leaves, ranging from light gray-green to bright green, and urn-shaped, white to pink flowers, which may be erect or drooping, and grow in clusters. The tiny apple-like fruits go from green to yellow to red/reddish brown as they mature; they are mealy upon ripening, very astringent when not yet ripe. Although they ripen in summer, they can persist on the plant into winter.

232   ]

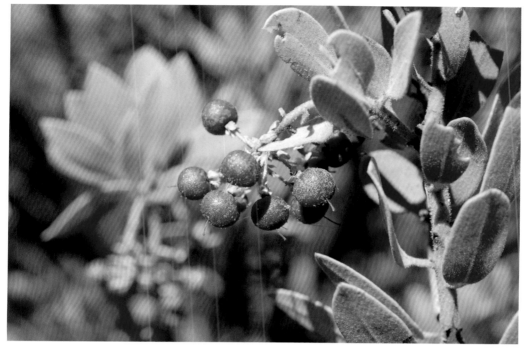

The berries of *Arctostaphylos pringlei* ripen from early to mid-summer.

Where, when, and how to wildcraft

Arctostaphylos uva-ursi is found where the Rocky Mountain habitat extends into northern New Mexico, further expanding north-northwest into Utah; it can be used interchangeably with our larger manzanita species, which inhabit the chaparral, a biozone that intersects with grasslands and oak woodlands, occupying huge mid-elevation swaths of southern Nevada, Utah, and California and occurring throughout Arizona and New Mexico as well as a bit into southwestern Texas. Manzanita is a resident of open, sunny sites as well as an understory shrub amid pine, oak, and juniper. Plants can dominate post-fire ecosystems; they survive fires well and colonize the area afterward. For internal medicine, gather the fresh leaf growth in late spring and early summer, optimizing for the highest arbutin content; prune the young leaf growth at the base of

the stem and set aside to dry. Berries, which are also mildly medicinal, should be gathered upon ripening in the early summer. Avoid gathering from the shrub when in flower.

Medicinal uses

Manzanita leaf is one of our primary urinary tract remedies. Its astringent, antiseptic, and antimicrobial properties make it quite useful for UTIs. As it tones and tightens the tissues of the urinary tract, it reduces alkalinity (not useful for acid urine infections). After the ingestion of a manzanita preparation, hydroquinone is derived from the endogenous plant compound arbutin. Hydroquinone effectively inhibits bacteria adherence to the mucous membranes of the urinary tract as urine is excreted through the ureters. It serves well wherever the genitourinary membranes are too lax and excretions are excessive, by toning and tightening the tissues. It is also useful for kidney inflammation, water retention, or bladder gravel. Use the leaf tea or tincture for UTIs; add the leaves to tea when menses is heavy and painful. Smoke the leaves to prepare the mind for stillness and meditation.

Manzanita is a classic ingredient in a post-partum sitz bath to reduce the likelihood of infection and promote tissue healing. The sitz bath is also useful for vaginitis and cervicitis, and can be combined with creosote bush, yerba mansa, and copperleaf for a post-surgical intervention of the female (or male) reproductive system.

The leaf tea can be applied topically to reduce the itchiness of a poison ivy rash, or to reduce body aches.

Future harvests

Manzanita is particularly abundant, so if we continue to gather with respect, it should be available for our use for a long, long time. If it doesn't grow in your area, consider intro-ducing it in your home landscape.

 Caution

This herb should not be taken for more than 2 weeks, continuously. Combine with mallow and other mucilaginous herbs to reduce its drying, astringent effects.

HERBAL PREPARATIONS

Leaf Tea
Standard Infusion
Drink 2–4 ounces, up to 3 times per day; pour 1 pint into a sitz bath, or combine in formulation for postpartum sitz bath.

Leaf Tincture
1 part dry leaf, by weight
5 parts menstruum (50% alcohol,
    50% spring water), by volume
Take 30–60 drops, up to 3 times per day, in water.

Leaf Smoke
Dry in the shade, then grind the leaf down into tiny pieces. Combine with other herbs such as wild tobacco or mullein leaf to create a smoke blend to aid in prayer and meditation.

Mexican palo verde

Parkinsonia aculeata

retama

PARTS USED leaf, flower

An often vilified "weedy" tree throughout the Southwest, Mexican palo verde holds some delightful surprises. This tree is used for food and medicine all over the world.

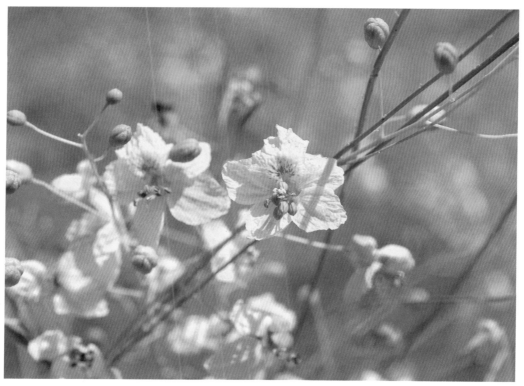

The top petal, or banner, of Mexican palo verde flowers has a splash of orange, and the flower buds are borne on long pedicels.

How to identify

The bark is smooth and yellowish green on young growth, facilitating photosynthesis even when no leaves are present; with age, the bark becomes fissured, furrowed, and gray-brown-beige. The long, slender leaves (or secondary rachis, more specifically) clearly separate Mexican palo verde from related species. Even when not present on the tree, the thin, needle-like leaf axis will litter the ground below it, as if someone had spilled a barrel of dry spaghetti. The numerous, tiny, elliptic green leaflets reach out like tiny thumbs from the rachis with moisture

Where, when, and how to wildcraft

Mexican palo verde is a weedy tree of waste places, disturbed ground, vacant lots, roadsides, fence lines, and underpasses. Its range has extended north, east, and west over the past century. Look to the southern rim of our region, moving up the eastern edge toward Dallas. It can flower almost any time of year, depending on moisture and warmth. Gather the leaves and flowers whenever they're available. A thin layer of green bark can also be gathered at any time; see "Gathering Tree Medicine" (page 25) for details.

Medicinal uses

A fascinating plant, as much for what it does as for the extent to which it is overlooked. Traditionally, leaf, fruit, and stem decoctions were taken orally to treat fever and malaria, and as abortifacients. Flower and leaf liniments are used topically to alleviate rheumatism. Because of its popularity in the folk medicine of Mexico, Nigeria, and India, it has been studied considerably of late.

Recent studies indicate that a tincture of the leaves may be effective against melanoma, in part due to its apigenin content. Its flavonoid content makes it useful for UTIs, and it has hepatoprotective properties as well. Studies also reveal its ability to help with obesity and insulin resistance, in part due to its effect on the mitochondria. The plant has also been shown to be effective against *Candida albicans*;

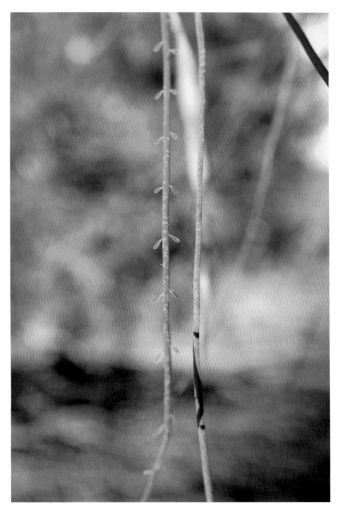

Super-tiny leaflets are oppositely arranged along a long, thin secondary rachis.

present, then quickly fall off, as drought arrives again. When fully verdant, these leaf features lend the tree an appearance similar to a sparsely foliated weeping willow. The yellow flowers contain a splash of orange on the top petal, or banner (rarely, the banner is solid orange); flowers often cover the entire tree, even when nearly leafless, in early spring. The pods clearly constrict around the maturing seeds within, splitting open once seeds are ripe.

therefore, it may be helpful in other types of fungal infections. Although the aforementioned studies were in vitro, or performed on animals, they do provide insight into how we may begin applying this herb, which is already widely consumed (beans, as food) and applied internally in local folk medicine traditions across the globe.

Future harvests

Mexican palo verde is an invasive plant in the Southwest. Its future abundance within our region depends, in part, on how well we treat our landscape. It is easy to grow below 4,000 feet, if you're so inclined.

 Caution

Avoid during pregnancy: it was traditionally used as an abortifacient.

HERBAL PREPARATIONS

Leaf and Stem Tea
Standard Infusion
Drink 4–8 ounces, up to 4 times per day.

Leaf and Stem Tincture
1 part fresh leaf and stem (and/or bark),
  by weight
2 parts menstruum (95% alcohol),
  by volume
Take 30–90 drops, up to 5 times per day.

mock vervain

Glandularia species
PARTS USED aerial

Mildly bitter and cooling, mock vervain is a relaxing remedy for the nervous system and the musculature of the upper back, neck, and shoulders. Restores deep, relaxed breathing, preparing one for sleep.

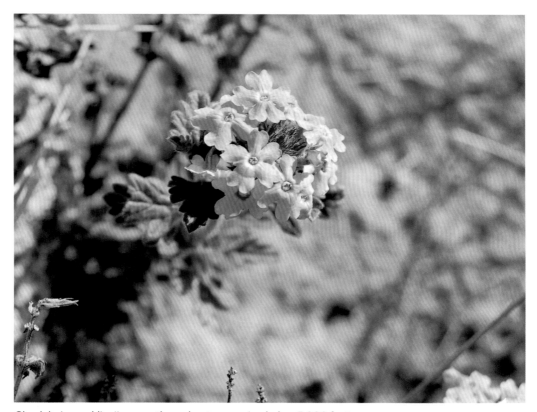

Glandularia gooddingii occurs throughout our region below 5,000 feet.

How to identify

Mock vervain is an herbaceous annual or perennial. The hairy opposite leaves, of various shapes, are dissected, toothed, deeply cleft, or cut to the midrib, and may possess a reddish purple margin, similar to the calyces. Some *Glandularia* species will root at the nodes of creeping stems. The pink, purple, blue, white, or lavender 5-petaled, symmetrical flowers with notched lobes grow in terminal clusters; calyces are hairy, with pointed, uneven teeth. The sharply hairy fruits contain 4 elongated nutlets. Rely less on botanical differences and more on taste and individual qualities of *Glandularia* species when determining their medicinal applications.

Where, when, and how to wildcraft

Found throughout our region in a variety of habitats, mock vervain likes disturbed soils near trails, roads, pastures, streambeds, dry arroyos, open woods, or post-forest fires, at 2,000–10,000 feet. Although variably abundant each year, it can be found in nearly all our environments. Look for flowers from early spring through early autumn. The entire aerial portions are used, gathered before or after flowering.

Medicinal uses

The tea or tincture is particularly relaxing to the nervous system (seeming to slightly stimulate the vagus nerve) and musculoskeletal system, making it a useful pain reliever and recovery aid after overwork or injury to the musculature. Also useful for alleviating nervous anxiety, coupled with insomnia and chronic tension in the neck and shoulders. Its relaxing effect on the liver may encourage menstrual flow that has been compromised by nervous tension and liver constriction. A relaxing and restorative nervine but not an overt sedative, it allows one to retain clear mental faculties while experiencing full-body relaxation. Drunk hot, the tea (or the tincture in hot water) is diaphoretic. Combine with estafiate in an evening chamomile tea for indigestion, stomach inflammation, liver constriction, nervous system excitation, or muscular tension.

Future harvests

Gather modestly in years of lesser abundance, or not at all. Consider inviting it into your home landscape.

HERBAL PREPARATIONS

Herb Tea
Standard Infusion
Drink 4–8 ounces, up to 3 times per day, or in the evening before bed.

Tincture
1 part fresh herb, by weight
2 parts menstruum (95% alcohol),
  by volume
or
1 part dry herb, by weight
5 parts menstruum (50% alcohol,
  50% spring water), by volume
Take 15–60 drops, up to 5 times per day. Note: the tincture occasionally turns into a starchy sludge; simply shake and continue to use.

monkey flower

Mimulus guttatus (*Erythranthe guttata*)

basómari

PARTS USED aerial

A cooling, moistening herb, taken internally for pain and applied topically to relieve hot, irritated skin conditions. It exhibits an affinity for the lungs, soothing irritated conditions of an acute or chronic nature.

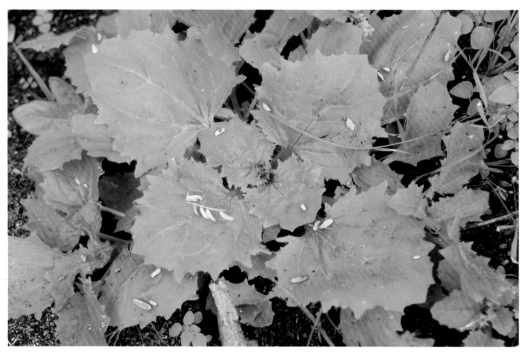

Monkey flower grows close to the ground, or within running or standing water. Its opposite leaves are irregularly toothed, and the leaf stem is often tinted red.

How to identify

Monkey flower is an herbaceous annual or perennial that grows close to the ground, often alongside or in water. Stem and leaf veins are often tinged pinkish red. The irregularly toothed, ovate, opposite leaves attach directly to the stem but may be alternate lower down on the plant. As the plant flowers, leaves can become perfoliate, looking as if the stem pierces up through them. The 5-lobed yellow flowers are said to resemble a grinning monkey, their throat often dotted with reddish brown spots. Paperthin fruits stick up at the ends of the flowering stems from autumn into winter. After the first frost, the leaves may turn purple and crinkle up. The related *Mimetanthe pilosa*, false monkey flower, which grows in similar habitats, is also a useful medicine; its leaves are narrow and hairy, and its corolla also bears maroon dots.

Where, when, and how to wildcraft

Monkey flower is scattered throughout the western half of our region from the Rio Grande westward, always near streams or dry creekbeds (arroyos). East of that point, *Mimulus glabratus*, roundleaf monkey flower, which can be used similarly, is found in the Hill Country, the Big Bend area, and in the Texas and Oklahoma panhandles. Monkey flower is just as likely to be encountered in a seasonal desert wash at 2,000 feet as it is at 8,000 feet in northern New Mexico, growing streamside among alder and willow. *Mimetanthe pilosa* is mostly found within the western third of our region in low-elevation desert washes and near springs. Gather the herb when abundant, with or without flowers, from early winter at lower elevations, mid-spring to early autumn at higher elevations. Simply pinch the fresh leaves off this delicate plant or prune back flowering stems. In large robust stands (which may appear seasonally, with abundant rains), one can pull whole plants up from the sandy soil, gently thinning out the stand.

Medicinal uses

Monkey flower is not only a food, it is a wonderfully effective and safe medicine. Apply the plant topically to relieve any hot, irritated conditions, such as burns, recently infected wounds, joint pain, or neuralgia. The tincture can also be taken internally for these painful conditions. Gargle or spray the tincture, and take internally for sore throat and other inflamed conditions of the larynx. The fresh plant tincture has a cooling and soothing effect on irritated mucous membranes of the lungs, making it a wonderful aid in recovering from lung inflammation.

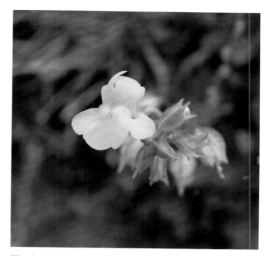

The lower lip of each monkey flower has a spray of red at the throat.

Herbalist Kiva Rose uses monkey flower for anxiety attacks and depression. Other *Mimulus* species are used as flower essence remedies; in Bach's original system, mimulus is used to calm a fear of known things.

Future harvests

Setting up strategic rainwater catchment systems in your home landscape can allow for more dependable cultivation of this ephemeral plant, which is dependent upon seasonal moisture.

HERBAL PREPARATIONS

Tincture

1 part fresh plant, by weight
2 parts menstruum (70% alcohol, 30% spring water), by volume
Take 10–30 drops, up to 4 times per day; or simply nibble the fresh plant.

Poultice

Mash up the fresh plant and apply directly to the body, as needed.

Mormon tea

Ephedra species
popotillo, joint fir, stick tea
PARTS USED stem

During allergy season, this ancient plant clears up and dries out stuffy sinuses;
it also serves as a urinary tract astringent and diuretic.

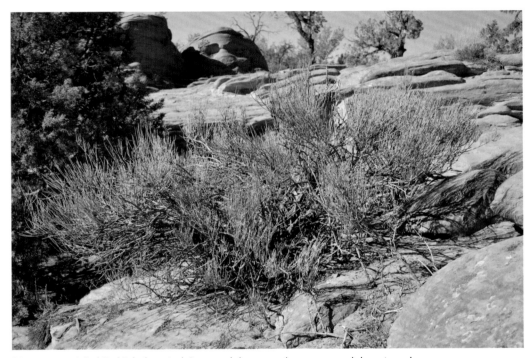

Mormon tea inhabits high desert plains, sand dunes, rocky mesas, and desert washes.

How to identify

A remnant of ancient coniferous forests, Mormon tea can be anywhere from 10 inches to 6 feet tall, depending upon the species and local conditions; plants may occur independently, or in clonal stands reproducing by underground rhizomes. The leafless stems are thin (less than 10mm) and yellow-green, bright or dark green, or bluish green; they are generally quite flexible and don't break or tear easily. Plants produce male and female cones (on separate plants) in late winter and spring; these are smaller than a pea in size and are borne at the stem joints in pairs or clusters. As the plant ages, it may develop a thick, gray to brown bark at its base.

Where, when, and how to wildcraft

Mormon tea occurs throughout our region (11 species total) as one of the most well-distributed perennial plants we have; it is found in abundance in the high sandy desert region of northern Arizona, southern Utah, and southern Nevada. Look to sand dunes in the high desert, or rocky canyons, arroyos, and bajadas in the desert grasslands and cactus forests. It's available for gathering year-round, although the winter foliage may be less potent. Search out fresh growth shortly after significant rains, and prune back from healthy stands that have recently put on growth. Cut just below the lowest green, flexible growth. Avoid gathering when the plants are actively coning ("flowering").

Medicinal uses

Mormon tea is a classic genitourinary tract remedy among various Native American tribes and contemporary folk herbalists alike. The tea of the stems is used to reduce kidney pain and inflammation, increase the output and volume of urine, and astringe the urinary tract. The stories that circulate to explain the root of the common name generally point to a Jack Mormon in an Old West mining town, selling the tea to his patrons after getting a tip from a local native about the effectiveness of this remedy for syphilis and the like.

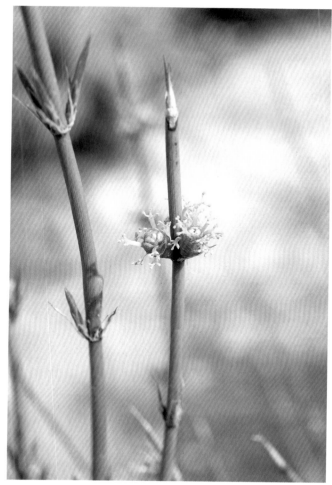

Mormon tea is dioecious. Pictured here are the male flowers of *Ephedra trifurca* (identified by the stems, which end in points, and the leaves and bracts in 3s) with stamens exserted from the scaled cones.

Although it's stated that no ephedrine can be found within our native Southwest *Ephedra* species (as opposed to its presence in *E. sinica*, ma huang, from China), indicating that there is no stimulant quality present, people who knew nothing of constituent studies frequently used the tea as a replacement for coffee, and very likely as a stimulant before coffee became popular in our area. This aspect of native *Ephedra* relates to its ability to decongest the lungs and relieve hay fever and rhinitis. Simply chewing the stems brings relief during allergy season. The tea or tincture is drying to the mucous membranes and improves blood flow to the lungs, boosting breathing capacity. Also, it is traditionally used for cough, pneumonia, and bronchitis. Consider using the tea or tincture in formulation for asthma or chronic obstructive pulmonary disorder (COPD).

The tannin-rich tea is also used to address intestinal complaints, being particularly effective for diarrhea. Topically, use to treat sores. Often enjoyed as a pleasing tea, the stems can be roasted before boiling. Mormon tea is high in calcium.

Future harvests

Gather with respect, and rotate your gathering locations annually.

HERBAL PREPARATIONS

Stem Tea
Standard Infusion
Drink 2–8 ounces, up to 3 times per day; low-desert species should be boiled to break down the tough protective coating.

Stem Tincture
1 part dry leaf, by weight
5 parts menstruum (50% alcohol,
   50% spring water), by volume
Take 30–60 drops, up to 3 times per day, in water.

mulberry

Morus species

mora cimarrona

PARTS USED bark, leaf, fruit

Mulberry holds a wide array of potent medicine well suited to modern disease states. Eaten when fresh, the deliciously sweet berries help to clear heat. A tea or syrup of the dried berries nourishes a weakened body.

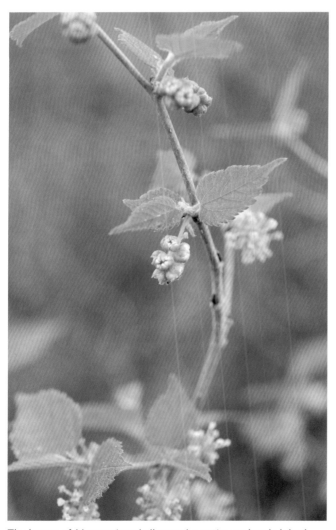

The leaves of *Morus microphylla* may be entire or deeply lobed with serrated margins; the female flowers are shown here.

How to identify

Mulberry is dioecious and deciduous; smooth gray bark, turning fissured with age, as well as the leaf scars and brown scales on the leaf bud, help to identify the leafless shrubs or trees during the winter months. Male and female flowers (thus, fruits) are usually on separate plants, occasionally on the same plant. The male catkins are rather small and inconspicuous. The female catkins hang down a bit and go from yellowish green to red and white as they mature. The leaves have toothed margins and a rounded base, and may or may not be lobed. *Morus rubra*, red mulberry, and *M. microphylla*, Texas mulberry, both native, are quite hairy on the backside of the leaf and are rough to the touch. *Morus alba*, white or Asian mulberry, is naturalized throughout our region; it is a larger, single-trunked tree with shinier leaves, which are less coarse on the underside, and produces vastly more fruit than *M. microphylla*, which generally appears as a multi-trunked shrub, less than 15 feet tall, with fruits ½ inch long at most.

Where, when, and how to wildcraft

Look to mid-elevation canyons or the shady side of boulders and hillsides to find Texas mulberry, growing alongside mesquite, willow, oak, or juniper, as well as other desert shrubs and cacti, from the desert grasslands to the high plains and into the Hill Country of central Texas, and up into Oklahoma. White mulberry is found at old homesteads or in disturbed areas within the eastern third of our region. Mulberry leaves can be gathered in early to mid-spring, and again after summer moisture arrives. The fruit is gathered in late spring or early summer. The bark is best harvested once the leaves have fallen off the tree, from late autumn to early spring; see "Gathering Tree Medicine" (page 25) for details.

Medicinal uses

The berries are a sweet treat, and when taken fresh (or from fresh preparations) they allay thirst and are cooling and soothing to an overheated body. Dried and used in tea, or boiled down to create a syrup, the berries are considered, in Chinese medicine, a warming rejuvenative tonic for the liver and kidneys. Indications include weak joints, premature gray hair, thirst, dizziness, deafness, poor vision, weakness, forgetfulness, and insomnia.

The leaves are used in Sonoran folk medicine as a tea for diabetes, high blood pressure, and high cholesterol, often combined with other local herbs.

In Chinese medicine, leaves gathered in autumn are used for their cooling and detoxifying properties; research shows that the oxyresveratrol content is highest at this time. Oxyresveratrol, a phytoalexin created by plants in response to local pathogens, provides medicinal benefit for us when ingested. Conversely, resveratrol, predominantly found in the stems, is likely to be more abundant in the new spring growth. Thus, we may combine preparations from both spring and autumn harvests. Recent studies have demonstrated that mulberry leaf extracts have the following array of effects on humans: antidiabetic, antibacterial, anticancer, cardiovascular, hypolipidemic, antioxidant, and anti-inflammatory.

I have utilized fresh mulberry spring leaf and stem tincture for my clients with chronic infections, metabolic syndrome, and an overall deficient condition.

Future harvests

Gather no more than a third of the fruits of Texas mulberry, as they are relatively sparse in production. Consider introducing this drought-tolerant plant to your home landscape, within a graywater or rainwater harvesting system.

HERBAL PREPARATIONS

Berry/Leaf Tea
Standard Infusion (combine with
  other herbs)
Drink 2–4 ounces, up to 4 times per day.

Leaf and Stem Tincture
1 part fresh leaf and stem, by weight
2 parts menstruum (95% alcohol),
  by volume
Take 30–90 drops, up to 5 times per day.

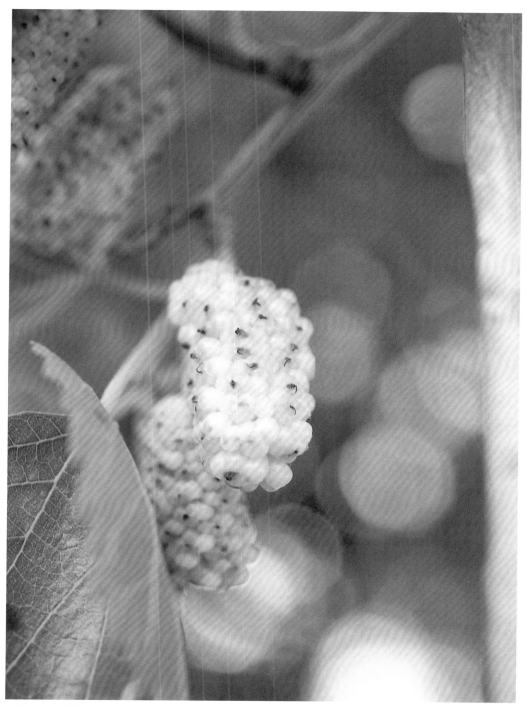

A ripe fruit of *Morus alba*, which is native to China but common in Southwest landscapes. The large leaves (entire or lobed) have a rounded base and a crinkly surface.

Verbascum thapsus
gordo lobo
PARTS USED leaf, flower, root

Native to Europe and now ubiquitous over much of the Southwest, mullein is an unsung plant ally with a wide range of medicine to offer the attentive wildcrafter.

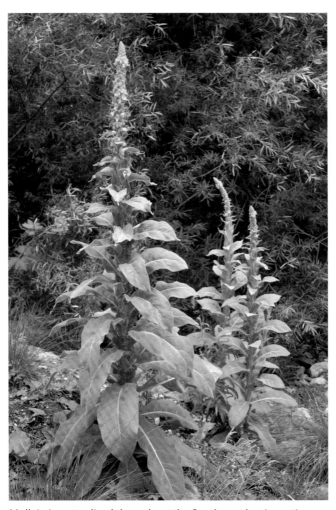

Mullein is naturalized throughout the Southwest but is particularly abundant in mid- to high-elevation conifer forests in the western half of our region.

How to identify

Before flowering, mullein can be difficult to spot among other ground-dwelling vegetation; however, once you become acquainted with its broad, velvety, frosted green basal leaves, it is easily distinguishable from everything else in its environment. Mullein leaves are characterized by vastly intricate venation, raised on the underside of the leaf. Although leaf stalks are present, they are well hidden in the basal rosette. When flowering begins in early summer, the center of the rosette of second-year plants extends upward, gradually revealing clasping leaves along the length of the central flower stalk. Stalks are usually 3–6 feet in height but may rise to 8 feet or more. The erect (and occasionally curved) flower stalk produces abundant 5-lobed yellow flowers, tightly packed along the length of the stalk in a nonlinear progression, with flower buds and seedpods in a mixed array. The light-colored taproot often tapers very quickly, branching off into numerous threadlike rootlets.

Where, when, and how to wildcraft

Mullein occurs, sometimes in tremendous abundance, throughout our range, excluding the high plains of Texas, Oklahoma, and New Mexico. It can colonize mountainsides at 9,000 feet after forest fires, or enter an urban garden at 2,500 feet in Tucson. Look for mullein where it may be abundant—in disturbed ground above 5,500 feet within the western half of our region. Forest clearings, roadsides, streamsides, vacant lots, garden beds, or other areas of significant disturbance are likely locations. The roots of this biennial plant are optimally gathered in spring of the second year, giving the root sufficient time to mature before it comes into flower. Root harvest requires unearthing the whole pre-flowering plant, so the leaves are gathered as well. Chop up the fresh roots and tincture, or otherwise dry for tea. Simply dry the leaves in the shade, or chop and tincture fresh. The flowers, or the entire stalk, are gathered early to mid-summer, depending on the location. In large stands, it's possible to gather abundant mullein flowers while gathering only the freshest portions of the flowering stalks; slice off the buds, flowers, and green seedpods with a long, thin knife, just as one may shave fresh corn off the cob. These are then tinctured, or infused in olive oil. The flowering stem is the most resinous part of the plant.

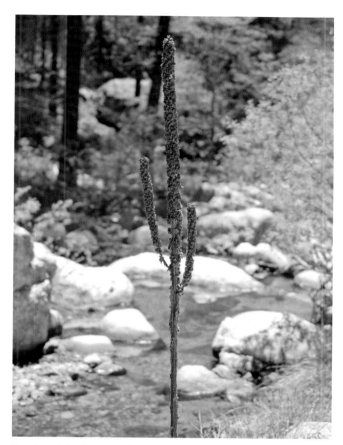

Dead mullein flower stalks often persist through several seasons. Here, its form is reminiscent of a saguaro cactus.

Medicinal uses

Each part of mullein—flower, leaf, and root—presents different applications, although there is some overlap. An oil infusion of the flowers can be applied to toughen tissues and relieve pain. Most commonly, oil drops added to the ear will relieve earache, but application anywhere on the body helps desensitize the tissue to pain. A fresh flower tincture taken internally will enhance the body's immune response to lung infections and can generate a significant response. Additionally, the flower tincture produces important effects in the lymph and cardiovascular systems, as well as affecting the emotional heart.

The leaf tea (or tincture) too is useful for acute respiratory infections and is soothing to the lungs when inflamed, but it is also specific for a sense of constriction within the chest. The leaves have a rich tradition of topical use as a poultice to resolve rashes, bites, stings, abscesses, wounds, and sores. They also relieve earache, sprains, and rheumatic joint pain as well as softening hard lumps (try steaming the leaves first in salt water).

The root tea or tincture helps restore proper function to the musculature of the bladder, when incontinence is experienced, whether caused by laxity or dampness in the tissue (from strain or lack of use) or injury to the nerve tissue enervating the muscle tone. Small doses of the root tincture can also bring full body relaxation after first enlivening the body.

Future harvests

Mullein capitalizes on disturbed habitats. Let's enjoy it while it's here—in abundance.

HERBAL PREPARATIONS

Leaf Tea
Standard Infusion
Drink 2–4 ounces, up to 3 times per day, or combine in formulation.

Root Tea
Strong Decoction
Drink 2–4 ounces, up to 4 times per day.

Flower Tincture
1 part fresh flowers, by weight
2 parts menstruum (95% alcohol),
  by volume
Take 10–90 drops, up to 3 times per day.

Root Tincture
1 part fresh root, by weight
2 parts menstruum (95% alcohol),
  by volume
Take 20–60 drops, up to 5 times per day.

Oil Infusion
1:4
Prepare flowers as a fresh plant oil infusion (see page 39); for earache, place 1 drop in the ear, up to 3 times per day.

Urtica dioica, U. gracilenta
ortiga
PARTS USED leaf, root, seed

Although chastised and feared for its ability to "burn" the skin when touched, nettle is one of our most cherished medicines. The leaf, seed, and root each provide distinct, nourishing remedies.

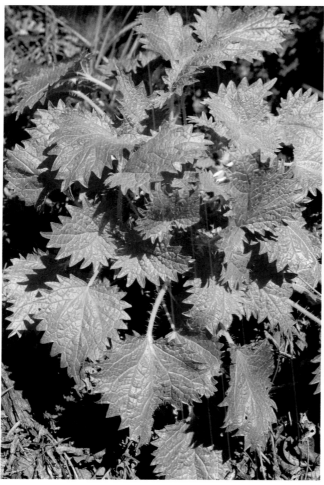

Urtica gracilenta is a native annual that inhabits shady canyons and oak woodlands below 6,000 feet in the western half of our region.

How to identify

Three species are found in the Southwest, but *Urtica dioica* is most common. It can grow to 7 feet tall in moist, shady locations. Its long, lance-shaped opposite leaves (sometimes broadly ovate) have distinctly toothed margins and are unscented. The classic "sting" of nettle derives from trichomes (or cystoliths, on older leaves), which are tiny, glassy, needle-like spines along the stems, leaf surfaces, and midribs of the leaves. Interestingly, the nondescript male (erect) and female (drooping) flowers can be found on the same (monoecious) or separate (dioecious) plants. When touched, all nettle species will cause a burning sensation, particularly in the pre-flowering stage. Broken cystoliths release caustic acids, irritate the skin, and induce urticaria (a red, itchy skin response). This is, in part, its medicine, however painful it may be.

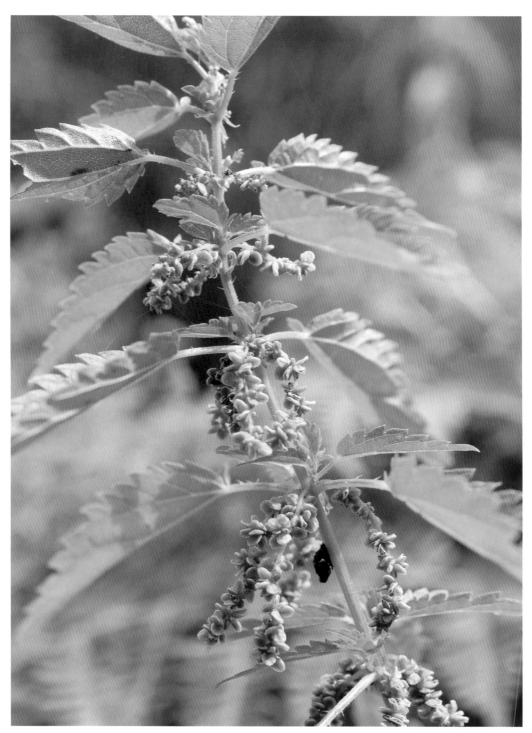

Urtica dioica occupies moist, shady areas throughout the Southwest.

Where, when, and how to wildcraft

Nettle is often associated with willow, alder, pine, and Douglas fir in the cool waterways of our region, occupying moist, shady areas, including canyons, oak woodlands, conifer forests, and, occasionally, disturbed areas and roadsides. It won't be found in our driest areas, or in the high plains and prairies of the panhandles. Nettle begins leafing out from its perennial rhizome in mid-spring (mid-winter for *Urtica gracilenta*, mountain nettle, in mid- to low-elevation disturbed areas) and begins to flower mid-summer. I prefer gathering the leaves before flowering, if possible, or at least before seeds begin to form. Harvest seeds in mid-autumn and the rhizomes after the seeds have ripened, until the ground freezes. Gather the leaves by cutting the stalks below the lowest green growth (skipping any yellowing leaves); the stalks may resprout from this cut. Since nettle stalks can be quite long, bring along a bed sheet to wrap up the harvest. Hang the leaves up to dry in the shade, or spread them out on screens or clean sheets. Simply strip the dry leaves from the dried stalk with gloved hands; despite what some say, the leaves can still sting after drying, particularly when handling the stems repeatedly. To gather the seeds, cut the upper stalks and place them directly into a paper or cloth bag to begin catching the seeds; then hang the stalks over a clean area, perhaps a sheet, which can catch the ripened seeds as they fall. Look for sandy ground, or rich deposits of soil absent of many rocks to dig the rhizomes, and coppice sections of an abundant root system for your harvest. This will stimulate new growth in the spring, causing the plant to regrow; this sort of "tending" is an important aspect of wild plant stewardship.

Medicinal uses

Nettle leaf is one of our most nutritious herbs, long utilized to help strengthen the blood, convalesce from long illnesses, and restore vitality; take as a food (eaten fresh or dried, ground, and added to smoothies, stews, soups, or baked goods), tea, or vinegar infusion to derive the greatest benefits. The tea is also a useful diuretic, especially in combination with other herbs; see "Diuretic Formula" (page 298). The leaf tincture is a wonderful hay fever remedy as it is exceptionally astringent and drying to the upper respiratory tract; in fact, it is specific for mucus discharge anywhere in the body.

The fresh leafy stems, used before going to seed, are a traditional counterirritant remedy for stiff, achy muscles, sore joints, and injuries to nerve tissue. Despite the pain and discomfort incurred from the procedure, the relief afforded by this therapy is substantial and long-lasting. Nerve damage, however long-standing, is a perfect candidate for topical nettle therapy. Slowly and incrementally, nerve sensation can be restored, even after decades. Apply the leaves topically to stop bleeding.

The root is a traditional remedy for internal bleeding of any kind. I find that it is also a nutritious remedy that is sweet and anabolic in nature, taken as tea or tincture, with an affinity for the male and female reproductive systems. It can improve libido, and it has been shown to inhibit aromatase. It is specific for benign prostatic hyperplasia and can improve nocturia quickly.

Herbalist David Winston uses the seed tincture as a restorative for diminished kidney function. The moistened seeds, applied to the scalp as a wash, are a tonic for stimulating hair growth.

Future harvests

One can transfer 6- to 10-inch sections of rhizome into suitable areas to expand nettle's presence in the wild. Robust forest fires, followed by scouring floods, have a similar effect, abundantly increasing a population by spreading the rhizomes to new areas.

HERBAL PREPARATIONS

Leaf Tea
Standard Infusion
Drink 4-8 ounces, up to 5 times per day.

Leaf/Root/Seed Tincture
1 part fresh herb, by weight
2 parts menstruum (75% alcohol,
　25% spring water), by volume
or
1 part dry herb, by weight
5 parts menstruum (40% alcohol,
　60% spring water), by volume
Take 20–60 drops, up to 4 times per day.

Leaf Acetum
1 part fresh leaf, by weight
3 parts menstruum (apple cider vinegar),
　by volume
Take ¼–1 teaspoon, up to 3 times per day.

oat

Avena fatua, A. sativa, A. barbata
PARTS USED leaf, stem, seed

Oats give us a classic nutritious tonic that calms and strengthens the nervous system, helps rebuild connective tissue, and is an aid in low libido or sexual debility.

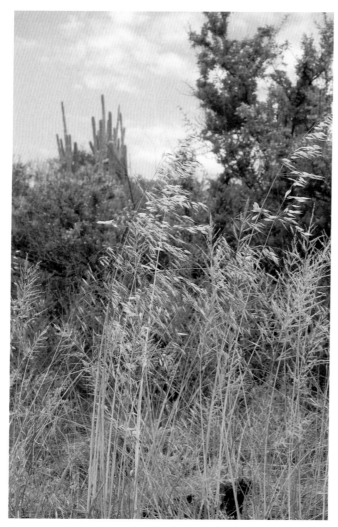

Avena barbata, slender oat, native to central Asia, is common in desert washes, roadsides, and hillsides in southern California, Arizona, and the eastern edge of our region in Texas.

How to identify

All *Avena* species on this continent are native to Europe and Asia. These annual tufted grasses grow in clumps and possess erect stems at maturity. The wide bluish green blades twist slightly, and their pointed tips often fall over; they're slightly rough to the touch, not as smooth as wheat and barley. Panicles of flowers open at the top of the stem upon maturity, revealing spikelets of 1–2 florets (2–3 in *A. fatua* and *A. barbata*). *Avena sativa* usually has no awns; *A. fatua* has 2 straight barbs. The calluses or covering of the seed are smooth in *A. sativa*, hairy in *A. fatua* and *A. barbata*. There's a particular heavy and glistening look to nearly ripened oat seeds that, once recognized, makes it much easier to consistently spot them from a distance. The seeds, then the plants, turn beige upon full maturity.

Where, when, and how to wildcraft

Oats are an introduced agri-cultural crop and a common naturalized weed throughout

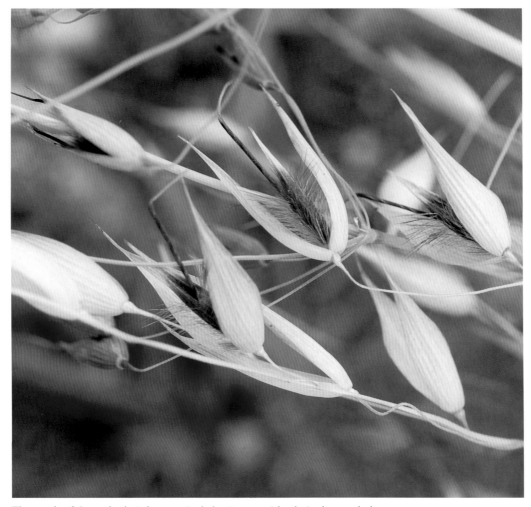

The seeds of *Avena barbata* have a single bent awn, with a hairy lemma below.

our region, in disturbed ground, roadsides, canyons, floodplains, bare hillsides, disturbed grasslands, Hill Country, and high desert. They are winter plants in the hotter, lower elevations, summer plants further north and at higher elevations. Gather the young, unripe seeds in "milky" stage by pinching the stem just below the barely ripe seeds, and pull out, stripping the spikelets. Since the seeds ripen from the bottom up, it's likely that either the bottom tier will be past the "milky" stage, or the top tier will

not yet be "milky." Rarely will you need to strip the entire inflorescence. The straw can be gathered just as flowering begins (for optimal nutrient content) or whenever it is still green.

Medicinal uses

Oat is one of our primary nourishing tonics. It is rich in silica (on par with horsetail, in some studies), as well as chromium, iron, magnesium, phosphorus, and selenium. Additionally, oats contain vitamins C and

A, a range of B vitamins, and several amino acids; these nutrients are readily available in a slow decoction or overnight hot infusion. The tea is restorative to the nervous system, bringing back a sense of calm and ease, giving one the ability to handle stress—and not be overwhelmed by life's challenges and stressors. In this way, oats can help an individual regain their sense of strength. Add cinnamon, ginger, or orange peel to the decoction in order to improve digestion and assimilation. A regimen of oatstraw tea can help improve or prevent osteoporosis.

Milky oat tincture, optimally tinctured fresh, works similarly. Depending on the severity of the burnout, it may take several days, or weeks, of several cups of strong tea or high doses of the tincture (5ml) daily for some folks to begin feeling the shift. As a nervine, it can help with insomnia, nervous restlessness, and depression. Historically, this therapy has worked well for the delirium tremens associated with withdrawal from alcohol. I've seen it do quite well for this purpose in combination with passionflower and anemone.

Future harvests
Gather this naturalized weed to your heart's content.

 Caution
Avenin, a protein found in oats, shares some peptide sequences with gluten, but the oatstraw tea is likely safe for all, even the gluten-intolerant, to consume.

HERBAL PREPARATIONS

Oatstraw Tea
Standard Decoction or Standard Infusion
Drink 4–8 ounces, up to 5 times per day.

Tincture
1 part fresh young "milky" seed, by weight
2 parts menstruum (95% alcohol),
  by volume
Pack the herb solidly to achieve the 1:2 ratio; take 10–60 drops, as needed, or up to 5ml, 2–3 times per day with moderate to severe burnout and fatigue.

Fouquieria splendens
PARTS USED bark, flower

Like a flaming torch when in flower, ocotillo connects us with the feelings and knowledge buried deep within our hearts.

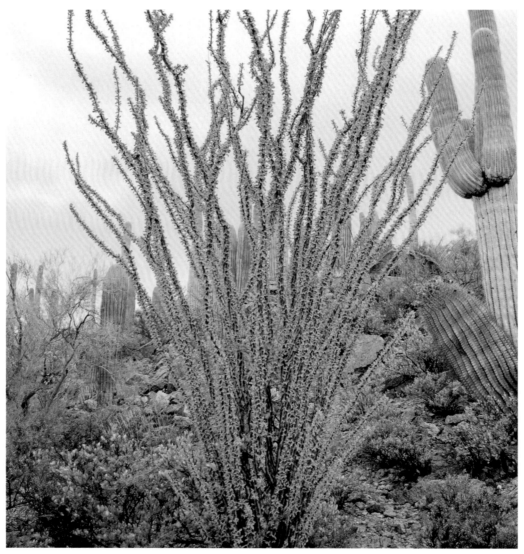

Ocotillo sprouts leaves year-round in response to rain. Although it is often confused with cacti, this woody shrub is not in the cactus family.

How to identify

Ocotillo, the sole representative of the Fouquieriaceae naturally occurring in the United States, is clearly distinguished by its numerous, spine-covered stems arising from a very short central trunk near ground level. The stout spines are more numerous toward the ends of the spindly stems. Bend a thin stem toward you and let go to witness how flexible they are. Plants may grow to 20 feet in height, their brilliant orange-red flowers borne in long terminal racemes. The thick bark is laid down in variable, overlapping layers of grayish brown and green; a thinner yellowish green layer of bark (where the resin is most concentrated) runs along the length of the branches. Tiny green spatula-shaped leaves appear all along the bark shortly after it rains. The common name derives from the Nahuatl word *ocotl* ("torch"), a reference not only to ocotillo's appearance when in flower but also to the tradition of bundling its branches to be used as torches when traveling through the desert at night.

Where, when, and how to wildcraft

Ocotillo exists in relative abundance throughout the Mojave, Sonoran, and Chihuahuan deserts. It prefers open, rocky hillsides, or otherwise exposed rocky areas below 5,000 feet. I have gathered ocotillo bark throughout the year and found it to be

Processing Ocotillo Bark

Gathering the branches of ocotillo is a sacred act. The heart-warming medicine this plant offers us is truly amazing. Its ability to create openings and heal wounds in places we did not know existed inspires our profound respect and gratitude.

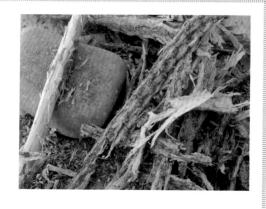

Ocotillo's inner bark is soft and flexible, but the outer resinous bark is stiff, thick and leathery, and resists cutting. A simple way to process the bark from fresh branches is to pound it with a hammerstone. Place a manageable length of fresh ocotillo branch, 2–3 feet in length, against a hard, slightly raised surface (a flat rock, brick, or concrete chunk on the ground). Select a hammerstone that fits comfortably within the palm and has a flat surface for pounding. The hammerstone should be thick enough that one's fingers don't extend beyond the pounding surface and can be kept tucked back, away from possible injury.

Place the branch on the larger flat surface, and pound the hammerstone onto the branch while turning the branch with the opposite hand. Take this opportunity to crush most of the spines, so the bark is easier to handle when chopping later. As the branch is pounded, the layers of bark will open up and begin to peel off. The bark can then be pulled off by hand. Some of the innermost, yellowish bark may adhere despite the pounding (possibly related to gathering during periods of extended drought); this can be scraped off with a knife. Finally, chop the bark into ¼-inch pieces (or less); this will ensure that a ratio of 1:2 is easily attained.

potent at any time; optimally, it's gathered immediately after the rain and before the leaves fully emerge (see the sidebar for full instructions on how to gather and process). The flowers are gathered in mid- to late spring; however, our lowest desert ocotillos may produce flowers in late autumn as well. Choose a raceme in which at least half the flowers are open; simply bend the spindly stem down and snap off the entire cluster. Unopened flowers are particularly astringent, thus won't taste as good in tea. Be sure to dry thoroughly before storing. Ocotillo flowers generally take 3–5 weeks to dry fully, even in our warm and dry season.

Medicinal uses

Ocotillo's main physical effect relates to lymphatic flow in the pelvic region—yet another important plant use that can be attributed to the work of Michael Moore. This effect may also help to resolve painful menses, abdominal bloating, or sciatica pain. I am aware of several women who were able to achieve an orgasm (or improve their experience thereof) only after using ocotillo tincture to relieve pelvic stagnation and associated emotional congestion. Use the tincture internally to resolve the sudden onset of hemorrhoids.

Its acrid taste (not present in all preparations) indicates its ability to break up congestion in the body (it clears dampness). A tea of the dry bark, which may be considerably more acrid than the tincture, is the preparation used internally by the Seri of northern Mexico against any type of infection. Another traditional remedy is as a gargle for sore throat. Use the more acrid preparations to relieve pain and restore mobility in congested or damaged joints (seemingly most effective where dampness is prominent). In similar fashion, the bark tea can be used in a bath to relieve musculoskeletal pain.

Emotionally, ocotillo connects deeply with the innermost feelings of our heart. This is perhaps the most profound quality of ocotillo. Much can be said of its healing ways, whether ingesting it in some form or simply being in the plant's presence. In an energetic sense, ocotillo connects us with what is lying just below the surface of our awareness, in our heart's center. By drawing our awareness there, it empowers us toward tremendous transformation, connecting with the ability to heal past wounds and to uncover emotions that are blocking our vitality and restricting us from being present with our true heart's desires. During these times, it is a very important and much needed ally in healing for us all.

Future harvests

If you should accidentally break a branch while gathering flowers, bury the base of the stem about 6 inches deep into the soil, or bring it home and place it in the ground or in a pot: it may come back to life. Ocotillo responds best when its stem is watered (don't just water the ground), especially in hot, dry weather.

HERBAL PREPARATIONS

Flower Tea
Standard Infusion or Sun Tea
Add dry flowers to other herbs in formulation or prepare as a sun tea for a cool, refreshing beverage.

Bark Tincture
1 part fresh bark, by weight
2 parts menstruum (75% alcohol, 25% spring water), by volume
Take 5-30 drops, up to 4 times per day.

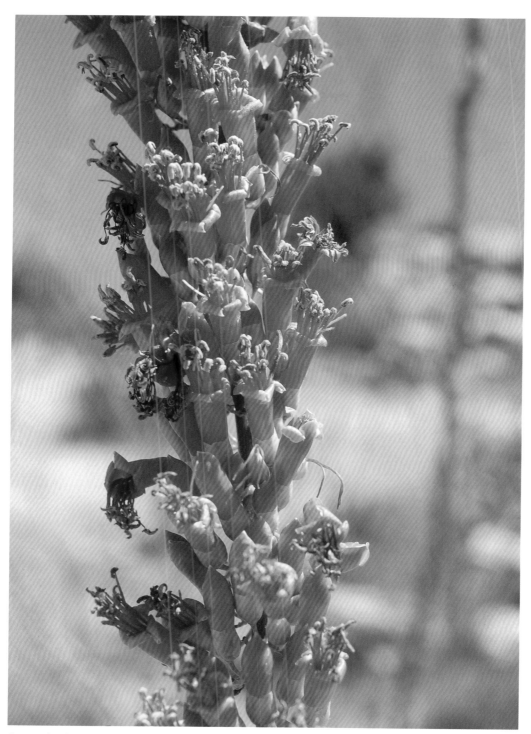

Across the deserts of the Southwest, ocotillo sets hillsides ablaze with its fiery red blossoms each spring.

oreganillo

Aloysia wrightii, A. gratissima
vara dulce, beebush, whitebrush
PARTS USED leaf, stem, flower

Makes a spicy, sweet tea that is delicious as well as stimulating and warming to digestion, while also relaxing the nervous system and relieving pain.

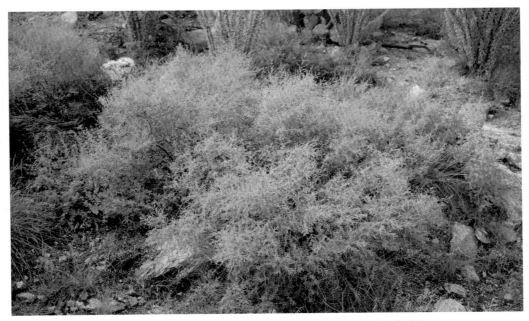

Aloysia wrightii can cover canyon hillsides from southern Nevada to the Big Bend of Texas.

How to identify

Absent leaves, these sparsely foliated woody shrubs can be difficult to notice: their thin, fragile beige stems are so well camouflaged by the surrounding rocky landscape. However, when in flower during the rainy season, oreganillo's fragrance often grabs your attention before you see it. Both stems and leaves are opposite, the deep green of the young leaves and the fuzzy white of the stems nicely contrasting near their tips, aiding in identification. The tiny, tubular white flowers of equal lobes are borne on terminal spikes.

Aloysia wrightii is 3–5 feet tall and wide; its leaves have rounded teeth along the margin, and their underside is as tomentose as the stem. *Aloysia gratissima* is generally taller, up to 10 feet; its olive-green leaves have mostly smooth margins and are rarely hairy beneath.

Where, when, and how to wildcraft

Aloysia wrightii occupies the western two-thirds of our region, beginning in the Big Bend of Texas and moving north up the Rio Grande valley; it then dips down below the Mogollon Rim heading into southeastern

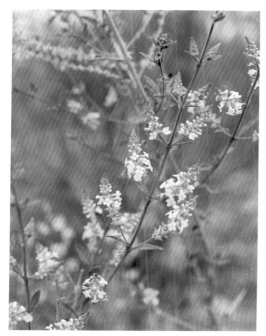

The tubular white blossoms of *Aloysia gratissima* are similar to but larger than those of *A. wrightii*.

conditions. Notice the mild liver relaxant effect as it enhances blood circulation throughout the body.

Aloysia gratissima, whitebrush, has similar attributes and is traditionally taken as a tea to relieve respiratory distress. In scientific trials, it has been shown to mediate the neuroinflammatory effects of amines; for example, it blocks the ability of MSG or aspartame, both common food additives, to trigger inflammation in the neural pathways of the brain, potentially provoking a migraine or cluster headache. It has also been shown to have an antidepressant effect, possibly through its neuroprotective actions, which may serve to modulate inflammation in the brain and/or gut lining. The properties of its essential oil are currently being studied in South America, where whitebrush has been used to treat dengue fever.

Future harvests

Choose large, healthy stands to gather from, and gather minimally from each bush.

Arizona, moves northwesterly toward Las Vegas, and finally reaches down into the Mojave and Joshua Tree National Park. Look to north-facing canyons, where it often covers rocky hillsides. *Aloysia gratissima* is abundant across Texas, from Dallas to the Big Bend, and is also found sparingly in southeastern Arizona near the border with Mexico. After seasonal rains, gather the tender, young, leafy shoots with or without flowers.

Medicinal uses

The warming and relaxing effects of *Aloysia wrightii* have various medicinal applications. Drink the hot tea for chest or head cold, seasonal allergies, sinus congestion, headaches, rheumatism, or as an analgesic in stomach or other gastrointestinal cancers. A hot tea will promote sweating in cold, deficient feverish states, or relieve pain and spasm during acute episodes of inflammatory bowel

HERBAL PREPARATIONS

Herb Tea
Standard Infusion
Drink 4–8 ounces, up to 5 times per day.

Leaf Tincture
1 part fresh leaf, by weight
2 parts menstruum (95% alcohol),
 by volume
or
1 part dry leaf, by weight
5 parts menstruum (50% alcohol,
 50% spring water), by volume
Take 10–30 drops, up to 3 times per day.

oshá

Ligusticum porteri
chuchupate, bear root
PARTS USED root, seed

The most revered herb in the Southwest, oshá's medicine is legendary. Use the root for acute viral infections, to enhance blood flow, or to treat venomous bites and stings.

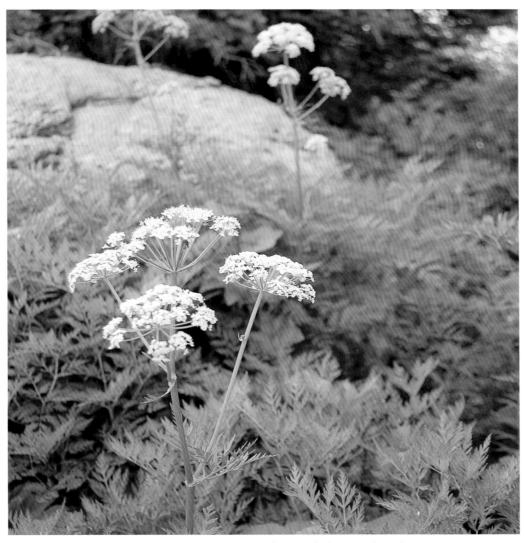

Oshá stands are more visible from a distance when in flower, which is usually mid-summer.

How to identify

Similar in appearance to those of carrot or parsley (other members of the Apiaceae), the irregularly divided leaves of oshá emerge annually, directly from the perennial rootstock. The overall shape of the ternately pinnate leaves is that of a semi-triangular rhomboid. Terminal umbrella-like compound clusters of bright white flowers appear on separate stalks, or emerge from the leaf axils; these flowers may ripen into ridged, beige seeds that are clearly compressed, laterally. The leaves begin to turn yellow in early autumn, causing the 2- to 4-foot-tall plant to stand out in its habitat. Thin "hairs," ½–2 inches long, are visible at the base of the stem at the exposed root crown; these are remnants of previous years' stalks. This is a *clear identifying feature of this plant*, distinguishing it from the very close lookalike, poison hemlock (*Conium maculatum*). An additional distinguishing feature, although less distinctive, is oshá's compressed (flattened on one side) seed; poison hemlock has *non*-compressed seeds. The fresh root of oshá smells strongly of spicy-sweet celery; the root of poison hemlock has virtually no scent. Oshá root comes in a variety of forms, including taproot, branching taproot, and rhizomatous runners.

Where, when, and how to wildcraft

Oshá is a plant of the higher elevations in the Southwest, rarely below 7,000 feet, often at 9,000–11,500 feet among aspen, Douglas fir, and spruce; it may also inhabit Gambel oak groves or sandy ponderosa pine forests. It is rare in Arizona but becomes most abundant in the higher elevations of southwestern Colorado, the southern Rockies of New Mexico, and the high elevations of southern Utah. Think "high, cool, and moist." Traditionally, oshá is gathered in early summer, as

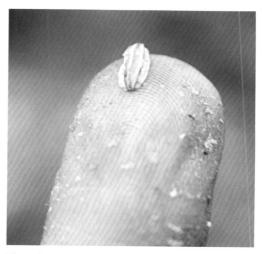

The ridged, beige seeds of oshá rest easily on the end of a fingertip: they are relatively flat, clearly compressed, laterally—in sharp contrast to the non-compressed seeds of poison hemlock.

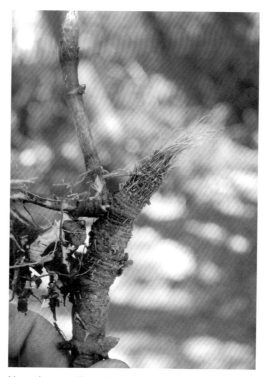

Note the root "hairs" at the top of the root crown (middle right). These are remnants of previous years' stalks and are a positive indicator for oshá.

the leaves first emerge from the ground, or in early autumn, as the leaves turn yellow; however, it does seem more potent when dug just as the leaves are emerging; see the sidebar for more details.

Medicinal uses

Oshá is an important sacred plant in the Southwest, often used ceremonially or for protection against malevolent forces. Take at the first sign of a cold, or during the febrile stages of influenza when energy is low and the person feels cold. Oshá aids the immune response in any influenza-like illness (respiratory viruses). One of the simplest ways to utilize oshá as medicine is to slowly chew the root. It is pungent and bitter (occasionally mildly sweet). Chewing the root also helps improve or prevent altitude sickness (combine with red root tincture).

Oshá Harvesting Guidelines

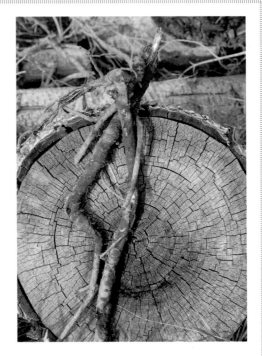

Oshá, or bear root, is one of the most popular herbs in the Southwest and has been for centuries. Its range is relatively secure (it mostly resides in national forests), but its habitat has been changing (becoming drier), and demand for this herb, commercially, is increasing. In northern Mexico, I have witnessed firsthand what overharvesting over an extended period can do to populations of oshá, which is now on the United Plant Savers' At-Risk list. Adhering to the following guidelines should provide ample oshá for everyone within this region seeking to use it as medicine.

Two traditional practices are in circulation. One is to *not* gather the root crown, but only coppice the side roots, leaving the root crown to resprout. The second is to dig up the root crown but leave behind distal segments of roots, many of which will resprout the following year; this second practice is common among the Tarahumara, or Rarámuri, in northern Mexico.

For the first practice (which I've gleaned from Hopi and Navajo gatherers), begin by clearing the ground around the root crown. Then dig a hole 2–3 feet from the base of the plant, all around the plant; continue to carefully dig out soil from around the plant, exposing side taproots and rhizomes. Depending on the size of the root crown, most of these side roots and rhizomes can be gathered. Although bears are known to dig oshá in the spring when they come out of hibernation, and don't bother to cover up their holes, we always refill the large holes dug to excavate the roots, often adding seeds, or creating a small berm to catch rainwater if on a slope.

The fresh root tincture is, arguably, more potent than the dry root tincture, and the dry root tincture is usually slightly less warming. Either form will be expectorant, diaphoretic, immune-stimulating, blood-moving, and locally and systemically antiseptic. Employ its immune-enhancing effects in any acute bacterial infections, or venomous bites and stings. Some herbalists have used oshá root internally to treat rattlesnake bite. Take larger doses, frequently.

A tea of the root provides more digestive stimulation and produces an emmenagogue effect, but much of the immune-enhancing and expectorant qualities are less apparent with a tea. A cold infusion may preserve the aromatic oils best. In Sonora, the fresh root, valued for its blood-moving qualities, is infused in olive oil and rubbed onto sore muscles, or any musculoskeletal injuries.

The fresh root honey infusion is fantastic for sore throat, hoarseness, laryngitis, dry cough, and as an immune stimulant at the onset of infection. The seed tincture has a particular affinity for the eyes. Use internally for any type of eyestrain, or to help clear minor opacities from the cornea; also quite useful for indigestion.

Future harvests

Kelly Kindscher of the University of Kansas led a 4-year study of oshá in the mountains of New Mexico and Colorado. For sustainably harvesting oshá root, he advocates a 20–30% harvest of a given area every 6–10 years. His study also showed that meadow sites (minimal tree cover) produced nearly twice the amount of plants and significantly more flowering plants; and the overall root mass harvested was 58% greater. The upshot? Oshá readily resprouts from partially dug roots. Follow the harvesting guidelines in the sidebar, and consider replanting oshá in north-facing, sloping meadow sites.

 Caution
Avoid internal use during pregnancy.

HERBAL PREPARATIONS

Root Tea
Standard Decoction or Cold Infusion
Drink 2–6 ounces, up to 5 times per day.

Root/Seed Tincture
1 part fresh root (or seed), by weight
2 parts menstruum (95% alcohol),
  by volume
or
1 part dry root, by weight
5 parts menstruum (65% alcohol,
  35% spring water), by volume
Take 20–60 drops, up to 5 times per day; take every 30–60 minutes in acute bacterial infections, or with venomous bites and stings; the seed tincture can be taken at 15–30 drops, up to 3 times per day.

Root Honey Infusion
Follow directions on page 37; take ½–1 teaspoon, as needed.

oxeye daisy

Leucanthemum vulgare
PARTS USED aerial

A nourishing, cooling herb with a pleasant taste and a mild anti-inflammatory effect, it also has specific effects on the female reproductive system.

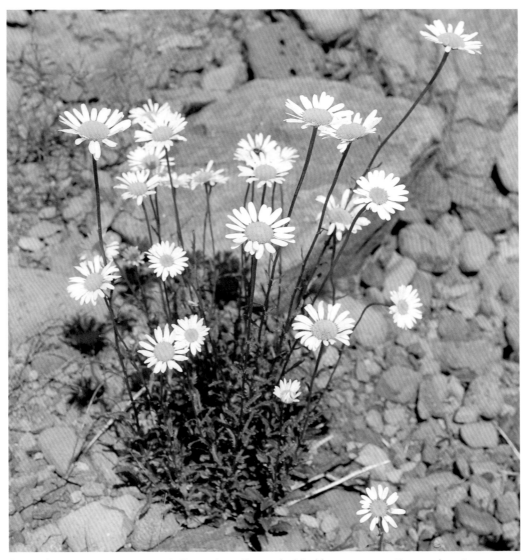

Oxeye daisy is easy to spot once in flower; its yellow and white blooms cover entire meadows in mid-summer.

How to identify

This rhizomatous perennial produces abundant, bright green basal leaves with toothed or lobed margins. The leaves vary in shape considerably, particularly along the stalk, as the plant ages. By late spring/early summer, flower stalks emerge from the center of the basal leaves, producing a brilliant display across open fields of individual, solitary heads of yellow (discoid) and white (ray flowers). The flower stalks are long and thin, and may turn a bit reddish with age. Turn over the flower head, and notice that the phyllaries (bracts below the flower head) are tinged with red at the margins.

Where, when, and how to wildcraft

Look for oxeye daisy in disturbed areas, roadsides, grazed pastures, canyon riverbeds, or ski resorts, mostly at higher elevations in the western half of our region. This naturalized Eurasian native may also be found at the extreme eastern edge of our region, near Dallas and further south. Oxeye daisy is easy to spot when it flowers in mid-summer, overtaking entire fields in a magnificent display, its bright white flowers shining like the full moon in midday sun. Clip the herb at its base and dry in the shade, bundled and hung, or laid out on sheets or racks to dry. Alternatively, high-grade your medicine by taking only the flowers within large stands by plucking them directly from the stem.

Medicinal uses

The tea has such a mild but pleasant flavor, it is a joy to drink it daily. The astringent, anti-inflammatory properties of oxeye daisy are experienced at the mucous membranes of the gut, respiratory system, and genitourinary tract. Its cooling energy helps allay hot, acute conditions, such as diarrhea provoked by intestinal inflammation, food poisoning, or giardia, or organic dysfunction in the tissues caused by chronic low-level irritation.

Consider the flowers in tea for children, or adults, with asthma or chronic bronchitis. Oxeye daisy clears heat from a uterus plagued by irritated tissue (e.g., from IUDs), energetic blockage or stagnancy, or poor blood flow generally. Apply a wash to burns, scrapes, and rashes or other atopic conditions.

Future harvests

Please, don't worry. It is considered invasive wherever it's found in North America (despite still being sold in "wildflower" seed mixes) so is evidently an apt survivor.

HERBAL PREPARATIONS

Herb Tea
Standard Infusion
Drink 4–8 ounces, up to 4 times per day; apply topically to affected area.

passionflower

Passiflora species
corona de Cristo
PARTS USED whole plant

Cooling and calming, passionflower is an excellent sedative to help relieve insomnia, anxiety, or palpitations. It can gradually dissolve the many layers of tension that cover traumatic emotional memories held within the body.

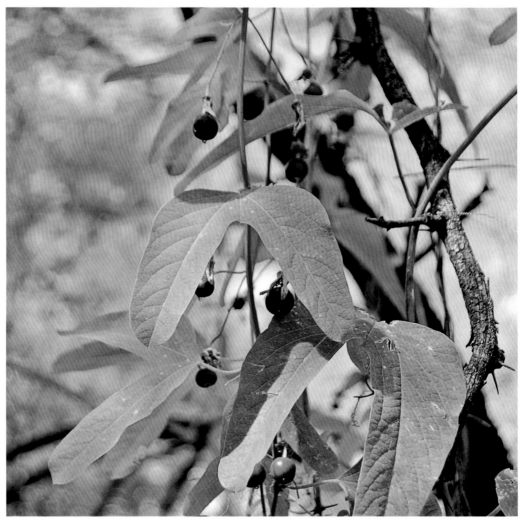

Passiflora mexicana, Mexican passionflower, clearly identified by its 2-lobed leaves and purple, marble-sized edible fruits, can be found in shady canyons in southeastern Arizona.

How to identify

Our *Passiflora* species are climbing perennial vines that may or may not grow a woody stem. The alternate leaves are palmate with deep, rounded lobes (2–5) and smooth (occasionally toothed) margins. The tendrils are in tight curls, like springs, opposite the leaves, distinguishing passionflower from other climbing plants. Pairs of tiny extrafloral nectaries are usually found on the leaf petiole. The perfect flowers are showy, their various parts in colors of white, purple, dark reddish purple, yellow, or green. The corona ("crown") is composed of long filaments radiating out just above the petals and colored sepals. At the very top of the inflorescence are 3 stigmas above 5 stamens. The egg-shaped to rounded fruits mature to green with white stripes, yellow, orange, or deep purple, depending on the spe-

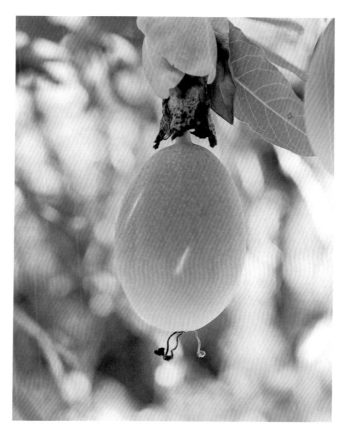

Passiflora caerulea, blue passionflower, has naturalized sporadically throughout the Southwest. Look for it in southern California, southern Arizona, and from Dallas to San Antonio.

cies. At least a dozen native and naturalized species occur within our region; all can be used as medicine.

Where, when, and how to wildcraft

Passionflower is found primarily across the southern tier of our region, yet it swoops up to central Oklahoma as well. In the Sonoran desert, look to waterways and canyons. In Texas, they may occur in mixed chaparral grassland, limestone outcroppings, oak woodlands, prairies, Hill Country, or the South Texas Plains. Begin gathering the herb in early summer as the flowers begin to appear (to aid in identification). Best practice is generally to cut back one to several feet of the young stem tips, including flowers if present. *Passiflora caerulea*, blue passionflower, from South America, can be found covering the native vegetation in some areas; when abundant (or perhaps before becoming so), consider digging whole plants of this species to help control the population. Every part of the plant can be used for medicine.

Medicinal uses

Passionflower is a well-known sedative and relaxing herb, employed for insomnia, anxiety, and palpitations; its affinity for the nervous system also makes it effective for relieving spasms, whether from coughing, muscle spasms, or trembling. Use it to help come down from a caffeine high. It can allay the pain of neuralgia, as well. Combine with hawthorn for mild to moderate episodic hypertension.

Interestingly, passionflower relaxes tonicity within the cardiovascular system, yet it can improve tone in the brain and nervous system (passionflower boosts GABA), elevating mood and creating a sense of relaxed alertness. When someone is extremely exhausted and cannot sleep, passionflower can tone the nervous system, adjusting it more toward the midline, so sleep is achieved. Passionflower has a subtle yet deep and profound effect on relieving shock in the body, both mental/emotional and physical.

Use passionflower in premenstrual formulas to help relieve pain and spasm, in addition to calming anxiety. It helps relieve congestion in the uterus or ovaries. When the liver is sluggish and menses is slow to start, or hemorrhoids are developing, passionflower helps tone the liver and improve vascular flow. It can be taken as a relaxant during pregnancy, labor, and breastfeeding.

The tea or tincture can open the lungs, relieving cough and dry constriction or irritation. Topical preparations have an antimicrobial effect.

Future harvests

Check into which *Passiflora* species grow well in your area and try them in the home landscape. Coppice wild plants moderately, and only from large, healthy stands.

HERBAL PREPARATIONS

Herb Tea
Standard Infusion
Drink 2–6 ounces, up to 4 times per day.

Whole Plant Tincture
1 part fresh plant, by weight
2 parts menstruum (95% alcohol),
  by volume
or
1 part dry plant, by weight
5 parts menstruum (50% alcohol,
  50% spring water), by volume
Take ½–2 teaspoons, up to 4 times per day.

---

pearly everlasting

Anaphalis margaritacea
PARTS USED aerial

A deliciously sweet aromatic herb useful in quelling inflammation, particularly in the lungs and on the skin. Add to a cold-and-flu-season tea for both its flavor and its effects.

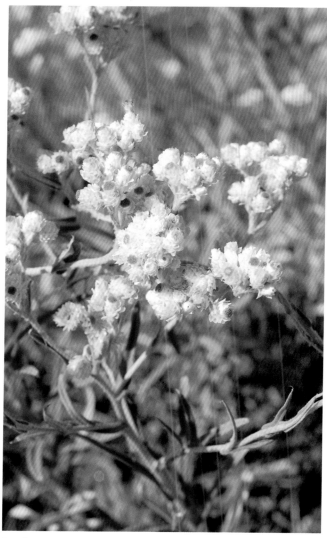

Pearly everlasting occurs in clearings of high-elevation conifer forests and disturbed habitats in wet desert environments.

How to identify

Single stems covered with soft white hairs and clasping leaves arise from a rhizomatous rootstalk. On their top surface, the linear to lance-shaped leaves are a lush green. In contrast, the density of soft white hairs on their undersurface causes this herbaceous perennial to stand out. Leaf margins are entire and curl under. Dense clusters of male (staminate) flowers with a yellow center and nearly translucent, papery white, broad phyllaries unfold at the top of the plant; just below, the female flowers (occasionally integrated with staminate flowers) occur in the leaf axils. The basal leaves and those on the lower stem die back upon flowering. Pearly everlasting is often confused with *Pseudognaphalium leucocephalum*, which, happily, can be used similarly.

Where, when, and how to wildcraft

It can be found in great abundance from mid- to high elevations in the western half of our region. Look to disturbed ground, streambanks or rises in seasonal arroyos, and openings in conifer forests. Flowering begins late summer and continues into autumn. Gather the plant whenever available, either prior to flowering or upon flowering. Dry in the shade, then strip the leaves and flowers for tea, or chop the whole leafy stem.

Medicinal uses

The tea of pearly everlasting tastes good, although its astringency may be too much for some to consider for regular use. Add to tea blends for its ability to reduce inflammation in the mucous membranes, which helps to improve recovery time from acute viral illnesses as well as reducing the severity of symptoms during the acute phase.

Great for stomach inflammation and gastric irritability, including acid reflux, the tea is also taken for hay fever and systemic fungal infections (combine with desert willow), and as a gum rinse.

Topically, the tea is used as a wash to soothe burns and heal cuts and scrapes. Use as a gentle face wash to cool and tone the skin.

Future harvests

Gather sensibly from large stands in disturbed areas, and it will continue to produce.

HERBAL PREPARATIONS

Herb Tea
Standard Infusion
Apply topically to affected area; drink 4–8 ounces, up to 5 times per day.

pecan

Carya illinoinensis
nuéz
PARTS USED bark, leaf, shell, nut

Both the bark and leaf preparations are warming and drying. Apply topically to fungal infections or wounds, and use internally to stimulate the appetite and to calm the nervous system.

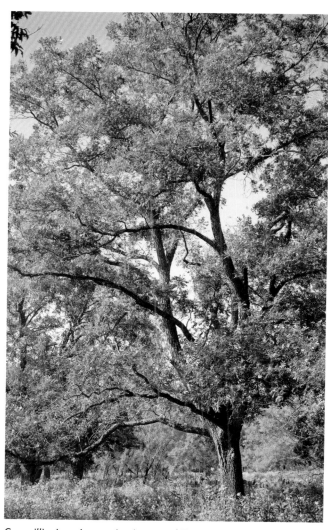

Carya illinoinensis, growing in central Texas.

How to identify

Pecan is a deciduous tree reaching heights of over 120 feet. Its bark is light gray to brown, and with age, develops deep yet narrow furrows that peel back at the ends of thin vertical strips. The 16- to 28-inch-long, oddly pinnate, compound leaves emerge from yellowish brown fuzzy buds with 4–6 scales; they're composed of oblong, lance-shaped leaflets with serrated margins. The stems and midribs of the leaflets are yellow, in contrast to the leaf blade's green, giving leaves a yellowish green look overall. The long male catkins are borne along the stem behind the more distal leaf clusters, within which the female flowers emerge. Female flowers may then mature into clusters of ridged, football-shaped green fruits that become streaked with brown, shriveling as the nut ripens within. The nuts are encased in a hard, light brown shell streaked and mottled with dark brown.

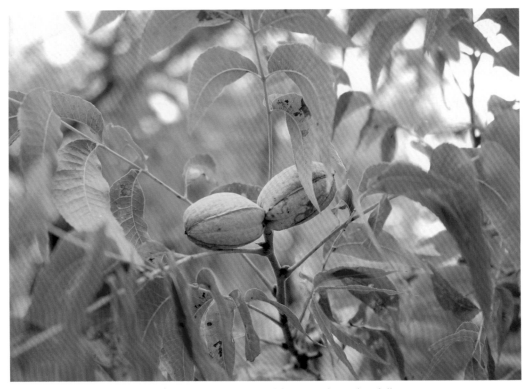

The nuts begin to ripen mid-autumn, and the husk will begin to split as they fully ripen.

Where, when, and how to wildcraft

Although pecan is cultivated in desert lowland orchards in the western half of our region, it occurs naturally in the riparian woodlands of central Texas and northward into Oklahoma. Gather leaves as they emerge in spring, or in late summer/early autumn as the nuts are ripening. Gather nuts from the ground in mid- to late autumn as they fall from their open husks, or when the whole ripe fruit falls to the ground.

Medicinal uses

Pecan has a rich tradition of use as a folk medicine in Texas and the Southeast. As a close relative of walnut, it shares its astringent property and affinity for the skin. Topical preparations of the leaf, bark, or shells have been used to address ringworm, bleeding wounds (powdered bark), thrush, and skin eruptions, and as a bath for backache (bark decoction). Internally, the bark is taken to "thicken" the blood (often indicated by weakness, lethargy, and an overall pallor) and to treat fevers, high blood pressure, and tuberculosis.

Recent scientific research indicates that a decoction of the shells can be used to treat diabetes, obesity, and hypercholesterolemia, as well as to induce apoptosis in certain cancer cell lines. This same remedy has been traditionally administered by the Mexican Kickapoo for hepatitis, stomachache, uterine hemorrhage, and leukorrhea.

The leaf tincture is a mildly sweet and aromatic aperitif. It has been shown clinically to be effective against mycobacterium and yeast infections; also useful in colds and flu. Use the leaf tincture within 3 years, as it tends to sour.

Several studies have shown that the regular consumption of high-antioxidant nuts such as pecan and walnut markedly decrease the occurrence of cardiovascular disease.

In the Southeast, the punk wood of pecan was the preferred substance for moxibustion.

Future harvests

Rather than wildharvest, contact your local pecan orchard about procuring shells, leaves, or bark from recent cuttings.

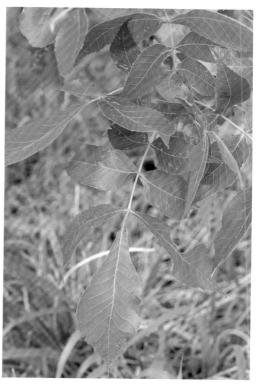

The leaves of other species (here, *Carya texana*, black hickory) can also be used as medicine.

HERBAL PREPARATIONS

Leaf Tea
Standard Infusion
Drink 2–4 ounces, up to 4 times per day.

Bark/Shell Tea
Standard Decoction
Apply topically to affected area; drink 2–4 ounces, up to 4 times per day.

Leaf Tincture
1 part fresh leaf, by weight
2 parts menstruum (75% alcohol, 15% spring water, 10% glycerin), by volume
Take 15–60 drops, up to 4 times per day.

pine

Pinus species
pino, pinabete
PARTS USED bark, needle, sap, pollen

Recent research indicates pine bark's usefulness for preventing cavities, improving cognition and attention span, and treating respiratory conditions, erectile dysfunction, and cardiovascular health.

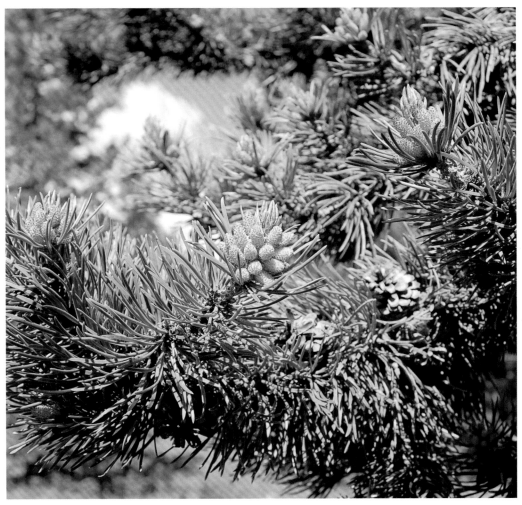

The open and pollinating male cones of *Pinus contorta*, lodgepole pine, growing in southwestern Colorado. The pollen can be gathered straight from the cone, or the whole cluster of cones can be snipped from the tree.

How to identify

Pinus species are the only conifers with fascicled, or bundled, leaves; in contrast, the leaves of fir, spruce, and other conifers attach directly to the stem. The leaves may occur in bundles of 1–5 needles within our region, aiding in identification of the individual species. Pines are evergreen conifers—the green needles are always present (unless the tree is exceptionally stressed)—and monoecious, bearing separate male and female cones on the same tree. The female cones

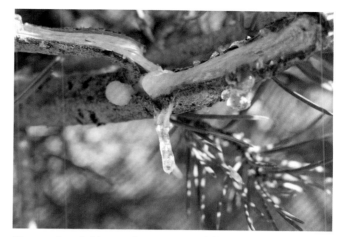

Pine sap (or pitch), one of our most useful topical remedies, is available to us year-round. As the summer heats up, this very sticky substance runs clear.

(which produce the seeds) remain on the tree after the relatively thin and small male cones (which produce the pollen) have fallen to the ground. Pine cones within our region are egg-shaped to elliptic and 2–7 inches long, depending on the species. Bark, which is often furrowed with age, ranges from cinnamon to gray and dark brown. The bark of *P. ponderosa* var. *scopulorum*, ponderosa pine, is light cinnamon-brown with darker brown furrows and occurs in layered plates, reminiscent of jigsaw puzzle pieces. The sweetly aromatic vanilla scent of ponderosa pine bark, especially when exposed to sun, is one of the finer pleasures of our mountain forests.

Where, when, and how to wildcraft

Pine trees are predominantly found in the mid- to higher elevations of the western third of our region. *Pinus edulis* and *P. cembroides*, the piñon pines, occur as low as 5,000 feet in canyons and rocky or exposed desert hillsides. All our other pines are found at higher elevations. The needles and the pitch can be gathered year-round. Look for chunks of dry, hard pitch adherent to the stem and trunk

or on the ground at the foot of the tree. Cut off the male cones just as they begin to open, around mid-summer, and tincture fresh. Gather pure pollen by shaking the open male cones into a plastic bag or wide, shallow bowl. See "Gathering Tree Medicine" (page 25) for details about gathering bark; scrape off the outer bark with a knife before processing.

Medicinal uses

The needles make a pleasant lemon-piney tea. This tea has been used internally to treat respiratory ailments from cough to tuberculosis. It is diuretic and can also bring relief to sore, aching muscles. Apply the needle tea directly to cuts and wounds to speed up healing.

The bark tea has been widely applied in folk medicine for relief from respiratory infections. Recent research points to its possible anticancer effects as well as effectiveness against hepatitis C and COPD; a mouth rinse of the bark tea (rich in antioxidants) shows promise against periodontal disease and reduces demineralization of the teeth.

The pitch, or sap, is a primary remedy for wounds, boils, burns, and infectious sores and abscesses. Simply warm some pitch until softened, and apply directly to the affected area. Cover with gauze to keep from sticking to clothing and leave on overnight. Attempt to peel it off, but if still stuck allow it to work longer. Once peeled, smell the pitch for any residue of infection; if noted, then reapply with a fresh piece of softened pitch. Repeat until the pitch no longer smells of anything but the pitch itself. This is a wonderful remedy. I thank my friend Gino Antonio for showing me this many years ago. I would consider using the pitch on sores with multi-drug resistant bacterial strains.

Although pine pitch tea is a traditional topical and internal remedy, the resins are largely insoluble in water, and only slightly more soluble in alcohol. Thus, an oil infusion can harness a different array of the pitch's medicine that can be applied topically. A decoction of the pitch yields a warming, bitter aromatic tea that quickly enhances circulation to the gut, lungs, and extremities. It is an enlivening circulatory stimulant and a quick way to help someone with the chills or who has been out in a cold wind. The pitch can also be dissolved in the mouth and eaten (or chewed like gum). Traditionally, it was used to treat fever, cough, colds, flu, indigestion, ulcers, intestinal parasites, and general debility.

Anyone wishing to enhance testosterone may benefit from ingesting pine pollen. The pollen can be combined with honey and eaten directly, or taken as a tincture to enhance testosterone in the body, thus improving energy levels, cognitive function, and circulation to the sex organs of males.

Future harvests

Strolling through a pine forest is uplifting and refreshing. Harvest with respect and gratitude, always.

⚠ Caution

If you decide to make tea with the pitch, your container (or pot) will have undissolved resin stuck all over it. It is best to use a dedicated pot or vessel for the decoction or infusion.

HERBAL PREPARATIONS

Needle Tea
Standard Infusion
Drink 2–4 ounces, up to 4 times per day.

Bark/Pitch Tea
Standard Decoction
Drink 2–4 ounces, up to 4 times per day; apply topically to affected area.

Ripe Male Cone Tincture
1 part fresh male cones, by weight
3 parts menstruum (60% alcohol,
   40% spring water), by volume
or
1 part fresh pollen, by weight
5 parts menstruum (70% alcohol,
   30% spring water), by volume
Take 30–90 drops, up to 4 times per day; halve the dosage for pure pollen tincture.

Inner Bark Tincture
1 part fresh inner bark, by weight
2 parts menstruum (95% alcohol),
   by volume
Take 30–90 drops, up to 4 times per day.

plantain

Plantago species
ribwort
PARTS USED leaf, root, seed

All the important skin-healing attributes in one humble plant. This nutritious herb soothes, cools, relieves pain internally, and helps restore fluid movement in the musculoskeletal system.

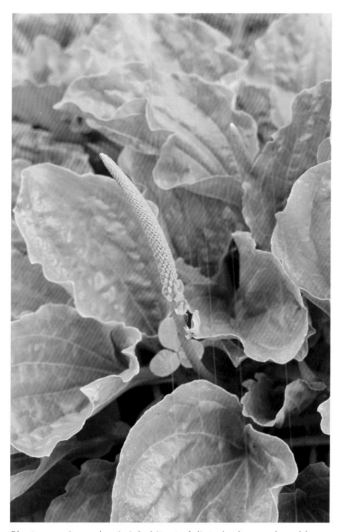

Plantago major, a classic inhabitant of disturbed ground worldwide, is naturalized here from Europe.

How to identify

Native and introduced *Plantago* species share similar characteristics. Arising from a taproot, the basal leaves may be narrow or egg-shaped, slightly toothed or not at all, woolly or nearly devoid of hairs, and often show prominent veins along their length. Our desert-adapted plants (*P. ovata*, *P. patagonica*) have much thinner leaves that appear gray-green, due to their covering of white, woolly hairs. Inconspicuous flowers, each framed by 4 colorless bracts, occur along an upright terminal spike (up to 13 cm long) that emerges from the center of the basal rosette (plantain's most telling trait). Viewed up close, the dark, mature fruits look like tiny acorns with a modified single-series cap; the several seeds contained within each capsule become mucilaginous when moistened.

Where, when, and how to wildcraft

It's hard to find a locale without plantain: it occurs throughout

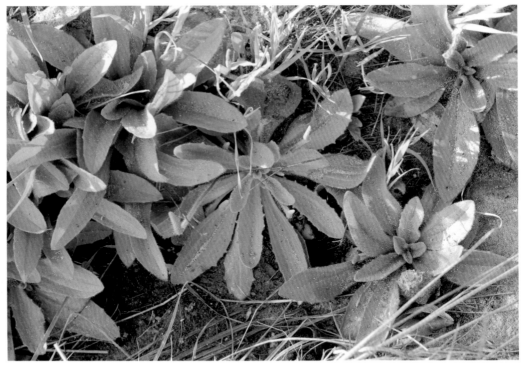

Plantago virginica is found along the eastern edge of our region as well as in moist areas of desert canyons. It is the best plantain for poultices in our desert areas.

the Southwest, in dry to wet climates, disturbed and undisturbed areas, at all elevations. *Plantago ovata*, Indian wheat, and *P. patagonica*, woolly plantain, both natives with thin, fuzzy grass-like leaves, are found in abundance and widely distributed across the lower desert habitats including cactus forests, grasslands, arroyos, and canyons. Gather the fresh leaves, spring through autumn, to use as a poultice. The fresh herb is tinctured, or can be dried for tea or oil infusion.

Medicinal uses

Plantain is a first-rate remedy for nearly any imaginable skin condition, including burns, infected or bleeding wounds, rashes, bites, stings, ulcers, or abscesses. It has the ability to act as a drawing agent, helping to raise splinters and the like out of the skin. Use a fresh plant poultice over the eyes, just within the ear, or over painful joints to relieve pain and soreness, and on the outer surface of the rectum when hemorrhoids are present. Plantain promotes healing by stimulating the laying down of new tissue, draws out and clears infection, soothes, cools, relieves pain, and helps prevent formation of scar tissue.

A plantain tea is a soothing, healing anti-inflammatory agent for the gut lining and can be used to resolve stomach ulcers and alleviate digestive discomfort; drink when blood is encountered in the urine, as it is broadly hemostatic, both topically and internally. Plantain also has an affinity for the female reproductive system and has been used to promote fertility and for menopausal support. I class it, with cleavers and violet, as a gentle cooling and moistening lymphatic herb that works slowly but deeply on the whole system (very phlegmatic in nature).

Use of the tincture can bring about greater mobility and fluidity of movement to the ribs and the musculoskeletal system in general. Take a small dosage of tincture (1–5 drops) and observe the sensations it elicits throughout your body.

The root is traditionally used as a blood builder, pain reliever, and for acute lung infections. The seeds are demulcent in action and can reduce intestinal inflammation. Taken in smaller doses (½–1 teaspoon), they are mildly laxative; at higher doses, they may relieve diarrhea.

Future harvests

Just go for a walk. You'll find it.

 Caution

Avoid plantain when using hormone replacement therapy: recent studies suggest it may bind to estrogen receptors and therefore potentiate exogenous estrogen.

HERBAL PREPARATIONS

Leaf Tincture
1 part fresh leaf, by weight
2 parts menstruum (70% alcohol, 30% spring water), by volume
or
1 part dry leaf, by weight
5 parts menstruum (50% alcohol, 50% spring water), by volume
Take 10–30 drops, up to 4 times per day.

Oil Infusion
1:5
Dry leaves and prepare as alcohol intermediate oil infusion (see page 38).

Poultice
Mash up the fresh plant and apply directly to the body, as needed.

Zanthoxylum hirsutum, Z. fagara, Z. clava-herculis
colima, toothache tree
PARTS USED bark, leaf, fruit

This warming and uniquely pungent herb increases circulation throughout the body. It's useful for toothaches, to improve digestion, and to help deliver the effects of other herbs throughout the body.

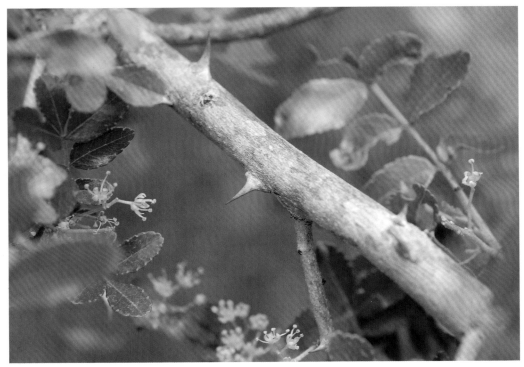

The smooth gray bark of *Zanthoxylum hirsutum* is studded with finely pointed spines; its leaves and flowers are similar to those of *Z. clava-herculis*.

How to identify

These are large deciduous understory shrubs (or small trees, in exposed areas). When young, they have smooth gray bark with prominent, short thorns. *Zanthoxylum hirsutum*, Texas prickly ash, has compound leaves of 5–7 shiny leaflets with wavy edges and rounded teeth, often with pairs of reddish thorns at the nodes. *Zanthoxylum fagara*, limestone prickly ash, has 9–13 rounded and shorter leaflets, also with rounded teeth on the margin, especially at the tips. *Zanthoxylum clava-herculis*, Hercules' club, is taller, with prominent stout, pointy spines all along the trunk. Each species produces clusters of tiny flowers with 4 yellow petals and stamens

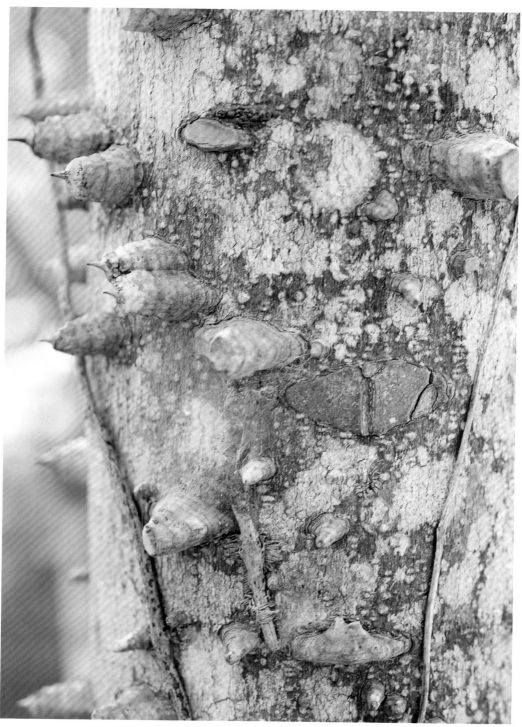

The short spines of *Zanthoxylum clava-herculis* are borne on corky projections.

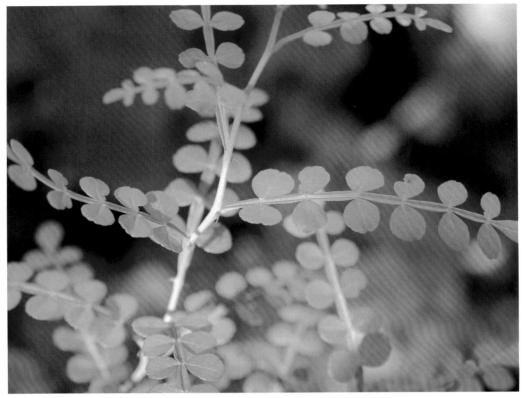

Zanthoxylum fagara, colima, possesses much smaller leaflets, and more of them than *Z. hirsutum*. Its thorns can easily blend in with the color of the stem.

that extend well beyond the corollas; the resulting tiny red fruits have a pocked surface, reminiscent of a citrus fruit. Upon nibbling any plant part, your mouth will tingle, then go slightly numb for a short time.

Where, when, and how to wildcraft

Within our region, prickly ash is found only in Texas and to some extent in southern Oklahoma. *Zanthoxylum hirsutum* occurs abundantly in the Hill Country, *Z. fagara* in the South Texas Plains, and *Z. clava-herculis* only in the wettest areas from Corpus Christi northward into Oklahoma. The bark can be gathered at any time, the leaves whenever available (mid-spring to late autumn), and the fruits in autumn.

Medicinal uses

Chewing on the fresh bark of prickly ash is one of my favorite herbal experiences. Tasting the fresh leaves, fruit, or bark provokes lively sensations in the mouth and is a wonderful local anesthetic, relieving a toothache; it stimulates saliva secretions, which promotes better gum health.

Including prickly ash tincture within a multi-herb formula is a classic example of a singular herb acting as a vehicle, or diffusive—an agent that actively transports and disperses the qualities of other herbs throughout the body. As a stimulant to peripheral circulation, prickly ash is wonderful in this role. Indeed, it is strongly indicated wherever circulation is sluggish.

Consider using this alterative herb in any cold, deficient, slow-to-change conditions (e.g., dampness), or chronic infections with poor circulation. I have cooked it up in apple cider vinegar with red root and inmortál, adding honey to make an oxymel for chronic infections. Prickly ash tonifies the digestion impeccably, enabling the body to optimally nourish itself.

Bark preparations are traditionally given for coughs, colds, sore throat, and damp respiratory problems, and to help relieve musculoskeletal pains, cramps, internal bleeding, or restrained urination. Leaf and bark oil infusions have been applied to injuries as blood movers, to promote healing (Coffman 2014).

Future harvests

Gather modestly, and spread your wildharvesting around to different locations each year. The fruits are relished by birds, which is why you will often find prickly ash beneath their perch sites (trees and fences).

 Caution

Beware of the sharp spines when handling the plant.

HERBAL PREPARATIONS

Bark Tincture

1 part fresh bark (leaf and fruit, also), by weight

2 parts menstruum (95% alcohol), by volume

or

1 part dry bark (and fruit), by weight

5 parts menstruum (65% alcohol, 35% spring water), by volume

Take 10–30 drops, up to 5 times per day, or combine in formulation.

Oxymel

Follow directions on page 38; take ½–1 tablespoon, up to 3 times per day, in water.

Opuntia species
nopál
PARTS USED flower, fruit, pad

Prickly pear exemplifies a perfect union of food and medicine.
Fruit, pad, and flower each carry potent healing.

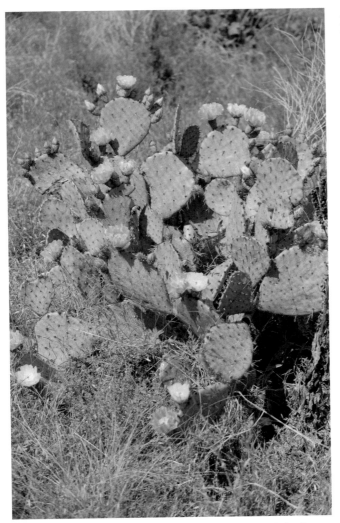

Opuntia species inhabit a wide variety of habitats and hybridize readily, yielding plants with variable size, form, and color. Pictured here in the Texas Hill Country.

How to identify

Prickly pear cacti readily show diverse characteristics across a small population. Pads may be round, elongated, or diamond- to egg-shaped, either concave or flat, and occasionally have wavy margins; they range in color from yellowish green to blue-green, and their areoles (little dots on the surface of both pad and fruit) may or may not have spines or glochids (tiny, modified leaf hairs). Pads begin to shrivel in response to drought and expand quickly after heavy rains. The cactus may be one pad high, running jointed along the ground, or several pads high, over 8 feet tall. The glochids are retorsed, so they are difficult to pull from the flesh once penetrated. Flowers, ranging in color from yellow to red, pink, or reddish orange, open and close within one day; once the tepals (not petals) close, they begin to shrivel on top of the ovary, which then develops into the fruit. Ripe fruits are likewise variable in color: light pink, copper-red, dark purple, and more. They

Gathering Prickly Pear Fruit

A pair of tongs is the most important tool; a comfortable pair with flat, non-toothed ends, with or without a spring in the handle, is optimal. A 5-gallon bucket with a reinforced handle (for when the bucket fills up) makes a perfect harvesting vessel; in fact, it is best to have two to balance the weight on both sides. As for selecting ripe fruit, it is not as easy as it

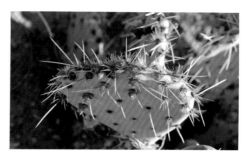

looks: fruits may reach the color of ripeness weeks before they are fully ripened. Suffice to say, a fruit that easily comes off the cactus (and often leaves a bit behind)—and is soft and at least somewhat sweet inside—is what we're after. Carefully reach out into the cactus (some are quite large) and pluck off a fruit with your tongs. Place it in one of the buckets and continue gathering.

may be elongated and fluted in form, or squat and barrel-shaped, tapering very quickly at the base. The fruits are covered with a thin skin, often covered in glochids (at the areoles) and occasionally spines. Beneath the skin, a layer of sweet, sour, salty, or bland flesh surrounds a pulpy mash of hard, flat, round, pale tan to gray seeds.

Where, when, and how to wildcraft

Prickly pear is found nearly everywhere: desert grasslands, oak woodlands, piñon-juniper forests, Hill Country, sandy prairies, rocky ledges in canyons, the South Texas Plains, high desert, high plains—even in conifer forests, up to 8,000 feet. The flowers are available mid- to late spring. Simply pinch the shriveled flower up and out of the cup in which it sits. Fruits ripen from mid-summer to late autumn, depending on the location and type of prickly pear; they come off quite easily with tongs when fully ripe (see sidebar for more details). The pads can be used year-round; however, the fleshiest pads are preferred for poultices.

Medicinal uses

One could consume pads and fruit of prickly pear on a daily basis, without conscious awareness of the medicinal effect it has. In a similar fashion, a person could ingest prickly pear daily as a medicine, able to target blood sugar normalization and insulin resistance, for example, and not even think of it as "food." It can nonetheless be safely consumed on a daily basis, for either purpose.

As a first-aid remedy, apply the pad poultice to venomous bites and stings, musculoskeletal injuries (including sprains and breaks), broken skin, sunburn, or any hot, itchy condition. The heated fruit can also be used topically to relieve pain. The fruit juice, taken internally, is one of our best musculoskeletal remedies for pain and stiffness. It allays arthritic pain as well as pain from injury or overuse. Take 1–4 tablespoons of the fruit juice daily to improve the various factors associated with metabolic syndrome, such as high blood sugar, high blood pressure, and excessive inflammation.

Prickly Pear Pad Poultice

This first-aid preparation can provide tremendous relief and benefit during a variety of wilderness or at-home scenarios. First, choose a terminal pad, still on the cactus, that appears full, fleshy, and relatively straight; a concave or undulating pad will be difficult to process. If it's a spine-covered prickly pear, find two flattish rocks that can be handled without your fingers extending beyond the edge of the rock. Grasp the rocks firmly and rub them on opposite sides of the selected pad, simultaneously, in a circular motion, gradually removing the spines and glochids from the pad. Now grasp the pad with one hand and, with a sharp knife (or sharp-edged rock, if necessary), cut it from the cactus at its base. Fillet the pad with a long, thin knife right down the center (if the pad is too large, cut in half, or to a smaller, more manageable size), exposing its white mucilaginous center. Apply this exposed section to the affected area. Keep in place until the drawing action has finished (30–60 minutes). Continue to apply fresh pads until the area has sufficiently cooled, or the pain and irritation has subsided.

A flower tea is demulcent and helps to heal irritated and inflamed tissue, both internally and externally. It is also a remedy for the genitourinary tract, specifically bringing relief to a painful and swollen prostate.

Future harvests

Return to where you gathered prickly pear fruit to scatter seeds. Clones are easy to propagate; simply cut a pad from a cactus with desirable properties, replant it in a favorable area, and supply with plenty of water.

 Caution

Excessive juice intake may provoke loose stool. Raw prickly pear fruit juice, in particular, can cause fever, chills, and body aches in sensitive individuals; as always, taste a small amount upon first consuming any medicinal that is new to you.

HERBAL PREPARATIONS

Flower Tea
Standard Infusion
Drink 2–6 ounces, up to 3 times per day.

Fruit Juice
Drink 1 tablespoon to several ounces, up to 3 times per day.

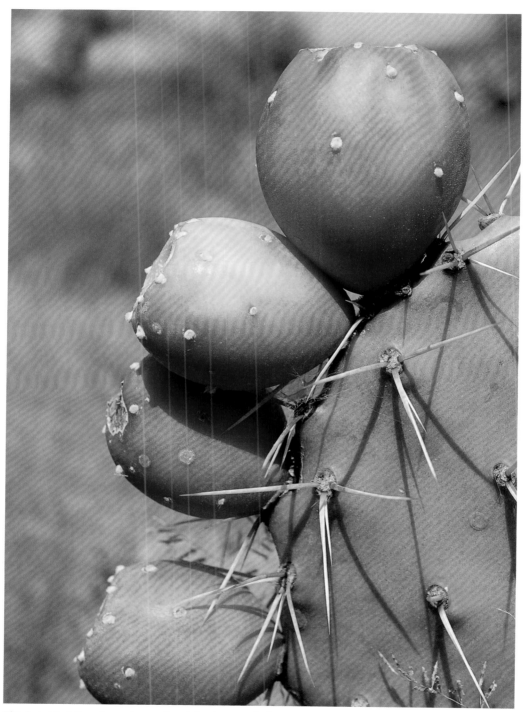

This hybrid of *Opuntia englemannii* and *O. phaeacantha* has fruits that ripen to a bright pink with greenish flesh inside.

prickly poppy

Argemone albiflora, A. pleiacantha, A. polyanthemos
cardo, cowboy's eggs
PARTS USED aerial

This poppy family plant is an excellent pain reliever, both topically and internally. It relieves nerve pain quickly and can allay cramping during menses.

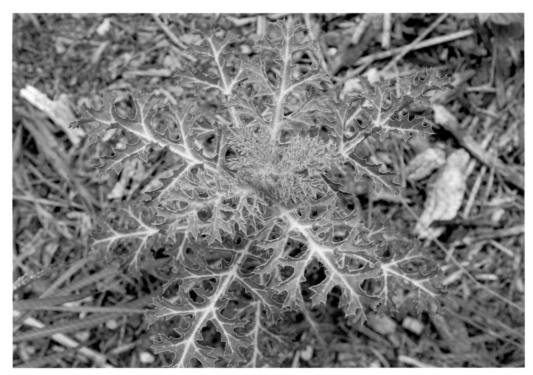

When first leafing out, prickly poppy can be identified by the clear contrast between the bluish green of its fleshy leaf blade and its lighter to milky white midvein.

How to identify

All parts of this annual or perennial plant (except for the flower petals) can have spines. The spiny, toothed leaves are more deeply lobed within the basal rosette. The flower stalks, emerging from the rosette's center, may be 2–7 feet in height. More shallowly lobed, alternate leaves occur along the stalk, which is covered in glistening white or golden spines. Flowers have 4–6 large, crinkly white petals (yellow in *Argemone mexicana*, red in *A. sanguinea*) surrounding a central boss of yellow stamens. The erect, elliptical seedpods are often covered in thick, bristly spines; they open no more than a quarter of the way down upon maturing and contain numerous dark seeds. Over a dozen species occur within our region. They can be used interchangeably.

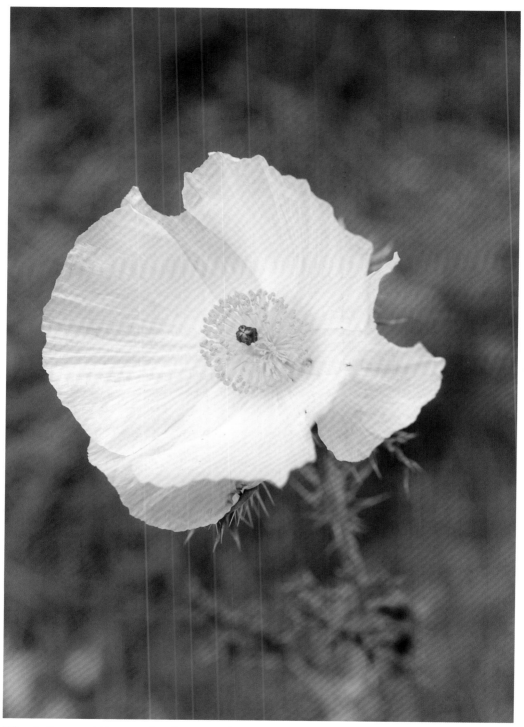

When in flower, prickly poppy is quite easy to distinguish: another name for the plant is cowboy's eggs.

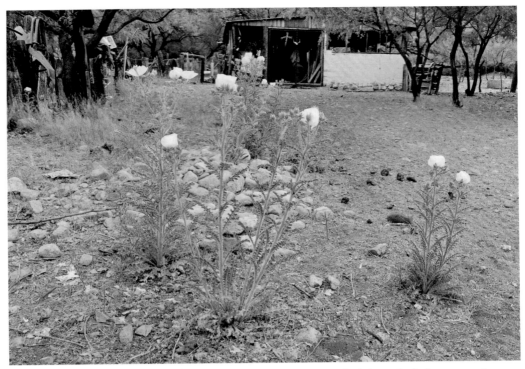

Pictured here is *Argemone pleiacantha*, southwestern prickly poppy, which is particularly common in Arizona and New Mexico below 7,500 feet. It is often found in abundance in overgrazed pastures.

Where, when, and how to wildcraft

Prickly poppy is found throughout our region. Find it in abundance in overgrazed pastures, mountain valleys, foothills and mesas of desert grasslands, and along roadsides or other dry, gravelly, disturbed sites. It is uncommon in the high desert. Gather the basal leaves and the flowering stalk from mid-spring through early autumn, when moisture is abundant. Use thick gloves when handling, and process outdoors to keep the spines out of your home. Touching this plant can be painful.

Medicinal uses

According to ethnobotanical records, the seeds were the most commonly used part of this plant, medicinally (but see Caution). Topical preparations were used to heal and relieve the pain of burns, cuts, sores, hemorrhoids, boils, and sore eyes. The fresh sap, which is mildly caustic, has been utilized on warts and corneal opacities.

Michael Moore (1989) states that the tea helps with palpitations from caffeine excess or during menopause. He also suggests using the tea of the leaf topically to relieve sunburn and internally for nerve pain, urinary pain, headache, and as an antispasmodic pain reliever for PMS (combine with silk tassel).

The leaf tincture works similarly to relieve pain. Consider it for any situation where pain has become overwhelming and interferes with basic functioning (eating, sleeping, sitting, lying down).

An oil infusion made from the aerial parts (stem, leaf, flowers, seedpods) can be applied topically to various nerve-associated pains (neuromas, sciatica, carpal tunnel, spina bifida, shingles; combine with California poppy) as well as joint pain or back pain, often to great effect.

Future harvests

Overgrazing in much of the Southwest has made this plant abundant. Consider spreading seed to disturbed soils in your area to see if it will take.

 Caution

The seeds should be consumed in moderation. They are emetic and cathartic, and in their industrially refined form, are potentially fatal when consumed. Ingest only dry plant preparations.

HERBAL PREPARATIONS

Flower/Leaf Tea
Cold Infusion
Drink 2–4 ounces, up to 3 times per day, or apply topically, as needed; strain well to avoid the potentially irritating spines.

Tincture
1 part dry plant, by weight
5 parts menstruum (50% alcohol,
    50% spring water), by volume
Take 10–30 drops, up to 5 times per day.

Oil Infusion
1 part dry leaf/stem/flower, by weight
5 parts extra virgin olive oil, by volume
Prepare as alcohol intermediate oil infusion (see page 38).

puncture vine

Tribulus terrestris
gokshura, goat's head
PARTS USED whole plant

This robust survivor is an important restorative and medicinal herb.
Drink the tea to help dissolve stones, or use the fruit powder, or tincture,
to help improve hormonal balance.

Puncture vine is nearly everywhere, including urban landscapes.

How to identify

This introduced annual produces pinnately compound leaves composed of 3–9 pairs of hair-tipped leaflets. The rachis, or central stem of the leaf, may be green or pale brown, similar to the finely hairy main stems of the plant. The solitary flowers have 5 yellow spatula-shaped petals; the segmented fruit that follows readily separates into 5 parts, each armed with a pair of stout spines capable of puncturing a wide variety of materials. Growth habit is prostrate and arachnid; plants sprawl out in all directions, close to the ground.

Where, when, and how to wildcraft

Look to disturbed ground below 8,000 feet, throughout our entire region. Puncture vine begins to appear with the onset of warm, moist weather. Gather the whole plant at any stage for tea. Gather the fruit separately for tincture; the exceptionally spiky seedpods are painful to the touch. Handle the mature

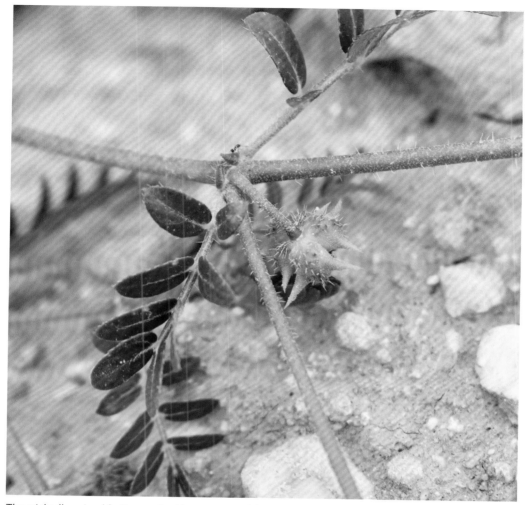

The wickedly spined fruits, a potent hormone modulator, form within 2-3 weeks of germination.

plant with gloves to prevent puncturing your fingers with the seedpods.

Medicinal uses

The tea of the whole plant holds value in UTIs and aids in dissolving kidney or bladder stones. It possesses diuretic and tonic astringent properties as well as soothing and antimicrobial effects, making it highly useful as a tea for the urinary tract.

It is also tonifying to kidney and liver function, secondary to lifestyle, chronic illnesses, or infections that may deplete these organs. A daily dose of the whole plant tea, accompanied by moderate exercise, can help moderate high blood pressure (even when moderate exercise alone doesn't help). This tea may also help to moderate high triglycerides and LDL levels and may help prevent gallstones. The whole herb can also be applied to eczema and other skin conditions.

The oft-cursed fruit has significant effects on our reproductive hormones. Ingested as a tincture, or powdered (mix with honey, in smoothies, etc.), it seems to improve the androgen/estrogen profiles in both males and females. This is experienced as enhanced fertility, increased sex drive and responsiveness, better energy level, enhanced cognitive function, or a reduction in menopausal symptoms. Benign prostatic hyperplasia can also be improved by puncture vine (combine with nettle root). The fruit tincture also possesses antifungal and antimicrobial properties, making it useful in both topical and internal applications.

Future harvests

Gather respectfully where it is already present, but think long and hard about introducing this "terror of the earth" anywhere else.

Diuretic Formula

Combine the following dry herbs, by weight, and prepare as a standard decoction; drink 1–3 cups per day. Also useful for hypertension.

- 4 parts puncture vine
- 3 parts cholla root
- 3 parts Bermudagrass rhizome
- 2 parts nettle leaf

HERBAL PREPARATIONS

Whole Plant Tea
Standard Infusion
Drink 4 ounces, 2 times per day; apply topically, as needed.

Tincture
1 part dry fruit, by weight
5 parts menstruum (60% alcohol, 40% spring water), by volume
Take 20–60 drops, up to 4 times per day.

Stillingia texana, S. sylvatica, S. linearifolia, S. paucidentata
pávil, queen's delight
PARTS USED root

This acrid herb is a wonderful cough remedy, useful for laryngitis and bronchitis. The internal and topical use of the plant resolves poorly healing wounds, tissue ulcerations, and red, swollen areas of the skin.

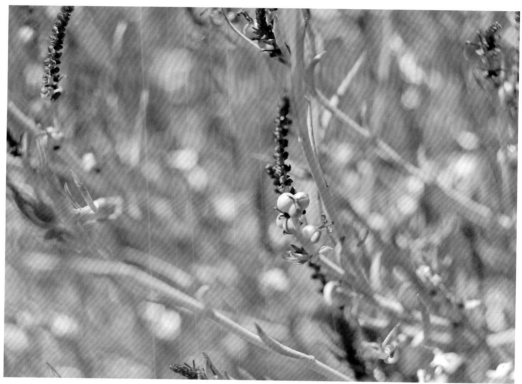

Stillingia linearifolia, as found in the deserts of southern California. This species is gathered in late winter, along with *S. paucidentata*. The flower spikes have separate male (here, purple) and female flowers (here, green 3-celled fruit).

How to identify

Stillingia species are herbaceous perennials that exude a clear or milky sap when broken. Plants are monoecious; the petal-less, green to greenish yellow inflorescences are borne on erect terminal racemes, with male and female flowers alternating along the spike. All species have thin, linear or lance-shaped leaves with margins toothed or entire. The inflorescence of *S. linearifolia* is green and purplish brown with ample spacing between the flowers; the inflorescence of *S. texana* is yellowish green, with flowers more densely crowded. The taproots have a thin, reddish brown bark and a white inner flesh.

Where, when, and how to wildcraft

Two distinct types of queen's root exist on each side of our region. *Stillingia sylvatica* and *S. texana* can be found in the eastern half, from the panhandles of Oklahoma and Texas, the Hill Country and westward across the high plains, and in sand dunes of New Mexico and Colorado; Michael Moore considered them the preferred species for medicine. In the far western region, *S. paucidentata* and *S. linearifolia* grow in the low desert plains and rocky slopes of southern California and along the side drainages of the Colorado River in Arizona and Nevada. The root of *S. paucidentata* and *S. linearifolia* is best gathered in late winter or early spring (following rains); the root of *S. sylvatica* and *S. texana*, in early spring or mid-autumn. Ultimately, either type can be gathered whenever needed or when an opportunity presents itself; see "Digging Roots" (page 26) for more details.

Medicinal uses

Use of queen's root is strongly indicated when the mucous membranes are red and inflamed, secretions are nearly absent, or fluid has built up within the tissues and become stagnant. *Stillingia* is a classic alterative, with an exceptional ability to remove waste products from congested tissues and improve the uptake of nutrition where inhibited. Its acrid taste is indicative of this quality of dispersing congestion. Its alterative and lymphatic properties may also be utilized in formulation for arthritis, eczema, psoriasis, fungal infections, chronic lung infections, or any red, swollen skin conditions.

Use the tincture topically or add to a salve preparation to stimulate healing in slow-to-heal ulcerous conditions (combine with figwort and copperleaf). A high-alcohol tincture of the fresh root is the best medicinal preparation of this plant.

Future harvests

Gather only from abundant stands. Replant seeds after digging the roots.

Alteratives

An unusual concept to those not versed in herbal medicine, alteratives were commonly used by Eclectics and other U.S. physicians in the 19th and early 20th centuries. Simply put, an alterative enhances the body's ability to take in nourishment (e.g., by clearing lymphatic stagnation in the gut) and eliminate wastes (e.g., by increasing sweating, stimulating kidney function). Alterative herbs have a significant impact on our digestive tissues and eliminative organs, such as the skin and kidneys. Each alterative herb is different, capable of affecting the body in subtle and specific ways; traditionally, many were classed as "blood purifiers."

Several herbs in this book are classic alteratives (queen's root, inmortál, golden smoke); others are mild alteratives (cleavers, red root). Studying a plant like queen's root lends deeper insight to this term than any definition could. Watch how it stimulates the mucous membranes to secrete, or how an accumulation of fluid will slowly dissipate upon ingesting queen's root. Alteratives are often valuable remedies during the stuck, stagnant, obstructed phases of chronic illness: they are known to go to the depths and shift what is immovable.

⚠ Caution

Stick to small, frequent doses. High doses can provoke nausea and painful vomiting. Queen's root is otherwise safe for continued use.

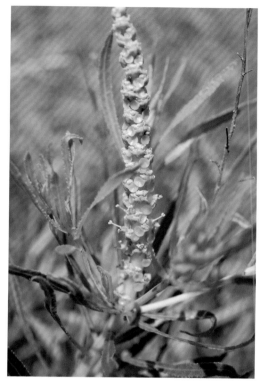

Stillingia texana is most abundant within the eastern third of our region.

HERBAL PREPARATIONS

Root Tincture
1 part fresh root, by weight
2 parts menstruum (95% alcohol),
  by volume
or
1 part recently dry root, by weight
5 parts menstruum (75% alcohol,
  25% spring water), by volume
Take 10–30 drops, up to 4 times per day.

Ceanothus species
buckbrush, deerbrush, Jersey tea
PARTS USED bark, leaf, stem, flower, root

This drying, astringent, and often acrid remedy, with a touch of wintergreen, dispels lymphatic congestion, addressing colds, flu, chest congestion, and digestive complaints.

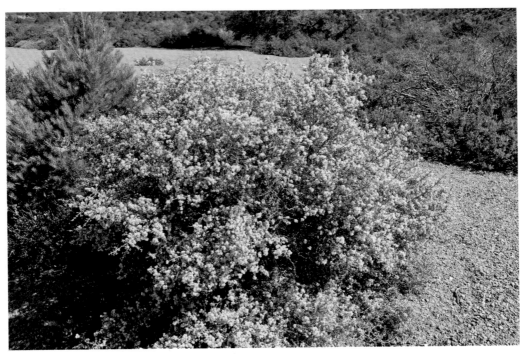

Ceanothus (greggii) pauciflorus, in full bloom, mid-spring.

How to identify

Ceanothus species may be evergreen or deciduous, upright or prostrate; all but *C. greggii* have palmately 3-veined leaves. Different parts of the plant, in different species, contain betulinic acid, thus smell strongly of wintergreen. All species within our region possess rounded clusters of tiny white blossoms and alternate stems and leaves, again with the exception of *C. greggii*, which clearly exhibits opposite stems. The relatively small leaves are egg-shaped to oblong lance-shaped. *Ceanothus integerrimus* and *C. herbaceus* have terminal flower spikes, in *C. greggii* the clusters are borne from the leaf axils, and the other species exhibit a combination of the two. The smooth bark is light gray, dark gray, yellow-green, or reddish brown. Small reddish brown capsules appear in mid-summer.

Where, when, and how to wildcraft

Red root occurs most abundantly in the western half of our region, at mid- to high-elevations. The most widespread species is *Ceanothus greggii*, desert ceanothus, found at 3,000–7,000 feet in dry, rocky desert areas from western Texas to southern California. Look for *C. herbaceus* in the high plains, Hill Country, and prairies in the eastern third of our region. *Ceanothus fendleri* reaches higher elevations, often accompanying pine, oak, and fir trees. Gather flowering branches in early to late summer. Roots are best gathered in mid- to late spring, before flowering, or in late autumn before the ground freezes. See sidebar for more details.

Medicinal uses

Red root is one of our best, most well-rounded systemic lymphatic remedies. Its toning astringency and mild acridity help to break up stagnant, congested conditions and increase organ function in a wide variety of chronic illnesses and acute infections.

Michael Moore discovered its ability to improve blood charge, which in turn enhances the movement of waste products throughout the body. Take the tincture in water, or tea, for swollen lymph glands, sore throat, tonsillitis, headache, cold and flu, chest congestion, or any infection where a heavy, full, or achy feeling is present. It's exceptionally valuable in formulation for

Gathering Red Root

Before you start digging, taste the plant. View the plants as individuals, because, as you'll find, they don't all taste the same, not even those of the same species, not even when they're growing right next to each other. I like to sample a leaf, or a sliver of bark; if it's acrid, producing a sharp burn at the back of the throat, and has both a wintergreen flavor and aroma, then you've found some great medicine. Yes, the root may taste stronger, but in my experience, the taste of the leaves and bark directly corresponds to a similar potency in the root. If you've found a potent-tasting bark or leaf, now you can make medicine out of that, too, perhaps saving a plant and saving yourself the time and effort of digging up a root, which can be rigorous work.

Once you've decided to dig (see "Digging Roots," page 26) and have exposed a plant's roots, judge whether the root is young and tender, or large, older, and fibrous. With older roots, use only the root bark, which, admittedly, will yield very little medicine. Consider, instead, coppicing older roots (thus, chopping up the peripheral rootlets gathered), or covering them up again and searching for younger roots to dig up elsewhere. Thin rootlets, or young taproots are often tinged with pink or red all the way through. These can be cut up and the whole amount used, not just the root bark. Additionally, where rhizomatous reproduction is happening, side runners going to new, younger plants can be easily pulled up from within 2 inches of the surface.

Some of the best-tasting and well-rounded red root tincture I've ever made has been from the stem bark of *Ceanothus integerrimus*. Simply strip all the bark with a knife, chop into small, ¼-inch pieces, and tincture. If the leaves taste potent, include them as well. Add 10% glycerin to all red root tincture preparations to considerably delay the precipitation of the tannins, which renders the tincture "chunky" over time.

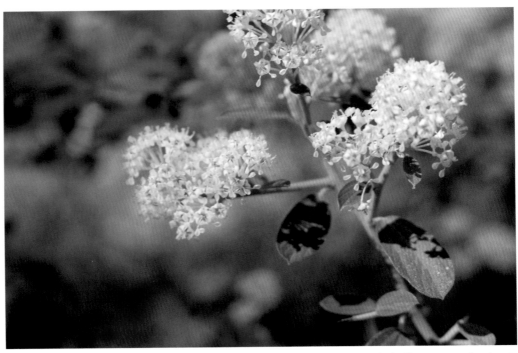

Ceanothus fendleri has alternate stems and leaves and the quintessential rounded inflorescence of red root.

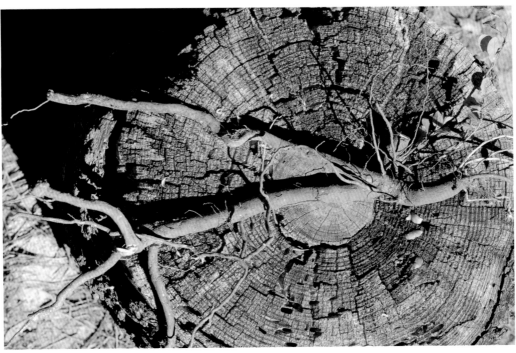

Young taproots are often red- or pink-tinged all the way through.

chronic lung insufficiency, asthma, or acute respiratory viruses (combine with oshá and yerba mansa). Combine with echinacea for bacterial infections and with ocotillo as a prophylactic or after eating a known or suspected food allergen. The leaves and twigs often make a delicious, astringent tea. Drink a flower tea for a week to help resolve boils.

Future harvests

Gather seeds in fall to drop into holes dug up when gathering the root in spring. Search for converging slopes, where natural check dams can form to catch nutrient-rich soils, and transplant or seed in these areas as well.

 Caution

Excessive use may provoke cold sensations.

HERBAL PREPARATIONS

Root Tea
Standard Decoction
Drink 2–4 ounces, up to 3 times per day, or use as a gargle.

Root Tincture
1 part fresh root (or root bark), by weight
2 parts menstruum (75% alcohol,
  15% spring water, 10% glycerin),
  by volume
or
1 part dry root, by weight
5 parts menstruum (50% alcohol,
  40% spring water, 10% glycerin),
  by volume
Take 15–150 drops, up to 5 times per day.

Flowering Stem Tincture
1 part flowering stem (including leaf),
  by weight
2 parts menstruum (90% alcohol,
  10% glycerin), by volume
Take 15–150 drops, up to 5 times per day.

Krameria species

cosahui

PARTS USED whole plant

A cooling and astringent herb with an affinity for the lungs and the blood, rhatany also helps tone up the gums and the whole digestive tract. It's a traditional folk medicine for diabetes and to promote longevity.

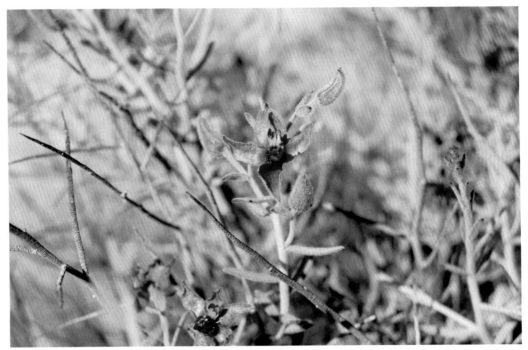

Krameria grayi can be found from the Big Bend of Texas to the deserts of southern California.

How to identify

From a sprawling, nearly prostrate herbaceous perennial (*Krameria lanceolata*) to a rounded shrub over 3 feet tall (*K. grayi*), the various species may appear to be quite different from each other at first glance. Overall they are generally a light grayish green. When leafless, these drought-adapted shrubs may appear to be dead; however, they quickly spring back to life with the return of the rains, putting out tiny, thin, pointed leaves covered with soft hairs. The flowers are all quite similar, reminiscent of an orchid in form, and their scent is divine; they're composed of 5 reddish purple sepals, and their tiny petals of similar color (some modified into oil-secreting glands that feed *Centris* bees) are attached near the ovary. The woolly rounded fruits, with reddish recurved spines, often persist on the plant for some time.

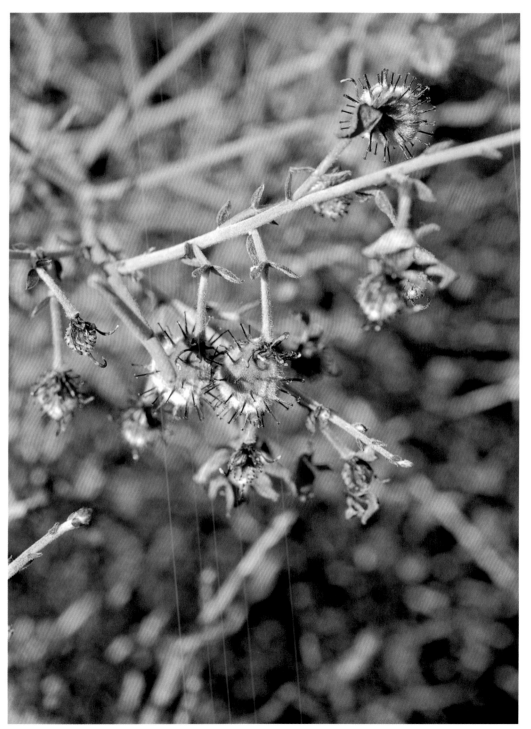

Rhatany's woolly seedpods, which are covered in recurved spines, easily stick to fur or fabric.

Rhatany is thought to be at least partially parasitic on surrounding plants.

Where, when, and how to wildcraft

Rhatany inhabits prairies, oak woodlands, and, in particular, mid- to low-elevation open desert and rocky terrain throughout the Southwest. *Krameria grayi*, white rhatany, and *K. erecta*, littleleaf rhatany, are common from southern Arizona to southern Nevada and California; both are also found in the Chihuahuan desert. *Krameria lanceolata*, trailing rhatany, is abundant in Oklahoma, Texas, and the high plains of Colorado and New Mexico, into southern Arizona. *Krameria ramosissima* is found along the Rio Grande in south Texas. Gather the flowering branches after heavy rains. Roots are best gathered from late winter to early spring, once the ground is well saturated. Practice root coppicing whenever applicable; don't dig up entire plants.

Medicinal uses

Rhatany is a cooling astringent herb with an array of uses. Toning and astringent to the gut mucosa, it relieves boggy gums, sore throat, swollen tonsils, diarrhea, ulcers, hemorrhoids, fissures, prolapse, and bleeding all along the digestive tract. Gargle the herb tea for swollen tonsils or a sore throat. In Mexico, the root tea is renowned for its ability to heal sores within the digestive tract and has been used to treat cancer of the mouth and other digestive organs.

Stories abound of how it has cured intractable cases of pneumonia and tuberculosis. Rhatany root preparations are indicated when an individual takes on a purplish hue and is under respiratory distress. The root tea or tincture can improve the exchange of oxygen in the lungs, alleviating these symptoms.

The Seri use the flower tea for colds and flu, cough, and diarrhea. The root tea, they say, is for diabetes, anemia, and to cleanse the kidneys and the blood. Michael Moore recommends rhatany for cystitis, urethral inflammation, ulcerative colitis, or heavy menstrual bleeding (possibly in combination with chaste tree). The tea is also drunk for arthritis.

Topically, the powdered root is applied to sores, even deep wounds, and as a wash for irritated or infected eyes, or swellings on the body.

Future harvests

Gather only from abundant, healthy stands. Consider introducing this drought-adapted plant into your home landscape.

Caution

Rhatany is rich in tannins, including polyphenols, and if taken in excess may provoke constipation or digestive discomfort. The cold infusions are particularly astringent.

HERBAL PREPARATIONS

Root Tea
Standard Decoction
Drink 1–3 ounces, up to 3 times per day, or use as a gargle; apply topically, as needed.

Herb/Root Tincture
1 part fresh herb (or root) by weight
2 parts menstruum (90% alcohol,
    10% glycerin), by volume
or
1 part dry herb (or root), by weight
5 parts menstruum (50% alcohol,
    40% spring water, 10% glycerin),
    by volume
Take 10–60 drops, up to 4 times per day.

---

rosemary mint

Poliomintha incana
bushmint, eagle medicine
PARTS USED leaf, stem, flower

Rosemary mint makes a delicious tea that is cooling and comforting, acting on the digestive system and calming the nervous system.

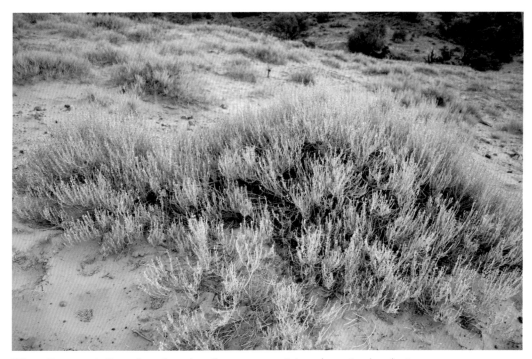

Where it occurs, in its preferred sandy soils, rosemary mint can be quite abundant.

How to identify

This multi-branched herbaceous perennial grows wide and low, to about 40 inches in height. The branches and fresh foliage are aromatic, slender, and upright, with a silvery bluish green appearance. The opposite leaves are thin and wispy, and they attach directly to the stem. The 2-lipped flowers grow in clusters of 1–3 on either side of the stem (1–6 total at each leaf node). The fuzzy calyces are green or purple and end in 5 sharp points of equal length. The lower lip of the corolla is often purple, pink, or lavender with slightly darker splotches dotting the throat.

Where, when, and how to wildcraft

Although rosemary mint is known from 6 states in the Southwest, its range is nonetheless quite limited: it's predominantly found in sandy soil from southern Utah to northern New Mexico. The optimal time for gathering is in the early summer (i.e., the hot, dry

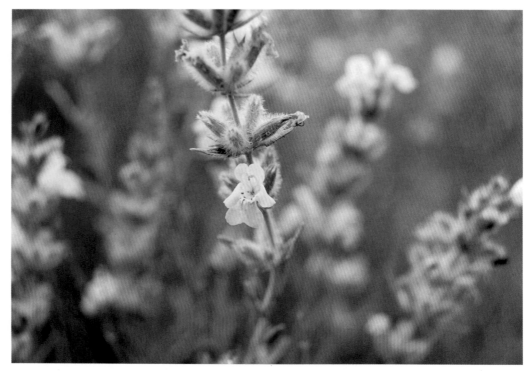

Rosemary mint blooms in late spring and early summer; flowers are white, purple-pink, or lavender, with noticeably fuzzy calyces.

summer), before the summer rains arrive. Clip flowering and leafy stems from healthy, robust plants, then dry in the shade.

Medicinal uses

Rosemary mint makes a delightful tea. It is very mildly bitter, fragrant, and slightly astringent with a cooling, invigorating sensation similar to peppermint. It's also anesthetic to the stomach and is undoubtedly anti-inflammatory (there is no published research on this plant). It is a food plant of the Hopi, so it's quite safe to use internally. Include it in evening tea blends to calm digestive discomfort, uplift the mood, and slightly relax the nervous system.

Traditionally, it's been applied topically to sores and rheumatic joints. Poultices have been applied to earache. Although I have only made tea with this plant, I'm sure a tincture could be applied with similar effect.

In my herbal apprenticeship with Diné healer Emerson Gorman, I learned that before they can be used in ceremony, feathers are cleansed by soaking them overnight in a cold infusion of eagle medicine.

Future harvests

Gather modestly wherever abundant, and consider bringing into your home landscape, in any of our middle to lower desert environments.

HERBAL PREPARATIONS

Herb Tea
Standard Infusion
Drink 2–8 ounces, up to 4 times per day.

---

sage

Salvia species
PARTS USED aerial

Sage possesses a wide array of healing applications. It stimulates the appetite and is useful in viral infections, night sweats, and high fevers.

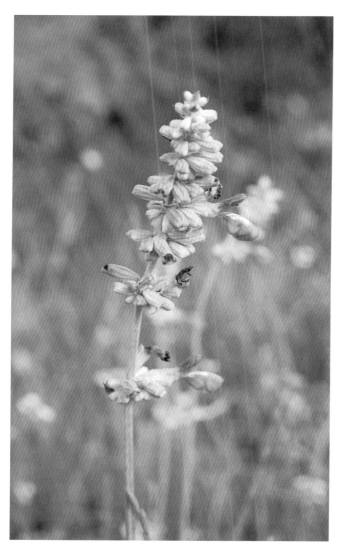

Salvia farinacea, mealy sage, found throughout Texas and into southern New Mexico, is characterized by long, thin shiny leaves contrasted with frosted stems.

How to identify

Many *Salvia* species found within our region have medicinal applications. Sage is in the mint family, so you can count on all plants having square stems and opposite leaves. The corollas, which may be red, blue, light blue, purple, white, or a combination thereof, will have 2 lips, the upper lip straight or arched and the lower often striped. The striated calyx is usually laterally compressed, with 1 or 3 lobes at the top, and 2 deeply cut lobes below. Each of the 2 stamens has a single anther sac. The flowers may appear in whorls, or opposite each other near the ends of the stems. Occasionally, you'll encounter a sage with a woody base (e.g., *S. pinguifolia*), but most of our sages are herbaceous perennials (no woody base).

Where, when, and how to wildcraft

Our sages (some introduced from the Old World, others Southwest natives) can be found in numerous habitats, including desert grasslands, high desert, oak woodlands,

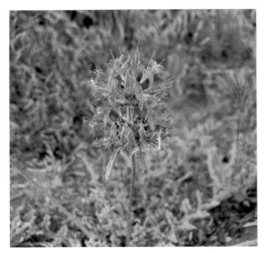

Salvia carduacea, thistle sage, is found in the deserts of southern California.

Hill Country, conifer forests, prairie, and South Texas Plains. Some flower in spring, others from late summer into early autumn. To assist in identification, gather the fresh growth when in flower, then dry in the shade.

Medicinal uses

I have used several *Salvia* species for medicine, including *S. apiana*, white sage, *S. columbariae* (see the chia profile), and *S. texana*, Texas sage. Texas sage, I've discovered, is specific for closed head injuries and other brain traumas. Not only does it relax post-accident musculoskeletal tension, it can also stop hemorrhaging, help reduce inflammation, and improve neuronal connections after the injury. White sage is widely employed as an incense for cleansing an individual or space. The tincture can be particularly relieving to prostate pain associated with swelling, which should improve with short-term usage.

In general, sage tea is strongly stimulating to the appetite. When drunk hot, sage tea promotes secretions, cooling the body through diaphoresis (sweating) and effectively relieving the general lethargy associated with viral infections. When drunk cold, more astringent qualities predominate, which serve to reduce night sweats (also improving other dehydrated conditions), milk flow, and digestive secretions.

Consider a tea or tincture for cough, runny nose, canker sores, sore gums, poison oak, postpartum uterine healing, fever, stomachache, laryngitis, or trembling with tight limbs. Apply topically to relieve dandruff, headache, varicosities, and sore breasts, or take as a hot gargle for a sore throat (combine with honey and lemon). Seed usage is covered under chia.

Future harvests

Gather only from healthy stands. Gather seed when ripe to cast in appropriate areas. Consider introducing native *Salvia* species to the home landscape.

HERBAL PREPARATIONS

Herb Tea
Standard Infusion
Apply topically, as needed, or gargle for sore throat; drink 2–4 ounces, up to 5 times per day.

Tincture
1 part fresh herb, by weight
2 parts menstruum (95% alcohol),
  by volume
or
1 part dry herb, by weight
5 parts menstruum (50% alcohol,
  50% spring water), by volume
Take 20–60 drops, in water, up to 3 times per day.

Herb Vinegar
½ cup fresh herb
8 ounces apple cider vinegar
Combine and apply topically to hot, irritated skin conditions.

Prunella vulgaris
heal all
PARTS USED aerial

A wonderful wound remedy, ready to use while on the trail. Relieving to conditions brought on by hot, humid weather and an excellent sore throat remedy.

How to identify

Found growing close to the ground, self-heal is difficult to see until it's flowering. Look for 1–3 sets of opposite leaves on the short, squared stems, which may possess tiny white hairs. Lanceolate to ovate-oblong leaves are mostly entire, occasionally toothed. The young leaves can resemble skullcap. The bracts, which hold the corolla, are green, purple, or a mix thereof; they can be quite a showy backdrop for the blue-violet, pink, or white corollas, of which the middle lobe of the lower lip is fringed—a distinctive feature. Beige-brown seedheads remain erect on the plant into autumn, at which time the leaves turn light yellow. Use the various subspecies and varieties interchangeably.

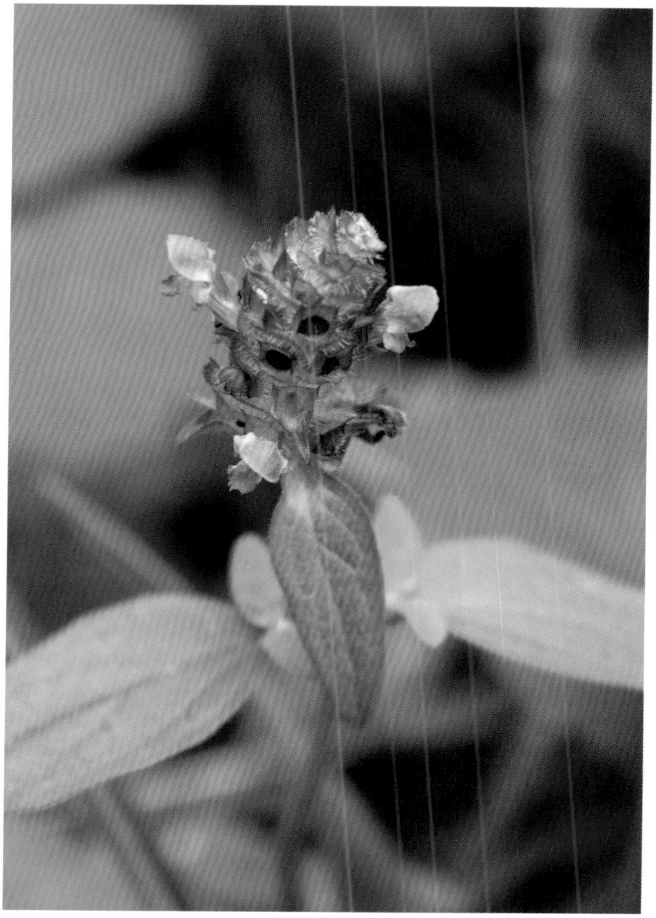

Where, when, and how to wildcraft

Found throughout the moister climes and higher elevations of the western half of our region, as well as its eastern edge, *Prunella* likes disturbed soil, trailsides, creekbeds, meadows, and forest openings. It can be found as a carpet in some locales; gather from these spots, clipping the green summer foliage (mid-summer for

Self-heal inhabits moist places throughout our region. Pictured here in southwestern Colorado.

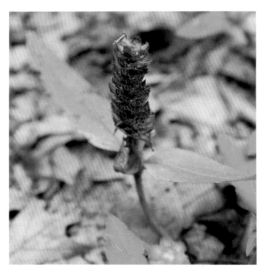

In Chinese medicine, the dry seedhead (here, of ssp. *lanceolata*) is gathered for medicine in autumn.

flowers), or return in mid-autumn to gather the dry seedheads (traditional Chinese herb).

Medicinal uses

The qualities of self-heal are cooling and drying. The tea is markedly astringent with a mildly sweet flavor. The tincture can be more sour and less astringent, making it more useful, taken by itself, on a regular basis. It is one of our primary topical remedies, as a poultice or tea, for poorly healing sores, cuts (it's styptic), scrapes, burns, boils, acne, hemorrhoids, bruises, mouth ulcers; and as an eyewash (reduces intraocular pressure).

It relieves heat throughout the body, or conditions that are worsened or precipitated by hot, humid weather (consider combining topically with creosote bush).

There's been some research into its antiviral activity, reflecting its traditional usage for cold, flu, cough, and chest congestion. Many consider it a top sore throat remedy as a gargle. Traditional Native American and Chinese usage points to its effects on the cardiovascular system, being indicated for high blood pressure with heat present; it is taken as a decoction of the flower spikes.

Taken internally, the tea can strengthen the womb and relieve excessive menses, possibly by alleviating constriction in the liver, where it can be particularly relaxing in its effects. Take the tea, or tincture, for backache, headache, migraine, shortness of breath, nausea, or sinus congestion. Apply a cool wash to soothe a hot, irritated infant.

Future harvests

Although often healthy where it grows, consider introducing it to appropriate new areas by transplanting rhizomes in the fall.

⚠ Caution

The tea is highly astringent: consider adding mallow to tea preparations.

HERBAL PREPARATIONS

Herb Tea
Standard Infusion
Apply topically as a wash, or douche; drink 4-8 ounces, up to 3 times per day, or use as a gargle for sore throat.

Tincture
1 part fresh herb, by weight
2 parts menstruum (95% alcohol),
  by volume
Take 15-60 drops, as needed; apply diluted to the affected area consistently until resolved.

Poultice
Mash up the fresh plant and apply directly to the body, as needed.

Herb Glycerite
1 part fresh herb, by weight
2 parts menstruum (100% vegetable
  glycerin), by volume
Take 1-5ml, as needed.

---

shepherd's purse

Capsella bursa-pastoris
bolsa de pastór
PARTS USED whole plant

With an affinity for the blood and the genitourinary tract, this astringent herb can help prevent bladder stones or resolve blood in the urine, gout, and high blood pressure.

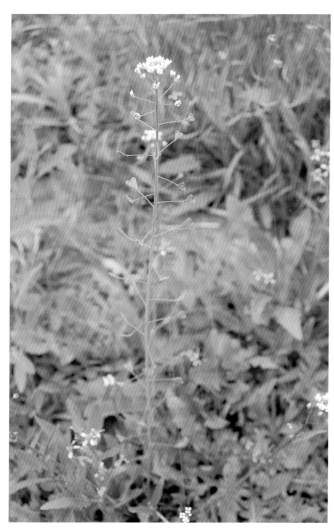

This mustard family plant, an annual "weed" from Europe, is naturalized throughout the Southwest.

How to identify

Shepherd's purse is an annual, 1–2 feet in height, with toothed and pinnately divided, or deeply lobed basal leaves, that look similar to arugula. The central flower stalk develops quickly, producing a few short, clasping leaves. A terminal cluster of white to pinkish flowers, each with 4 petals, leads the way for little heart-shaped seedpods (silicles, to be precise), a clear identifying feature, each on the end of a long green stem radially surrounding the main flowering stem. Shortly after seeds mature, the plant turns light beige.

Where, when, and how to wildcraft

Although it's not everywhere, it can be found just about anywhere. Shepherd's purse inhabits disturbed soils, trailsides, roadsides, agricultural fields, parks, yards, horse corrals, and forest clearings throughout our region, east to west. Appearing in late autumn in our low-elevation and warmer areas, it progresses higher in elevation and further north through the progression of spring. Gather the whole plant when in flower to tincture fresh, or dry the plant for tea or poultice.

Medicinal uses

Any passive discharge may be astringed by shepherd's purse. It has a significant impact on the genitourinary tract as an astringent diuretic, helping to resolve UTIs, the formation of stones, or blood in the urine. In these situations, the tea form is best. It can also be used both topically and internally for bleeding hemorrhoids.

Fresh plant preparations are preferred, but tea, capsule, tincture, and poultice can all be prepared from the recently dry herb. Use internally to relieve diarrhea and enteritis. Pure seed preparations are preferred for gas, bloating, stomach pain, to stimulate digestion, or to treat intestinal worms. A fresh tincture of the tops of the plant in seed is useful in clearing uric acid, thus improving gout. Shepherd's purse has also been used to lower blood pressure and as a general sedative nervine.

Shepherd's purse contains capillary-strengthening rubinosides and vasoconstricting bursinic acid (Moore 1989). The presence of these plant constituents may explain this herb's ability to resolve midcycle bleeding, excessive menstrual flow (bright red), and vaginal discharge. It is a first-aid remedy of repute, employed in birthing to arrest sudden uterine hemorrhaging.

The fresh plant poultice or tea can be used as a topical antimicrobial for skin infections or infected wounds and to alleviate inflammation from bruises, sores, rheumatic pains, and poison ivy rash. A seed poultice is applied as a counterirritant to relieve painful joints or open up chest congestion. The tincture is used similarly, as a topical liniment.

Future harvests

This introduced plant, although often abundant, is not considered invasive. Scatter some seeds in late autumn, within your home landscape.

 Caution

Avoid during pregnancy or in cases of hypotension.

HERBAL PREPARATIONS

Herb Tea
Strong Infusion (fresh or recently dry herb)
Drink 4–8 ounces, as needed.

Tincture
1 part fresh herb, by weight
2 parts menstruum (95% alcohol),
   by volume
or
1 part recently dry herb, by weight
5 parts menstruum (50% alcohol,
   50% spring water), by volume
Take 20–60 drops, as needed.

Poultice
Mash up the fresh plant and apply directly to the body, as needed.

Siberian elm

Ulmus pumila
PARTS USED inner bark

The inner bark of Siberian elm is nutritious and soothing to the digestive tract, making it a great remedy for acid reflux, indigestion, and constipation.

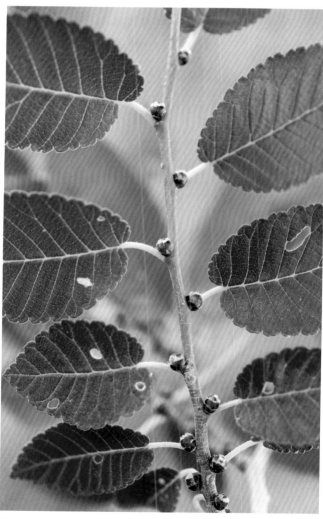

The round, reddish brown leaf buds of Siberian elm, a common "weedy" tree throughout the Southwest, are present from autumn (here, in October) through to the following spring, when they open. Flower buds are very similar but larger.

How to identify

This rapidly growing deciduous tree with an open crown grows up to 100 feet tall in optimal conditions. Flowers open before the leaf buds in early to mid-spring. Leaves are singly serrated, alternate, and entire; they are quintessentially asymmetrical at the base (as in all *Ulmus* species). Round-winged seeds (samaras) occur in clusters along the stems, arising from inconspicuous, greenish female flowers; male flowers occur separately on the same tree. The samaras ripen to a light tan. Bark is somewhat smooth and light gray, becoming rough and furrowed with age. *Ulmus americana*, American elm, *U. crassifolia*, cedar elm, and *U. rubra*, slippery elm, are all naturally occurring within the eastern quarter of our region and may be used similarly.

Where, when, and how to wildcraft

Siberian elm is a drought-resistant shade tree native to Eurasia; it was introduced to North America to serve as a windbreak and is now naturalized throughout the continent. Look to roadsides, old orchards, homesteads, and agricultural areas, where it may become prolific. Gather the bark in spring (before leaf-out), when it is sweetest. See "Gathering Tree Medicine" (page 25) for more guidance.

Medicinal uses

The bark decoction is mildly sweet, mildly astringent, and demulcent, making for an excellent healing and relaxing digestive aid. It is tonifying to digestion, moistening to the digestive tract, and slightly relaxing to

Powdered Elm Bark Lozenges

When young branches are freshly gathered, scrape off their thin outer bark with a knife angled at 90 degrees to the bark; this will reveal a brown inner bark beneath the gray outer bark. Then make circumferential cuts every 12 inches or so along the branch, and peel the bark off in strips. Once fully dry, break the bark down into smaller pieces to fit into a blender. Blend on high for 5–10 seconds to break up the fibrous bark and powder the starches. Pour into a fine sieve and shake out the powder. Retain the bark fiber for decoctions (it will retain its demulcent healing properties).

To make the lozenges, mix approximately equal parts of the powdered bark and organic honey and stir together. If the honey is stiff or cold, warm slightly for better blending. Mix thoroughly until it becomes a stiff dough. Quickly roll out into long, ½-inch-thick rolls on wax paper, and cut into pieces ½–¾ inches long. Once cut, toss in more powdered bark (may also use licorice root powder) to coat the lozenges and prevent them from sticking to each other. Take orally, as needed; melt and apply directly to sores or poorly healing wounds.

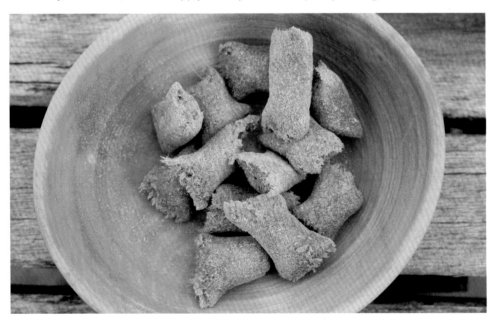

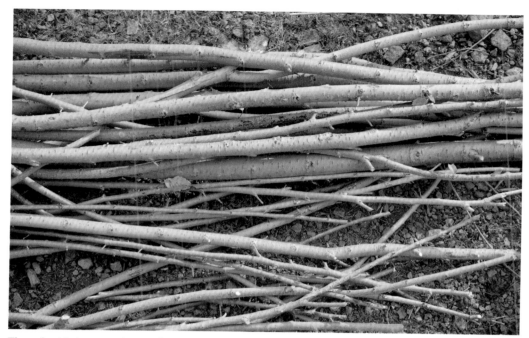

These freshly harvested young branches of Siberian elm still have relatively smooth bark.

the nervous system, making it an excellent remedy for acid reflux. Use this nourishing herb in soups, smoothies, and tea blends to help recover from surgeries affecting the digestive system or long-standing illness, or as a postpartum recovery aid.

Apply the tea topically to soothe burns, wounds, boils, or irritated skin. Traditionally, bark poultices of other *Ulmus* species have been applied to broken bones and sprains. Elm bark lozenges make a wonderful cold and flu season "treat" for children. They soothe and coat the mucous membranes of the throat, aiding in the body's immune response.

Future harvests

This naturalized "invasive" is calling itself to our attention. Take note of it now, gather abundantly but with respect, and share with friends.

HERBAL PREPARATIONS

Inner Bark Tea
Standard Decoction
Drink 2–8 ounces, as needed; apply topically to soothe irritated skin.

silk tassel

Garrya flavescens, G. *ovata*, G. *wrightii*
cuauchichic
PARTS USED bark, leaf, stem

A reliable antispasmodic, acting on larger smooth muscle cramps, and a first-rate remedy for dysentery as well. While relaxing the liver and enhancing blood flow, it stimulates digestion.

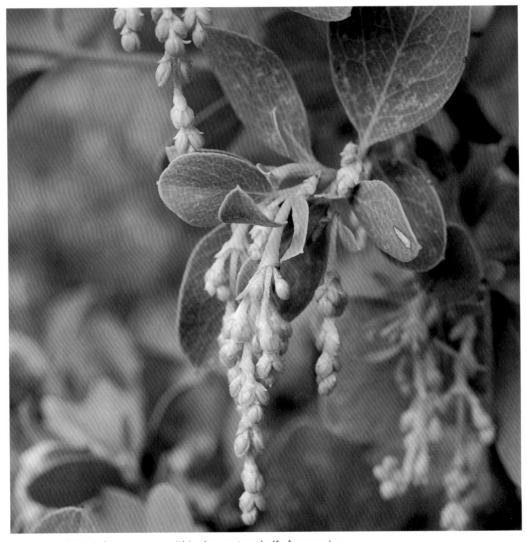

Garrya wrightii inhabits canyons within the western half of our region.

How to identify

This evergreen shrub (up to 20 feet in height) has an overall light grayish green look (*Garrya ovata* is a brighter, shiny green). Mostly multi-branched, occasionally single-trunked in the understory. Bark is light gray to grayish brown. Leaves are simple, opposite, and entire—thick, stiff, and covered in soft fuzzy hairs (*G. flavescens*), sometimes with wavy or curling margins (*G. ovata*). On new growth, the yellowish green stems (*G. wrightii*) or pinkish red stems (*G. flavescens, G. ovata*) stand out against the green leaves. The inflorescences are dangling (much longer in *G. flavescens*) and covered with fine silky hairs (hence the common name); male and female flowers are on separate plants. The fruits of *G. wrightii* are dark purple, brown, or black; those of *G. flavescens* and *G. ovata* are dark blue. The bitter fruits can persist into winter.

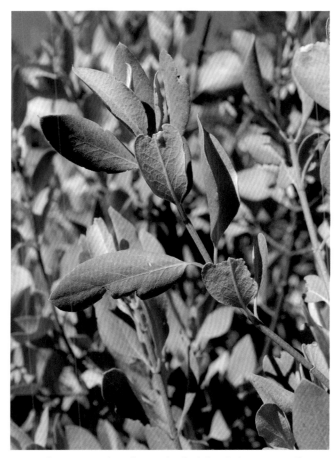

Garrya flavescens, ashy silk tassel, which has lighter, more silvery leaves and reddish stems, occurs primarily within the western third of our region.

Where, when, and how to wildcraft

Silk tassel occurs throughout our region. *Garrya flavescens*, ashy silk tassel, extends into southwestern Utah, southern Nevada, and southern California, as well as Arizona, where *G. wrightii* is abundant. From New Mexico to the Texas Hill Country one may find *G. ovata*. Look to mid-elevation canyons, boulder-strewn north-facing hillsides, and riparian woodlands. Although leaves are present year-round, they are best gathered in spring or autumn, once ample rains have arrived. Stem bark preparations, although considerably stronger, can be prepared from autumn or winter harvests of the smooth-barked branches.

Medicinal uses

This is not our most diverse medicine, but what silk tassel can do is particularly important. As an astringent for the digestive tract, it makes a very useful remedy for acute diarrhea or dysentery. Nibble the fresh leaf in the field, or take the tea or tincture internally. The strong bitter flavor of the leaf stimulates digestive secretions and may also slightly drop the blood sugar; it can induce hunger quite rapidly.

Despite its tonifying effects on the digestive tract and the salivary apparatus, it provides a significant relaxing effect to the liver. This relaxation enhances blood distribution throughout the body, possibly also generating a subsequent bile release. For some people (who are directly experiencing liver tension), this effect may bring a sense of ease and quiet, even to the point of inducing sleep. Others (perhaps those with ample relaxation already present in the liver) may feel lethargic, slightly nauseous, or develop a frontal headache as a result of taking even a small dose. When applied to the right person, this relaxant effect can relieve menstrual cramping and other large muscle spasm throughout the body. Traditionally, the leaf tea has been used for colds, stomachaches, and as a laxative.

Future harvests
Gather modestly and with respect from large stands, and this hearty shrub will continue to provide medicine for many years to come.

 Caution

Avoid during pregnancy. If the liver-relaxing effects produce a frontal headache or nausea, simply discontinue usage. In all cases, short-term use is best.

HERBAL PREPARATIONS

Leaf and Stem Tea
Cold Infusion
Drink 2–3 ounces, up to 4 times per day.

Leaf and Stem Tincture
1 part fresh leaf and stem, by weight
2 parts menstruum (95% alcohol),
  by volume
or
1 part dry leaf and stem, by weight
5 parts menstruum (50% alcohol,
  50% spring water), by volume
Take 45–60 drops, up to 5 times per day; can be taken in teaspoon doses, 3 times per day, for dysentery.

Scutellaria species

PARTS USED aerial

A cooling sedative that relaxes and restores the nerves, it is specific for exhaustion, depression, anxiety, and insomnia. It relaxes muscular tension and relieves nerve pain.

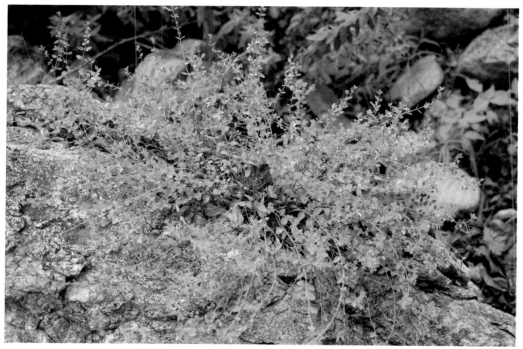

The dryland *Scutellaria potosina*, Mexican skullcap, is found across southern Arizona and southern New Mexico.

How to identify

This scentless mint family perennial comes in two basic types within our region. One is taller (up to 3 feet), thinner, and more upright, with no woody base, and grows in moist soils (marsh type). The second grows in shorter compact mounds with smaller leaves on relatively drier, exposed soils, and develops a woody base with age (dryland type). The former grows from slender rhizomes, the latter from somewhat fleshier roots covered in thin brown bark. All our skullcaps have opposite leaves with square stems and violet-blue and white flowers emerging from the leaf axils, in pairs. The oft-hairy corolla possesses a hooded upper lobe, a broad lower lobe, and a pair of smaller side lobes with the tube extending upward from the rimmed calyx, which is often magenta or reddish purple. Each seedpod looks like two mouths calling for food.

Where, when, and how to wildcraft

Our marsh skullcap type grows in or very near water from the headwaters of our great rivers, high in the conifer forests, to the seasonally wet prairies and grasslands of our northeastern quadrant. More abundant within our region, the dryland skullcap type grows in the Hill Country, the high plains of Texas and Oklahoma, oak woodlands, desert grassland riparian areas, or sandy grasslands of the South Texas Plains. Depending on the type of skullcap and location, flowering skullcap can be found from mid-spring to early autumn. The dry herb quickly degrades, so gather fresh (taking no more than 2 in 10 flowering stems from any one plant) and dry in the shade for use within 6 months.

Medicinal uses

A wonderful remedy for all things nervous system and brain-related, use the tincture for insomnia, irritability or depression with exhaustion, anxiety, or disturbed sleep with agitation and exhaustion. Also helpful for restoring the nerve tissue in acute injury and relaxing tension to promote better blood flow to the area. Consider skullcap with any form of spasm, tic, tremor, or convulsion. Its antispasmodic action is specific for the genitourinary tract, for pain associated with the female reproductive system, or breast pain. This nervine is safe to use during pregnancy (combine with passionflower). The tea is useful, but the dry herb quickly degrades, so gather fresh and dry in the shade for use within 6 months. Apply the tea directly to gums to soothe teething infants. Consider combining with other relaxants (oreganillo, beebalm, desert lavender, wild mint) to improve its bitter flavor.

Future harvests

Gather modestly, from large stands only.

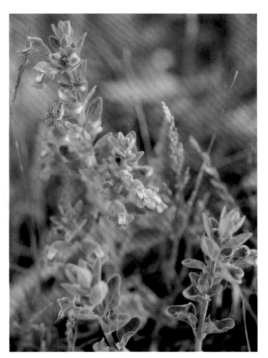

Scutellaria drummondii is very common in central Texas.

HERBAL PREPARATIONS

Herb Tea
Standard Infusion
Drink 2–6 ounces, up to 3 times per day; use recently dry herb only.

Tincture
1 part fresh herb, by weight
2 parts menstruum (95% alcohol), by volume
or
1 part recently dry herb, by weight
5 parts menstruum (50% alcohol, 50% spring water), by volume
Take 25 drops to 4ml, up to 3 times per day.

snakeweed

Gutierrezia species
escoba de la víbora, broom snakeweed
PARTS USED aerial

Ubiquitous and highly useful, snakeweed can be used both topically and internally as a tea to relieve pain.

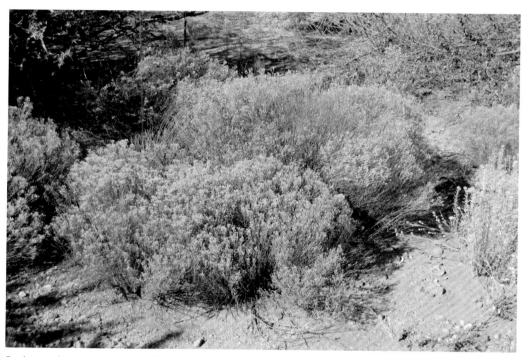

Snakeweed is a common and often abundant shrub throughout the Southwest.

How to identify

This herbaceous perennial, 10–24 inches tall, forms a rounded mound of thin, wispy green stems and linear leaves atop grayish brown woody stems from previous years' growth. The resinous leaves have a piney scent and are very thin, disappearing from the bottom of the stems as the plant produces small inflorescences of ray and disc flowers (3–8 per head), subtended by 2–3 rows of whitish phyllaries with green tips. As with other aster family plants, the tiny beige achenes are scarcely visible upon maturation.

Where, when, and how to wildcraft

Snakeweed is found throughout our region in nearly every habitat up to about 7,000 feet, primarily on exposed slopes and open plains, or rangeland. The related *Amphiachyris dracunculoides*, prairie broomweed, is found from eastern New Mexico into Texas and Oklahoma. Make bundles of the flowering stems in late summer/early autumn and hang up to dry in the shade.

Medicinal uses

Snakeweed is a traditional pain remedy that's been used for generations throughout the Southwest, both topically and internally. The topical application of any *Gutierrezia* species is safe and useful for musculoskeletal pain and injuries. It has also been used for stomachache, excessive menstruation, and to relieve cuts, scrapes, and rashes. As a bath tea, you can't go wrong. Its relatively mild aromatics seep in through the skin, working on aches and pains as well as mild skin infections. Bring to boil a small bundle of chopped, dry herb in a quart of water and add to bath water while sipping on a half cup of the tea.

Future harvests

This plant is incredibly abundant on historically overgrazed lands and too ubiquitous to pass up. It is best we make friends with it.

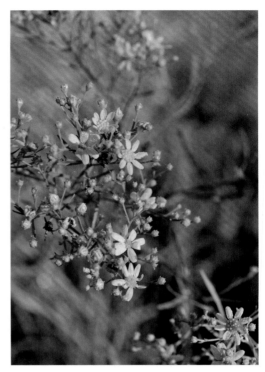

Amphiachyris dracunculoides, abundant within the eastern half of our region, can be used (topically) very similarly to snakeweed.

> ### HERBAL PREPARATIONS
>
> **Herb Tea**
> Standard Decoction
> *Drink 2–4 ounces, 1–2 times per day; take a bath in the tea.*

Sonchus asper, S. oleraceus, S. arvensis
chinita
PARTS USED whole plant

This highly nutritious and cooling plant works on the liver, digestive tract,
reproductive system, nervous system, lungs, and more. Too abundant to pass up,
you should get to know this weedy plant as both food and medicine.

How to identify
Basal leaves with sparsely or intensely spined margins and red to pinkish midribs appear in whorls, arising from a lightly colored taproot. The leaves of the annual or biennial *Sonchus asper*, spiny sow thistle, are usually deeply cut to the midrib with rather prickly margins. A hollow flower stalk ascends in the first or second year; the alternate stem leaves curve beautifully where they clasp the stem. *Sonchus arvensis* is a perennial herb, flowering each year. The bright yellow composite flowers appear in corymbs, relatively spread-out clusters of 4–12 inflorescences, each flower beginning as a squared-off barrel-like bud and ending in the shape of a Hershey's Kiss once the inflorescence has closed. Plants exude a milky latex when broken. The white and densely fuzzy spherical seedheads are easily blown from the plant.

The leaves of *Sonchus asper* can be deeply or shallowly lobed; the leaf margins are covered in tiny spines, and the midrib is often reddish purple.

Where, when, and how to wildcraft
Sow thistle is nearly everywhere, with three different species, naturalized from Europe, spread throughout our region. Look to disturbed soils, waste places, pastures and lawns, at

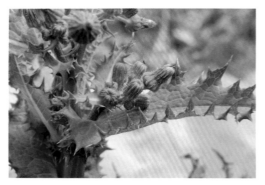

The flower buds of *Sonchus asper* have tiny spines along the phyllaries.

all elevations. Beginning in late autumn/early winter, the leaves sprout in our warmest environments. This plant can be found in the higher elevations and colder climates by mid- to late spring. Either gather the root and basal leaves prior to flowering and consume, or dry for tea, or harvest the entire flowering plant for fresh tincture.

Medicinal uses

Although often considered as an alternative to dandelion, sow thistle stands alone in its attributes. From anti-quorum sensing, to bitter tonic, to insulin-sensitizing, the plant is broadly active. There's a strong resonance with the liver, but the digestive and respiratory systems are two areas of considerable focus in the traditional applications of the herb. The leaf tea or tincture stimulates digestion, bringing enhanced blood flow to the digestive organs while allaying inflammation and calming the nervous system.

Many cultures have successfully applied it for bronchitis, asthma, cough, and pertussis. Consider using it to relieve delayed menses that presents with concurrent liver constriction. It has been used to reduce postpartum inflammation in the womb and the perineum, and is applied to the gums to relieve the pain from teething. Consider it a pain reliever and relaxing remedy for musculoskeletal injuries.

Future harvests

This abundant, naturalized plant is practically begging us to gather it.

HERBAL PREPARATIONS

Leaf Tea
Standard Infusion
Drink 2–4 ounces, up to 3 times per day; apply to the affected area consistently until resolved.

Root Tea
Standard Decoction
Drink 2–4 ounces, up to 3 times per day.

Whole Plant Tincture
1 part fresh plant, by weight
2 parts menstruum (95% alcohol),
  by volume
or
1 part dry plant, by weight
5 parts menstruum (50% alcohol,
  50% spring water), by volume
Take 10–30 drops, up to 4 times per day.

Aralia racemosa
PARTS USED leaf, root, fruit

This warming and stimulating herb enhances the senses and lifts the mood. It is pain-relieving, clears mucus from the lungs, and can help to rejuvenate the lungs, kidneys, and adrenals.

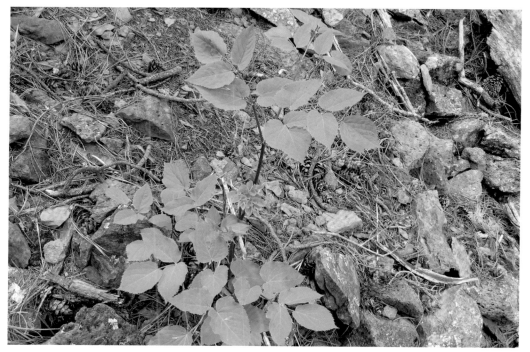

Spikenard is a forest-dwelling plant that enjoys shady, moist areas at mid- to high elevations in the Southwest.

How to identify

Each spring, this elegant herbaceous perennial grows to a height of 3–6 feet on stout green and red stems, each with a deep groove running along one side. Deep green leaves are once or twice compound, with delicate, doubly serrated leaflets in groups of 3–5. The small, 5-petaled creamy white flowers, arrayed in umbrella-like terminal racemes, mature into reddish purple berries. The aromatic roots (which look something like swollen, rheumatic fingers or limbs) have a smooth, thin, light brown bark.

Where, when, and how to wildcraft

Spikenard inhabits moist and shady canyons and mountainsides at 4,000–9,000 feet in the western half of our region. Gather the leaves prior to flowering (mid- to late summer). Gather the fruits in late summer (birds

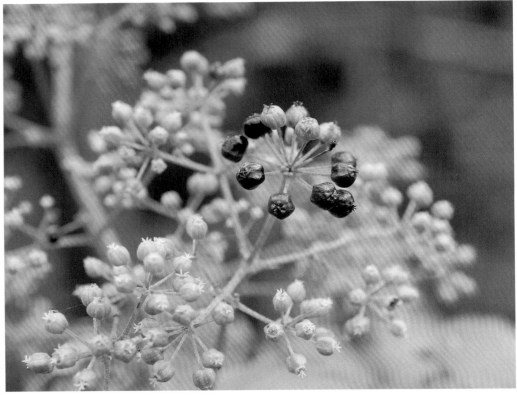

Spikenard berries ripen in late summer. They are a favorite food of local birds, so gather only a modest amount, if any at all.

also relish them). Dig roots (see page 26) in early autumn when the leaves begin to turn yellow, or in spring, just as the leaves begin to emerge from the ground.

Medicinal uses

Spikenard acts on the human body in various ways, once ingested: it immediately opens up and stimulates respiration, enhances digestion and eliminative functions, calms the mind and senses, and supports neuro-endocrine function. The continued use of the herb, on its own or in formulation, has a cumulative effect in the nourishment of our whole being.

The leaves are best used as a tea or tincture to help dissolve phlegm and improve the blood supply to the lungs; this stimulates immune function in chronic or acute respiratory conditions. Chew on the fresh aromatic leaf stalk for a little pick-me-up while sauntering through the forest. Leaf preparations are more warm and dry in nature than other parts of the plant.

The berries, eaten fresh or tinctured, have a mood-altering effect. This sweet and pungent remedy can allay anxiety, lift depression, and improve our relationship with the world around us by opening our senses, when dampened, and bringing a greater sense of ease when distraught or tense.

Conversely, the root preparations ground and strengthen us, connecting us to our deepest reserves and unlocking the tension that often covers a reservoir of stamina lying deep within us. Through continued use, the root preparations (tea, tincture, or honey infusion) are restorative to the neuroendocrine system, in particular the adrenals and nervous system, imbuing a sense of deep calm and sense of strength in the face of adversity (combine with American licorice). Root preparations are moistening in nature. Additionally, spikenard is a remedy for mastitis and cystitis.

Future harvests

This plant grows in very sensitive areas within our region. Spend several seasons observing it within its habitat before digging any roots, and dig only in areas of abundance. Practice root coppicing and replant root crowns to maintain or spread the population. In years of ample production, berries can be carried to appropriate areas for planting before the first snow.

HERBAL PREPARATIONS

Leaf Tea
Standard Infusion
Drink 4–8 ounces, up to 4 times per day.

Root Tea
Standard Decoction or Cold Infusion
Drink 2–4 ounces, up to 4 times per day.

Root/Leaf/Berry Tincture
1 part fresh root, leaf, or berry, by weight
2 parts menstruum (95% alcohol; 75% for
  berries), by volume
or
1 part dry root or leaf, by weight
5 parts menstruum (50% alcohol,
  50% spring water), by volume
Take 10–60 drops, up to 4 times per day; take 20–60 drops of leaf tincture.

Root Honey Infusion
*Follow directions on page 37; take
½–1 teaspoon, as needed.*

Melilotus species

trébol

PARTS USED aerial

Wonderfully aromatic upon drying, sweet clover is a beautiful addition to herbal tea blends even in very small amounts. It possesses pain-relieving qualities that can be applied both topically and internally.

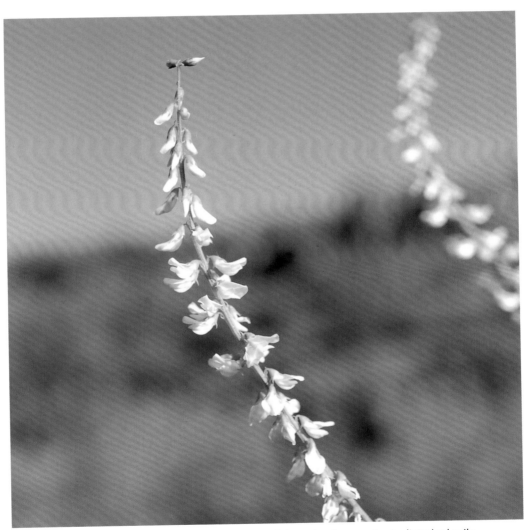

Melilotus albus is a naturalized plant from Europe found throughout our region in disturbed soils. The tiny white flowers on terminal racemes resemble those of American licorice, a pea family relative.

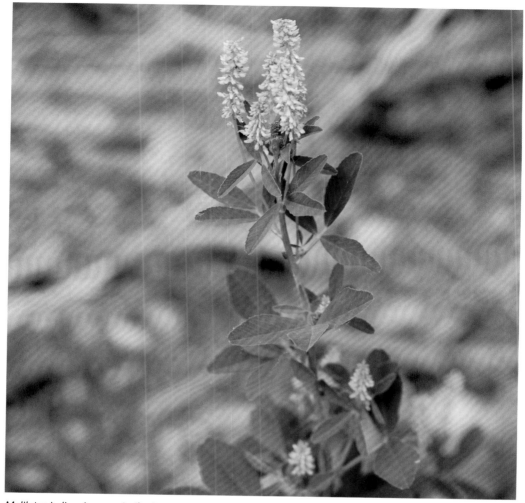

Melilotus indicus is very similar in appearance to *M. officinalis* but is shorter and occurs at lower elevations.

How to identify

These weedy, naturalized pea family plants are annual (or biennial) and upright, with 3-part leaves. The smooth, flat leaflets are oblong to lance-shaped with tiny teeth along the margin. *Melilotus albus*, white sweet clover, produces abundant racemes of white pea flowers with the classic keel, long banner, and somewhat tucked-in wings; *M. officinalis*, yellow sweet clover, has yellow flowers. White and yellow sweet clover are usually 3–5 feet tall, to 7 feet or more in optimal conditions. *Melilotus indicus*, sour sweet clover, an annual, is under 3 feet tall.

Where, when, and how to wildcraft

Sweet clover is found throughout our region except for the driest desert locations. These are all plants of waste places—roadsides, washes, fields, floodplains, agricultural fields—as well as pristine meadows. Sour sweet clover flowers in mid-spring at lower, warmer elevations. In the eastern portion of our region, white and yellow sweet clover can also flower in mid-spring; in the western half, just past mid-summer (white first, then yellow). In large stands, pull the whole stem from the ground, or prune back near the ground. Hang to dry in the shade.

Medicinal uses

Adding sweet clover to almost any herbal tea blend will improve its flavor. Simply add a ¼ teaspoon per cup of tea, or 5–10%, by weight, of your formula. It has been used for centuries, bundled and hung within a home, to lend its sweet scent and relieve any dank aroma; the scent of the plant grows stronger upon drying.

Traditionally, a tea or poultice of the plant is applied to the skin to relieve inflammatory conditions and ulcers, and pain in the joints or abdomen. Taken internally, it is warming and stimulating; it has been used to relieve nerve pain, the chill in viral illnesses, and headache or pain resulting from a cold, congested state. The herb has an affinity for the female reproductive system and can relieve pain when taken internally; consider it whenever a part of the body is tender to the touch and cold in sensation.

Future harvests

These plants, all nonnative, may be considered invasive (or at least "weedy") in your area; they are likely to survive wherever they are established. Nevertheless, gather respectfully, taking no more than you need.

 Caution

Avoid when taking blood-thinning medications.

HERBAL PREPARATIONS

Herb Tea
Standard Infusion
Drink 2–4 ounces, up to 3 times per day; apply topically, as needed.

Herb Acetum
1 part fresh herb, by weight
4 parts menstruum (apple cider vinegar), by volume
Take ½–2 teaspoons, daily; apply topically, as needed.

Cirsium species and *Carduus nutans*
PARTS USED whole plant

Both food and medicine, thistle is often associated with tenacity. Plants are widespread and abundant, offering a wide variety of simple solutions for our ills.

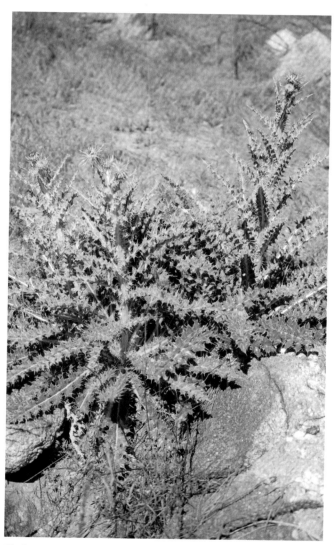

Cirsium neomexicanum flowers in early to mid-spring in the western half of our region. Note the red tips of the upper phyllaries in the center of unopened flower buds.

How to identify

Both native and nonnative *Cirsium* species (about 24 in our region) as well as *Carduus nutans*, musk thistle, are included here as one entry. Although slightly variable in their appearance, and to some extent their application, there is much interchangeability in their medicinal applications. Plants may be annual, biennial, or perennial forms, but what they all share in common are bristly-tipped, lobed or toothed alternate leaves (some have spiny stems as well), the absence of ray flowers, spine-tipped phyllaries (just below the open flower head), and a fluffy seedhead of pappus. Flowers can be red, purple, pink, yellow, or white. Roots may be fleshy or fibrous taproots, or, less commonly, interconnected rhizomes. Thistles range from about 18 inches to nearly 7 feet tall.

Where, when, and how to wildcraft

Thistles are widespread in the Southwest, skipping only some of our lowest and driest desert areas (below 1,000 feet). Find the basal rosettes throughout

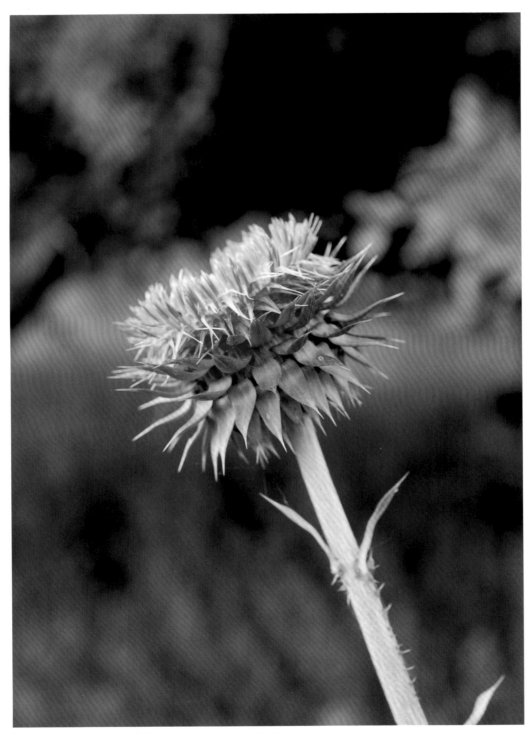

Carduus nutans is a naturalized "invasive" thistle with a long tradition of use throughout Eurasia.

the winter (or early spring at our highest, snow-covered elevations) to identify before they begin flowering. Some traditional preparations call for just the root, which is gathered before the plant goes to flower. Otherwise, gathering the entire plant, when flowering, works well for making tincture. Outside of the flowering season, in large stands, dig the whole plant for tea or tincture, or simply trim several basal leaves and leave the root to leaf out again, and flower later on.

Medicinal uses

There is a global legacy of using thistles for medicine but a very limited practice for the same in North America. Several species have been used as an eyewash, poulticed onto aching joints, or as a topical wash for sores, burns, or bleeding hemorrhoids.

Cirsium ochrocentrum, yellow spine thistle, is applied as a root decoction for diabetes by the Zuni in New Mexico. *Carduus nutans* is used similarly in Turkey, in addition to being a bitter tonic. Scientific studies have shown various thistles to be antioxidant, and to improve fatty liver disease by improving lipid metabolism; this corresponds to the traditional uses of sow thistle and other related, bitter thistle-types such as artichoke and milk thistle.

As a nutritious food plant, thistle is very safe for internal consumption. I find the whole plant tincture of *Cirsium neomexicanum*, cardo santo, to be a wonderful restorative for the stomach and spleen, grounding and sweet in its flavor yet also astringent. Several *Cirsium* species have been used to allay stomachache and improve digestion.

Future harvests

Gather roots only from large stands of 25 plants or more. Gather seeds from early summer to autumn and sow them whenever you dig up roots.

HERBAL PREPARATIONS

Root Tea
Standard Decoction
Drink 4–8 ounces, up to 3 times per day; apply topically, as needed.

Whole Plant Tincture
1 part fresh plant, by weight
2 parts menstruum (95% alcohol),
  by volume
Take 10–40 drops, up to 4 times per day.

Bidens species
aceitilla, Spanish needles
PARTS USED aerial

*This cooling, antimicrobial and antiviral herb with hepatoprotective and
neuroprotective properties occurs abundantly in our region. Useful for allergies,
arthritis, UTIs, and asthma, this relatively unknown plant awaits your discovery.*

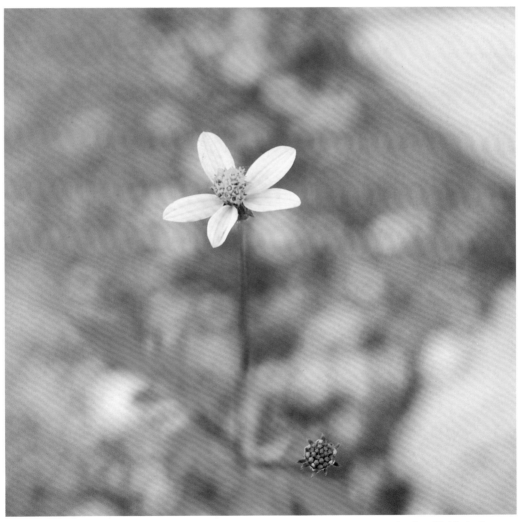

Bidens pilosa, the most commonly known and thoroughly studied species, is easily identifiable by its
white petals.

How to identify

All *Bidens* species are 1–4 feet tall, with opposite, toothed or divided leaves. The solitary inflorescences are composed of yellow to yellowish orange disc flowers and yellow or white (*B. pilosa*) ray flowers (ray flowers sometimes absent) that are followed by their namesake, the tic-like seeds. Barbed awns (1–8 per seed) enable dispersal; by autumn, as our pant legs collect vast amounts of the seeds, plants never fail to grab our attention. Most are annuals, and they grow in large colonies, covering the ground, but there are exceptions; *B. aurea*, for example, is an herbaceous perennial. Tickseed leaves are highly variable—and similar in appearance to many other, unrelated plants. The yellow disc flowers and opposite leaves, along with the "tic seed," are instrumental in identification, until you know your local stands well.

Where, when, and how to wildcraft

Look for tickseed in any disturbed ground, particularly silt deposits along watercourses beneath the shade of trees. Both native and introduced *Bidens* species occur throughout our region, except in the lowest, driest deserts (and only sparsely in the high plains of Texas and New Mexico). Everywhere else is fair game. The optimal time for harvest varies, depending on the location. This is determined by when the plant forms its flower buds, beginning mid- to late summer and extending into early autumn at the higher elevations. Gather entire annual plants, but trim only the flowering tips of perennials. Prepare the fresh plant tincture immediately, or save some herb to dry for tea.

Medicinal uses

Very little ethnobotanical evidence is available for this plant. Yet through the efforts of herbalists Michael Moore and Stephen Harrod

Buhner and scientific researchers across the globe, it has been shown to have a wide array of important effects. Tickseed is effective against numerous pathogens, including herpes (HSV-1 and HSV-2), *E. coli*, *Bacillus*, *Cytomegalovirus*, *Plasmodium*, *Salmonella*, *Staphylococcus*, *Candida albicans*, *Mycobacterium tuberculosis*, *Leishmania amazonensis*, *Serratia marcescens*, *Pseudomonas aeruginosa*, *Enterococcus faecalis*, *Klebsiella pneumoniae*, and *Shigella flexneri*. Fresh leaves have the most potent antimicrobial effects (attributed to the presence of polyacetylenes). Make a fresh plant tincture, in the flower bud stage for optimal strength. Buhner (2014) recommends application of the fresh leaf juice to infectious wounds and eye infections; it may also be taken internally. Consider the fresh plant tincture for any respiratory or urinary tract infection, as well as genitourinary inflammation.

Michael Moore first noted that tickseed leaf tea is a mucous membrane tonic, with effects similar to those of yerba mansa. The tea is also anti-inflammatory, antiallergenic, toning to the mucous membranes, immune-modulating, and heat-clearing. The heat-clearing effect corroborates other cultures' traditional applications of the tea for both acute infections and reducing swelling and inflammation. Consider tickseed for UTIs unresponsive to antibiotics.

Tickseed has an affinity for the red blood cells, protecting them from the effects of certain infections, such as the tick-borne Babesia (often concurrent with Lyme disease). It's also hepatoprotective and neuroprotective.

In addition to reducing histamine release, thereby improving hay fever, the tea or tincture may also allay asthma, cough, and whooping cough, or serve as an expectorant. It has traditionally been used for rheumatism, arthritis, sprains, and bruises, both topically and internally.

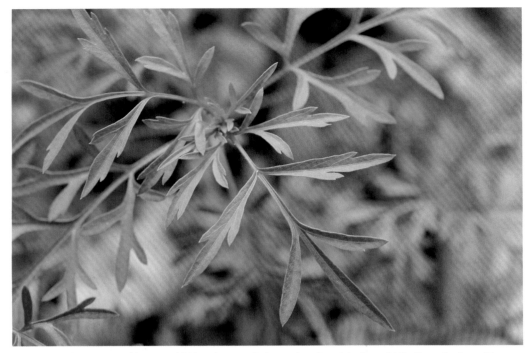

The pinnately compound leaves of *Bidens leptocephala* are deeply cut to the midrib. It can be found from the Big Bend westward into the mountains of central Arizona.

In my experience, what tickseed does, it often does slowly and subtly. It is capable of affecting our entire system, addressing complex, systemic issues as well as organ- and tissue-specific conditions or infections.

Future harvests

Just wait for summer rains to arrive. Tickseed spreads tenaciously, and some have come to regret introducing it and its barbed seeds into their home landscape.

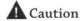 Caution

Consult a health practitioner if you are taking blood-sugar-lowering medications.

HERBAL PREPARATIONS

Herb Tea
Strong Cold Infusion
Drink 8 ounces, 2–4 times per day.

Tincture
1 part fresh herb in bud, by weight
2 parts menstruum (95% alcohol),
  by volume
Take 30–90 drops, up to 4 times per day; double or triple dosage for acute infections, up to 6 times per day; high dosage can continue for up to 4 weeks.

Ailanthus altissima
PARTS USED bark, leaf, fruit

This bitter remedy is useful for giardia and other gut parasites as well as inflammatory asthma and other histamine-related conditions.

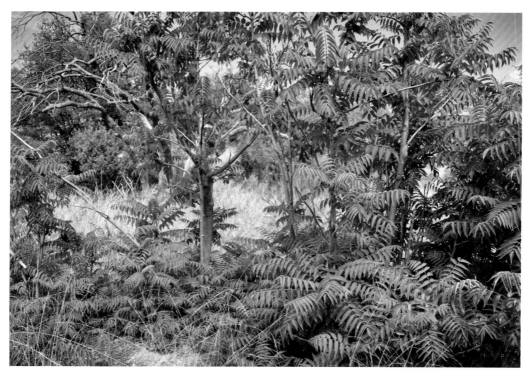

Tree of heaven, naturalized in the Southwest, is a common sight in disturbed ground in urban areas and old mining towns.

How to identify

Fast-growing and deciduous, tree of heaven reproduces vegetatively from creeping rhizomes, creating large colonies in disturbed areas. It normally reaches a height of less than 30 feet but may grow taller. Its winter twigs are thick and smooth, light brown to light gray. Long, hanging, pinnately compound leaves are reddish copper-brown at first, with either an odd or even number of serrated, entire leaflets. The leaflets have a pair of teeth near the base, or coarse teeth along the margin. The central leaf stem is yellowish green to reddish brown. The shape and size of the leaves resemble those of walnut, which is unrelated botanically. The winged samaras have twisted ends; they appear in late summer and change from yellowish green or red to tan upon maturity. A commonly described trait of this tree is

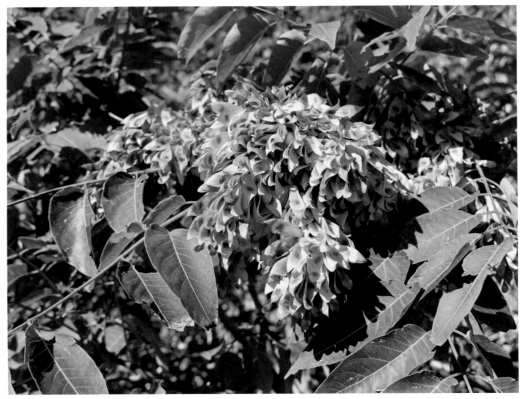

The large clusters of greenish yellow seeds (samaras) that develop at the branch tips make it easy to identify tree of heaven from late summer through winter.

its pungent odor, with a hint of peanuts and rotted food mixed in.

Where, when, and how to wildcraft

Roadsides, waste places, canyons, and old homesteads are where you'll likely find this tree, which was introduced from China in the 1700s and is now widely naturalized across the continent. It is less common within the eastern third of our region. Gather the bark in early spring before leaves emerge, or in late autumn once the leaves have fallen. The seeds and leaves can be gathered whenever present.

Medicinal uses

This overlooked and often-cursed tree is a complex and potent medicinal plant. As with goatbush and several other of its simarouba family relatives, its tincture is quite bitter. Bark or leaf preparations treat giardia and other intestinal parasites. It's a reputed remedy for dysentery resulting from acute intestinal infections, and it relaxes griping. Bark tincture has been shown to be a stronger medicine than that of the leaf.

It's also useful with asthma or other high-histamine conditions. Eclectic physicians applied the tincture for palpitations and as an antispasmodic (it inhibits cAMP-dependent phosphodiesterase) in doses of 5–20 drops. It has a significant cardiac effect, increasing the volume of blood pumped through the heart and the heart rate. It also dilates the vasculature, reducing blood pressure. Research indicates it is effective against Epstein-Barr virus as well as *Plasmodium falciparum*, the infectious agent in malaria. Related species (e.g., *Ailanthus excelsa*) are used for malarial infections in India and Southeast Asia. The seeds can be used similarly to the inner bark.

The leaves are applied topically to treat boils, abscesses, acne, and skin rashes. Recent research suggests that a bark tincture administered topically may be useful against multi-drug resistant bacteria; it is certainly worth exploring whether a tea of the bark, fruit, or leaves may topically address MDRB infections.

Future harvests

Giggle, or sneer, depending on your disposition.

 Caution

May cause skin irritation. Excessive doses may cause nausea, vomiting, or dizziness; symptoms resolve quickly upon stopping the dosage. Start at the low end of the suggested dosage range and work up, as needed.

HERBAL PREPARATIONS

Bark/Leaf/Seed Tea
Standard Infusion
Apply topically, as needed; drink 1–4 ounces, up to 5 times per day.

Bark Tincture
1 part dry, powdered inner bark, by weight
5 parts menstruum (50% alcohol,
  50% spring water), by volume
Take only 5–20 drops if you have a cardiovascular condition; otherwise, take 30–90 drops, up to 3 times per day; for giardia, take ½–1 teaspoon, 3 times per day.

Viola species

PARTS USED aerial

Beautiful violet works on the whole body, enlivening our detoxification pathways, calming the nervous system, and supporting the heart (hence another of its common names, heartsease).

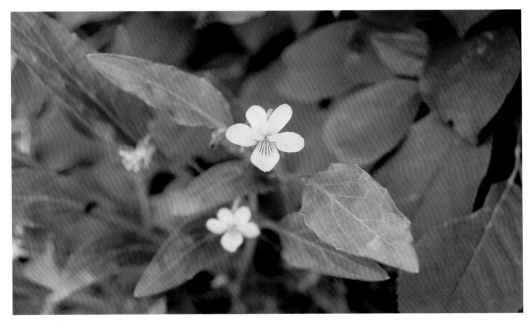

Viola nuttallii is a perennial herb that flowers in early summer in the Southwest.

How to identify

All our violets are low-growing herbaceous annuals or perennials, generally less than 10 inches tall. The simple basal leaves arise from a vertical rootstock or from creeping rhizomes. The leaves may have tiny teeth or scalloping along the margins and are often heart- or kidney-shaped at the base, coming to an elongated (or short) point. The showy spring flowers—in various shades of blue, purple, and violet (of course) but also white (*Viola canadensis*) and yellow (*V. nuttallii*)—are 5-lobed (2 upright, 2 spreading, 1 downward), with the lower lobe often possessing veins of purple, and bearded at the throat; they often emerge directly from the ground and may be infertile. The closed, self-fertilizing flowers of autumn (sometimes kept within the soil) produce the viable seed. The 3-valved seedpods burst open upon ripening, ejecting the seeds some distance.

Where, when, and how to wildcraft

Violet inhabits shady, moist locations throughout the Southwest. In the western two-thirds of our region, it can be found at

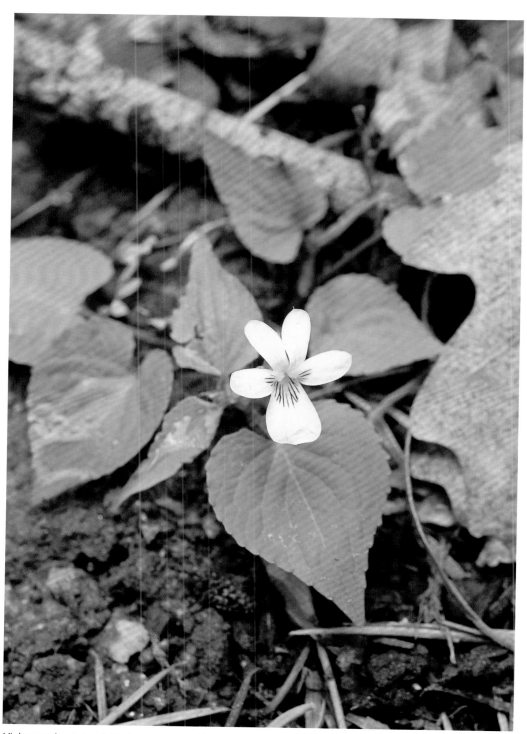

Viola canadensis is relatively common in high-elevation conifer forests in moist, shady areas.

mid- to high elevations along streambeds, in canyons, and under the canopy of trees in oak woodlands or conifer forests. It is largely absent from the high plains and high desert areas along our eastern edge. Get to know your local populations of violet before gathering; if found in abundance, gather the leaves and flowers to tincture fresh or dry for tea. Dried violet should be used within several months.

Medicinal uses

Violet is a pleasant alterative with mild yet profound effects throughout the body. Its mildly acrid flavor indicates its ability to disperse congestion, but violet is not irritating in the way that queen's root, walnut, and other acrid alteratives may be. Cooling and moistening, it calms and sedates hot, irritated tissues.

Use as a tea, alone or with other herbs, to soothe and cool irritated mucous membranes of the digestive tract, respiratory system, or genitourinary tract. Externally, place a fomentation over sore eyes or the temples to relieve a headache that is hot and tense.

Derived from a tea of the flowers, violet syrup is a classic remedy for calming and quieting a child's cough. It's also used as a spring tonic and to treat colds.

Traditionally classed as a "blood purifier," violet is used internally for skin eruptions, acne, and catarrhal (phlegm) conditions of the lungs and intestines. Continual application of the hot tea may help to resolve boils (combine with red root flowers or Bermudagrass). The tea or tincture can be used to relieve bladder pain, joint pain, or stomachache, as the plant contains analgesic properties.

Future harvests

These plants can be part of a robust and vibrant ecosystem. Gather immature seedpods and store in a paper bag; once seedpods open, scatter the seeds in an appropriate area in late autumn.

HERBAL PREPARATIONS

Herb Tea
Standard Infusion
Drink 2–5 ounces, up to 3 times per day; apply topically, as needed.

Whole Plant Tincture
1 part fresh plant, by weight
2 parts menstruum (95% alcohol),
  by volume
Take ½–2 teaspoons, up to 3 times per day.

walnut

Juglans major, J. microcarpa, J. nigra
nogál
PARTS USED bark, leaf, fruit

A traditional digestive remedy, useful for both constipation and diarrhea. The warming aromatic flavor of the leaf tea produces an appealing beverage with healing qualities.

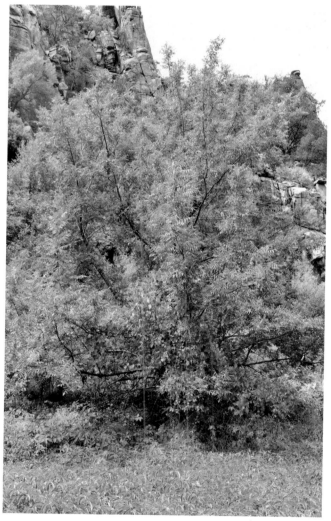

Arizona black walnut, *Juglans major*, mid-summer, in a lush, green canyon setting.

How to identify

Our main species, *Juglans major*, is a tall tree (occasionally shrub) of desert riparian habitats. It has alternate, aromatic, pinnately compound leaves with 9–15 serrated leaflets; both leaflet midribs and rachis (where all the leaflets attach) are yellow. With age, its grayish brown bark becomes furrowed in long strips. Both male and female flowers are green. The female flowers, tucked in neatly at the center of terminal leaf clusters, may ripen into walnuts. Walnut leaves turn black rapidly upon freezing, whether in spring, autumn, or early winter.

Where, when, and how to wildcraft

Look to riparian areas and moist canyons throughout most of our region (generally absent from the South Texas Plains and high desert). The leaves begin appearing in mid-spring and are best gathered before fruits form in late spring. Gather entire leaves, but leave some leaves in each cluster. Be careful not

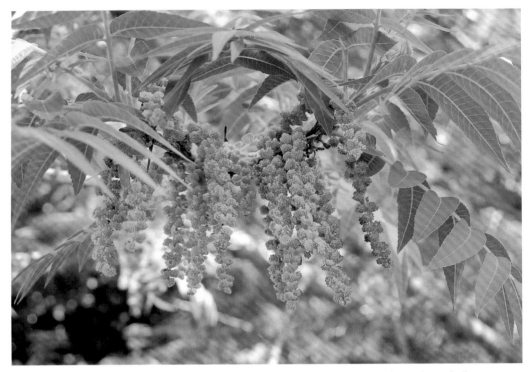

Walnut is monoecious: separate male and female flowers occur on the same plant. The male flowers (pictured here) are in long racemes and occur along the branch, behind the terminal leaf clusters and small female flowers.

to injure the female flowers when gathering. The immature fruits (green hulls) are medicinal and can be gathered in early summer, just as the first ripened fruits begin to turn black and fall off; pull and twist the green fruits off the tree when encountered near ground level, or climb the tree to harvest them. Gather ripe nuts from the ground; they fall from the tree in mid- to late summer.

Medicinal uses

The leaf preparations are milder than those of the bark, and the hull preparations are significantly more astringent and reserved for fungal infections (and gut parasites), used both topically and internally. Walnut's alterative actions stimulate the slow and gentle release of bile from the liver and tone the intestines,

making it an excellent remedy for slow digestion or dampness and heat in the lower intestines (combine with ash). Use the leaf tea (1 cup) or tincture (30 drops) as a laxative; double the dosage for chronic diarrhea.

Use walnut preparations topically and internally for inflammatory skin conditions that are long-standing and eruptive (acne, eczema, impetigo, lichen planus). In stubborn cases, use bark preparations.

Recent research points to the internal use of walnut tincture to improve weight loss and lower blood pressure. Male flower preparations have been shown to reduce ultraviolet radiation damage to the skin.

Walnuts are considered brain food and have been shown to improve mood (particularly in males). The oils and polyphenols

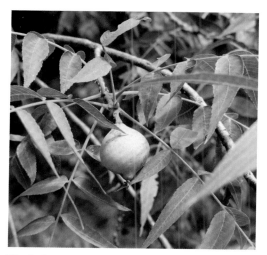

The fruits appear within the terminal leaf clusters. We gather them when green, just before they mature and turn black, to use as medicine. Green fruit can also be found on the ground.

present in the nut are used to treat BPH and improve lipid profiles. The use of walnut as an internal medicine has ranged from eating them directly to ingesting an extraction of the nut in the form of a tea or tincture.

Future harvests

Again, try not to disturb the female flowers when gathering leaves, so the nuts have a chance of maturing.

 Caution

Use disposable gloves when processing the fresh hulls for tincture, as they readily stain skin a brownish yellow, with a duration of several weeks.

Eriogonum species
colita de ratón, skeleton weed, sulphur flower
PARTS USED whole plant

These versatile plants can be found in great abundance. Use wild buckwheat to relieve lumbar pain in pregnancy or as a postpartum bath. The tea is drunk to strengthen the blood and the heart, or relieve headache or stomachache.

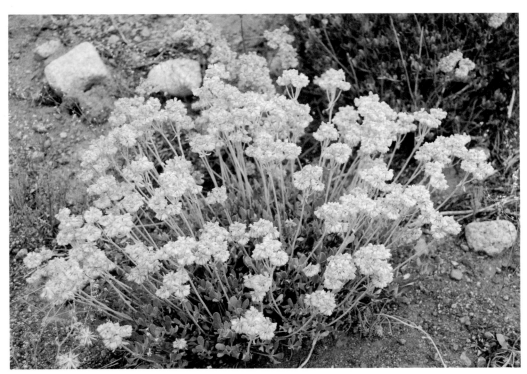

Wild buckwheat flowers may be white, pink, yellow, or a combination thereof. Pictured here is *Eriogonum umbellatum*; it and other yellow-flowered species are also known as sulphur flower.

How to identify

The name of the genus helps describe the general appearance of its plants (*erion*, "woolly"; *gonu*, "knee," "joint"). Many of our *Eriogonum* species (3 dozen are known to have been used as medicine) do have a woolly covering on their leaves and stems, lending a grayish green appearance, but those with jointed stems are rarely seen in the Southwest. These plants are both annual and woody perennials within our region, with a great deal of diversity among them. The tiny white, pink, or yellow flowers occur in clusters, which may be spread open or relatively tight. Leaves are entire, often a bit fuzzy, and may be round, ovate, lance-shaped, or

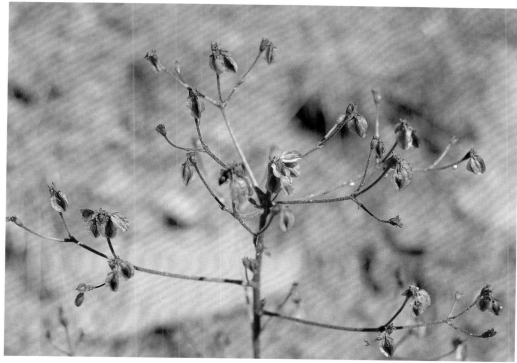

The seeds of *Eriogonum alatum* are clearly winged.

spatula-shaped. The seedheads (and often the whole plant) turn brick-red upon maturity. *Eriogonum fasciculatum*, flattop buckwheat, a wide, rounded shrub about 2 feet in height, is commonly used in landscaping. *Eriogonum alatum*, winged buckwheat, is tall (up to 6 feet) and thin, with winged seedpods that resemble those of curly dock (a knotweed family relative).

Where, when, and how to wildcraft

Wild buckwheat is scattered throughout our region but is particularly common and abundant in the western half. Look to rocky hillsides, disturbed ground, desert washes, desert grasslands, canyons, oak and juniper woodlands, and clearings in conifer forests. The plant can be gathered somewhere within our region nearly all year long; even the dead, standing annuals have value in winter. Begin

by gathering some leaves and flowers. Once the species name is confirmed, explore the local ethnobotany (or ask a local herbalist or ethnobotanist) to learn how that particular species was used.

Medicinal uses

These diverse plants were used in equally diverse ways by indigenous inhabitants of the Southwest. Several species were not only food plants but were used during pregnancy and postpartum, and given to infants, thus they are exceptionally safe to use. The whole plant can be used as a tea, internally, or topically as a poultice, fomentation, oil infusion, salve, or powder.

A primary internal application is for inflammation and stagnation in the genito-urinary tract. Michael Moore emphasized wild buckwheat's use as an anti-inflammatory and antioxidant tonic for the kidneys. The whole plant can be used, but the flowers are most appropriate for the kidneys, lending a soothing and cleansing action. Root preparations are used to reduce lumbar pain in pregnancy, ease labor pains, and relieve pain postpartum. The whole plant can be used as a sitz bath to promote healing and relieve pain, postpartum. The tea is used to relieve premenstrual symptoms (pain, bloating, cramping). The whole plant decoction is traditionally used as a blood tonic, to relieve stomachache, to treat tuberculosis, coughs, colds, and high blood pressure, and to prevent hardening of the arteries. The leaf infusion is drunk to relieve stomachache, headache, and other pains. In addition to soothing and cleansing the kidneys, drink the flower tea to relieve food poisoning and to promote heart health (root tea, as well).

Topically, this plant is highly useful. Apply a wash to burns, cuts, wounds, acne, rashes, bites, and stings. The powdered plant too works well on wounds and bites. It is pain-relieving as a wash or poultice for swollen, rheumatic joints and was traditionally used for leg paralysis, backache, and snakebite, both topically and internally. The flower infusion makes an effective eyewash. Chewing on the plant or a root decoction tones and tightens the gums and cleanses the mouth.

Diné healer Emerson Gorman uses several *Eriogonum* species for internal bleeding and for lung and kidney disorders.

Future harvests

Gather with respect, from large stands of common species only.

HERBAL PREPARATIONS

Root/Leaf Tea
Standard Decoction
Drink 2–4 ounces, up to 3 times per day.

Flowering Tips Tea
Standard Infusion
Drink 2–8 ounces, up to 3 times per day.

---

wild mint

Mentha arvensis
poleo, Indian mint
PARTS USED aerial

Aromatic and stimulating, the pungent flavor of wild mint is uplifting to the mood and anesthetic to digestive discomforts. Use wild mint to relieve respiratory viruses or to enhance the effects of antibiotic pharmaceuticals.

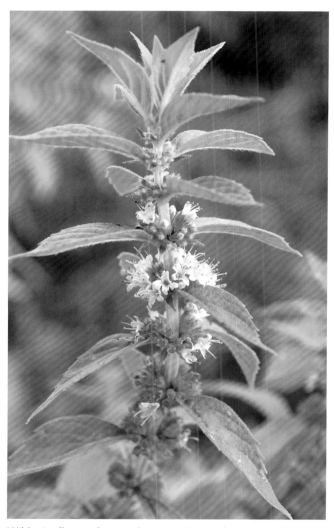

Wild mint flowers from mid-summer into early autumn, along high-elevation creeks in the western half of our region.

How to identify

This native perennial herb grows erect from creeping rhizomes, or stolons. A quintessential mint family plant, the stems are square in cross section, the foliage quite aromatic, and the white to pink flowers (corollas) are 2-lipped. The whorls of flowers occur at the leaf nodes, not above the leaves as in spearmint, peppermint, and other *Mentha* species. The opposite leaves are lance-shaped, with serrated margins. Other than aroma and fine differences in leaf appearance, very little distinguishes young wild mint plants from young skullcaps in early to mid-summer, and plants often grow intermingled or right next to each other. You'll find that serrations on wild mint leaves diminish toward the base, whereas serrations on skullcap leaves diminish toward the tip.

Where, when, and how to wildcraft

Wild mint is quite limited in the Southwest, confined to mid- to high-elevation waterways in the western half of our region and nearly absent from Texas and Oklahoma. Begin looking for wild mint in early summer, and gather when coming into flower in late summer/early autumn. Michael Moore has pointed out that the location within a stand, its growing condition, and the shape of the plant can be indicators for the type of chemical cocktail you may anticipate from a wild mint. Lush plants in the center of large stands are more likely to have more menthol; therefore, they taste better (at least some think so) and are more pain-relieving and antispasmodic in their effects. Peripheral, somewhat solitary, or many-branched specimens are more likely to have a pulegone scent (think pennyroyal) and perhaps more carvone (spearmint). Spearmint-scented plants are best utilized for a pleasant-tasting tea; those with pulegone, for herpes infections and applications involving the female reproductive system. Gather from large stands on alluvial floodplains or adjacent to streams and rivers by clipping at the base of the stem. Tincture the herb fresh, or dry for tea.

Medicinal uses

Wild mint is more pungent than garden mints but is nonetheless safe for use with infants and children. It was traditionally employed as a hot tea in cases of fever, colds, flu, stomachache, gas and bloating, nausea, indigestion, and diarrhea. The tincture may be useful with nausea during pregnancy (combine with algerita leaf).

Although normally considered for digestive issues, wild mint makes a wonderful remedy for acute respiratory conditions, including severe cough, sharp pain upon breathing, constricted breathing, and pneumonia and other bacterial lung infections. Topical preparations (poultice, tea, tincture)

can be applied to aching joints, arthritis, or swollen rheumatic joints. Crushed leaf poultices can be applied to the head for headache or to insect bites to reduce pain and itching.

If taking a pharmaceutical antifungal, consider taking the tincture of wild mint, concurrently, as it has been shown to potentiate the antifungal's effects. Similar potentiating effects are found when taken with antibiotics, also reducing resistance to the antibiotics.

Future harvests

Wild mint spreads itself via flooding. When gathering the herb, simply drop segments of its creeping rhizome into the river, so they may be deposited in rich, moist soil somewhere downstream. These short segments can also be transplanted to a home garden, but beware—mint can take over wide areas.

Caution

Avoid during pregnancy (potentially high pulegone content). Excessive use of mint tea may cause incontinence; decrease usage to restore normal bladder function.

HERBAL PREPARATIONS

Herb Tea
Standard Infusion
Drink 2–8 ounces, up to 4 times per day.

Tincture
1 part fresh herb, by weight
2 parts menstruum (95% alcohol),
   by volume
or
1 part dry herb, by weight
5 parts menstruum (50% alcohol,
   50% spring water), by volume
Take 10–30 drops, as needed; best to use
within 2 years as aromatics can break down.

wild oregano

Monarda fistulosa var. *menthifolia, M. citriodora* var. *austromontana, M. pectinata*

orégano de la sierra, beebalm

PARTS USED aerial

This warming herb increases circulation, thus relieving pain, promoting diges-tion, and stimulating sweating when feverish. Through its effects on the nervous system, it relaxes the mind and restores proper function throughout the body.

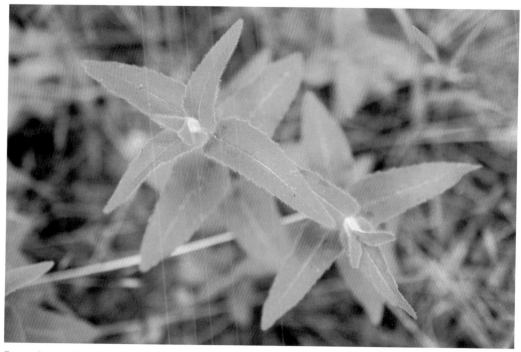

Even when no flowers are present, wild oregano can be identified by the serrated leaf edge, the reddish midrib, and the distinctive spicy scent of its leaves.

How to identify

Wild oregano is a fragrant herbaceous perennial growing on stiff, square-sided stems with opposite, serrated, and entire leaves on short petioles. The pink to purple corollas of *Monarda fistulosa* var. *menthifolia* normally occur in a single whorl (occasion-ally 2–3 whorls) in a terminal cluster; *M.* *citriodora* and *M. pectinata* produce multiple flower clusters along the stem. Large bracts just beneath the flower clusters are occa-sionally tinged pink. Plants often leaf out again from the base in early to mid-autumn. Rounded mounds of beige seedheads help identify wild oregano from late autumn to early spring. A unique "citronella" race

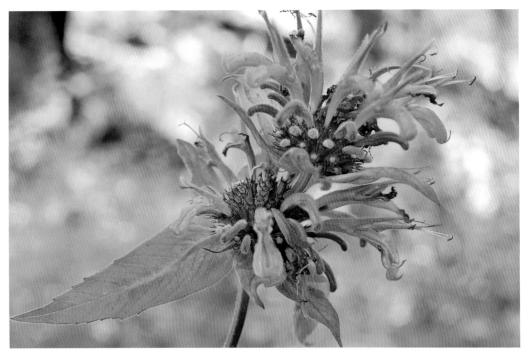

The upper lip of the corolla is narrow, and the lower lip is broad.

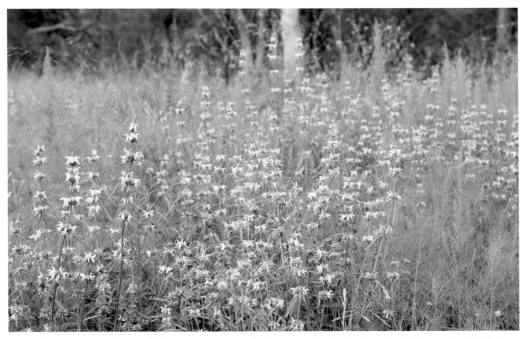

Monarda pectinata, orégano de la sierra, can grow in large stands in pine forests in the western half of our region.

occurs randomly throughout the Southwest; it is obvious when encountered—its smell permeates the air.

Where, when, and how to wildcraft

Find wild oregano at mid- to high elevations throughout Arizona, New Mexico, southern Utah, southern Colorado, southwestern Texas, and sporadically along the eastern edge of our region into southwestern Oklahoma. A widespread herb that prefers rich, moist, shady soils predominantly along creeks, it has adapted to be relatively drought tolerant in the western half of our region. Wild oregano emerges in mid-spring and flowers at the height of summer, usually preceding the summer rains (occasionally following) in the western half of our region. Cut the entire flowering stem, as both the stems and leaves are useful food and medicine. Alternatively, the top cluster can be plucked from each stem of Monarda citriodora and M. pectinata, leaving 1–4 clusters on the plant.

Gather the terminal flower clusters of M. fistulosa var. menthifolia only from very large stands that can sustain the loss of dozens of flower clusters (meaning hundreds of flower clusters are present).

Medicinal uses

Wild oregano offers a unique combination of warmth and stimulation, as well as relaxing qualities. Specifically, the tea has a calming effect on the nervous system while also benefiting digestion. "Citronella" wild oregano, similar in taste to lemongrass, is less oregano-and-thyme spicy and particularly relaxing to the nervous system; it acts upon the heart/mind in a beautiful way, essentially preparing the body for healing.

Thanks at least in part to its high thymol content, the hot tea or tincture can be taken to stimulate the immune response during acute viral or bacterial infections of the respiratory, digestive, or genitourinary tracts. It is also a traditional arthritis remedy, applied

Wild Oregano Flower Honey Infusion

Gather only a small portion of wild oregano flowering stems in a given area, and make efforts to expand your gathering area to reduce the pressure on a single population. Once stems are gathered, pluck off enough flower clusters to fill a jar (5–6 ounces is enough for a quart canning jar). Fill the jar about a third full with whole, fresh flower clusters. Then pour some honey over the top. Add more flowers, then more honey. It may at first appear as if the honey won't cover the flowers, but the flowers gradually shrink. There will be plenty of honey (some 3 cups total in a quart canning jar). Screw the lid tightly onto the canning jar. As the flowers rise to the top, turn the jar upside down to allow for the honey to cascade back over the flowers. Repeat daily over a 2-month period, as the flowers macerate out of direct sunlight. To strain out the flowers, place some cheesecloth over a kitchen strainer fitted to a bowl with space underneath to receive the honey. Pour the contents of the jar onto the cheesecloth, and let the honey strain through the cloth for several hours. Reserve the honey in dark jars; it will last for years. Just a bit of wild oregano honey will abruptly halt a dry cough; take ½ teaspoon to 1 tablespoon, as needed. The honey-soaked flowers can be chewed for relief of a sore throat, laryngitis, or the onset of a cold; they can also be made into a cup of hot tea.

topically and taken internally. *Monarda* species have been used to address kidney ailments and may be of benefit in conditions characterized by histamine release.

A honey infusion of the flowers, which has a lovely sweet and spicy flavor, is a remarkable remedy for a dry cough or sore throat. Apply the honey infusion to slow-healing wounds or staph infections to speed up healing.

Future harvests

Gather sensibly from large stands after walking the area to assess the local population. Bring seedheads into areas that seem suitable for propagation.

HERBAL PREPARATIONS

Herb Tea
Standard Infusion
Drink 2–8 ounces, up to 4 times per day; gargle for sore throat.

Tincture
1 part fresh herb, by weight
2 parts menstruum (95% alcohol), by
  volume
or
1 part dry herb, by weight
5 parts menstruum (50% alcohol,
  50% spring water), by volume
Take 10–30 drops, up to 4 times per day.

wild tobacco

Nicotiana species

tabaquito

PARTS USED aerial

Smoked for individual prayer and during ceremony, wild tobacco is also used topically for painful joints, hemorrhoids, eczema, boils, or dandruff.

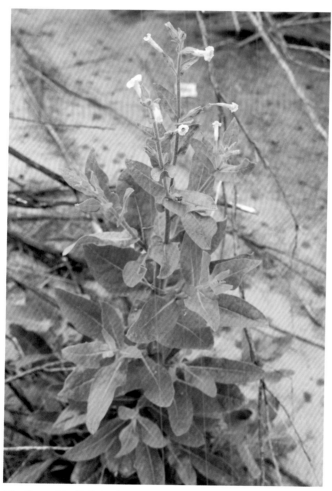

Nicotiana obtusifolia is abundant in drainages throughout our low and high desert habitats. It's sticky to the touch.

How to identify

Our several native species in the Southwest are relatively similar in appearance, especially upon flowering. *Nicotiana glauca*, tree tobacco, a naturalized plant from South America, has a distinctly different presentation: it has much larger bluish green, smooth leaves on long petioles, yellow flowers with non-distinct petals—and can grow to a height of 15 feet, with a trunk 3–6 inches in diameter. All other species are 2–5 feet tall and produce lance to linear, or oblong basal leaves covered with glands, making them greasy/sticky to the touch. The pointed leaves, often with undulating or wavy margins, clasp the flowering stalk. The white corollas have 5 lobes (rounded or pointed) with shorter or longer tubes (narrow or fuller) and 5 calyx teeth, which may be equal or unequal in length. Upon maturity, small black seeds can be found in the egg-shaped beige capsules.

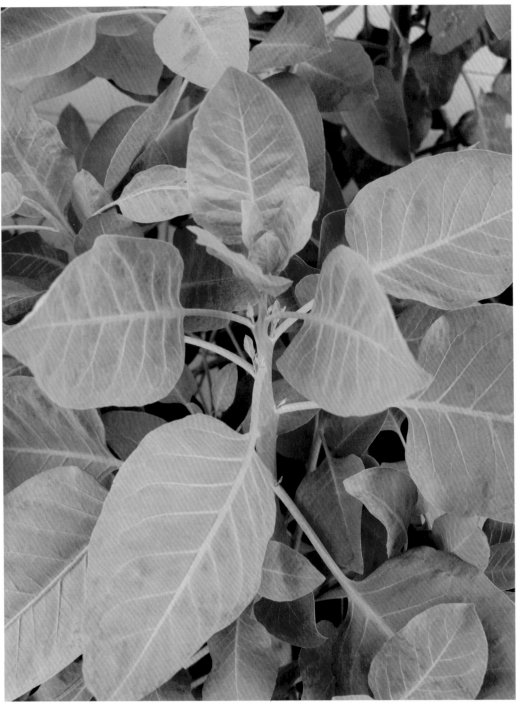

Nicotiana glauca produces the largest leaves of all our local species; they make excellent poultices for swollen, inflamed conditions.

Where, when, and how to wildcraft

Wild tobacco grows throughout our region with the exception of the high plains and much of the high desert. Look for it in the disturbed soils of roadsides and desert washes, ravines, canyons, and sandy slopes; in the lower desert, wild tobacco may also be found amid large, dark boulders from autumn to mid-spring. Tree tobacco is particularly fond of disturbed areas along the southern tier of our region. The leaves can be gathered whenever present, nearly year-round. When in flower, cut the flowering stems back and dry in the shade for topical applications (oil infusion, fomentations). Process the leaves in the sun to reduce their potency.

Medicinal uses

Wild tobacco is still widely used—primarily smoked—by the indigenous peoples of the Southwest during sweat lodges and other ceremonies. It is smoked during personal prayer in order to clear malevolent forces and to ensure a journey is begun in a positive way. Tobacco represents honor and respect. It is often offered to someone as a gift or gesture of respect, as when, for example, one approaches an esteemed healer for assistance.

Smoking the dried and pulverized leaves and stems was a treatment for headache, colds, asthma, cough, or other lung afflictions. The smoke also be blown into the ear for earaches. The powdered leaves were often moistened and dried in the sun as small cakes or balls to be smoked later.

The aerial portions of the plant (leaves, stems, flowers, seeds) are made into a tea by decoction and applied to injured or aching joints as a soak or fomentation. This tea is also used as a wash for hives, eczema, dandruff, or other skin irritations. A fresh plant poultice is used similarly. One can directly apply the dried and powdered plant to sores or suppurating wounds. Test the skin with a small amount of the tea first, and wait 20 minutes to watch for potential adverse reactions. The seeds were also pulverized and applied to rheumatic swellings.

Future harvests

Tobacco grows abundantly where conditions are to its liking. Consider scattering seed over disturbed soil in late autumn or mid-spring to cultivate a new patch.

 Caution

Do not consume tobacco internally. It is toxic and may bring on abrupt nausea. Traditionally, tobacco was used as an emetic in very small amounts.

HERBAL PREPARATIONS

Wash or Fomentation
Standard Decoction
Apply topically, as needed, to painful joints, injuries, insect bites, stings, etc.

Oil Infusion
Dry leaves and flowers and prepare as alcohol intermediate oil infusion (see page 38); use topically on painful joints or combine with yarrow oil for hemorrhoids.

---

willow

Salix species
saúce
PARTS USED bark, leaf, stem, flower

A classic herbal remedy used for its pain-relieving qualities by both humans and animals alike.

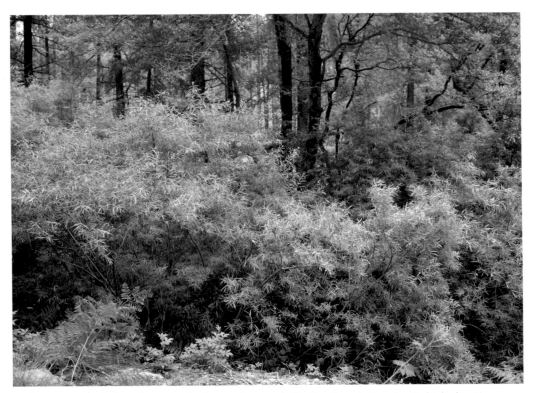

Willow is commonly found as a shrub along waterways in the Southwest, from low to high elevations. Pictured here is *Salix lasiolepis*, arroyo willow, growing along a creek at over 8,000 feet in Arizona.

How to identify

Like all willows, our Southwest species are taxonomically challenging and highly variable, growing into shrubby or tall trees with entire, alternate leaves of variable shapes—the classic form being lance-shaped with a long, narrow tip. Willow leaves have smooth or toothed margins and are most often smooth and shiny. Flowers may emerge before, during, or after leafing out (least common), depending on the species. But one may easily recognize the fuzzy willow flower buds in spring, as they all resemble the "pussy willows" sold by florists. Aiding in winter identification, willow leaf buds have one scale (separating it from cottonwood,

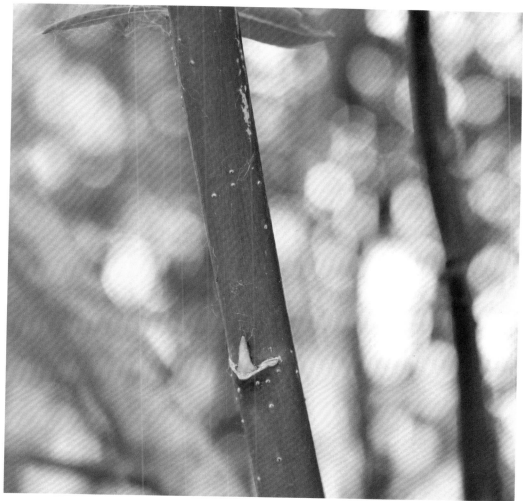

The young stems of willow are often green, yellow, red, or some combination thereof. Notice the leaf bud has but a single scale—a trait of all *Salix* species.

which has several scales). Willow bark ranges from smooth in most species to furrowed and split with age in such species as *Salix gooddingii*, black willow, and may be gray, yellow, green, or reddish brown.

Where, when, and how to wildcraft

With dozens of species, willows are among the more widespread plants in our region (with the exception of our driest desert habitats). Willows like waterways but may be found in wet meadows or on the margins of lakeshores, prairies, bogs, or wet lowlands. Gather the bark in the early spring or late autumn; see "Gathering Tree Medicine" (page 25) for details.

Medicinal uses

Most well known for its pain-relieving effects, willow can be used both internally and externally to this end. The tea of the bark, stems, and/or leaves can be applied for recent injuries, painful joints, skin eruptions, cuts, bites, stings, ulcerous wounds, bleeding hemorrhoids, sores, or eczema.

The leaf or bark tea is useful in relieving pain and irritation in various genitourinary conditions (enlarged prostate, kidney infections, UTIs) while also promoting urination. Use the tea as a gargle for sore throat and to allay fevers that are dangerously high or have been deemed to be too long in duration. The tea or tincture may quickly stimulate the appetite.

The tincture of the fresh willow flowers (aments) is considered a sexual sedative (reduces arousal) and allays irritation of the genitals. Some herbalists have also used this tincture to ease hormonal fluctuations in menopause.

Future harvests

In order to sustain our relationship with this tree medicine, gather with respect and gratitude, however abundant the stand.

 Caution

Avoid if you tend to experience low blood sugar.

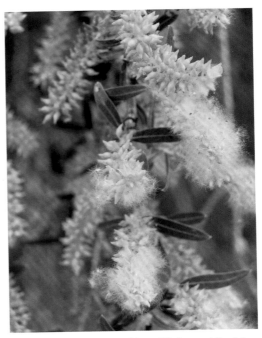

The maturing female catkins of *Salix gooddingii*, in mid-April in southern Arizona.

HERBAL PREPARATIONS

Bark/Leaf Tea
Standard Decoction (bark) or Standard Infusion (leaf)
Drink 2–4 ounces, up to 4 times per day; apply topically as a wash or fomentation, as needed.

Bark Tincture
1 part dry bark, by weight
5 parts menstruum (40% alcohol, 40% spring water, 20% glycerin)
Take 15–60 drops, as needed.

yarrow

Achillea millefolium
plumajillo
PARTS USED whole plant

This aromatic bitter tonic is both stimulating and relaxing, offering applications for nearly every body system. Yarrow is one of our most diverse remedies.

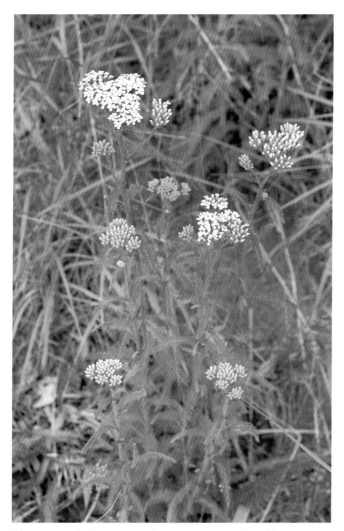

Along our region's eastern edge, yarrow flowers in mid-spring; in the western half, at the higher elevations it inhabits, it flowers from mid-summer to autumn.

How to identify

The finely dissected and divided leaves of this herbaceous perennial form feathery basal rosettes, which in spring may be no more than 1–3 inches tall. At various spots along its rhizomatous, aromatic root structure, it may push up a pubescent flower stalk, about 18 inches tall, with alternate leaves. An umbrella-like terminal cluster of broad, white (rarely pink) ray and disc flowers helps bring this inconspicuous plant into focus. The light brown rhizomes extend on their pink to white meristem growth and produce a tingly sensation on the tongue when tasted.

Where, when, and how to wildcraft

You'll find yarrow throughout the Southwest, save for mid- to low-elevation deserts in the west and the South Texas Plains; and it occurs only sparingly throughout the high plains. Look to meadows, roadsides, streamsides, and disturbed areas in our conifer forests, or alongside mesquite

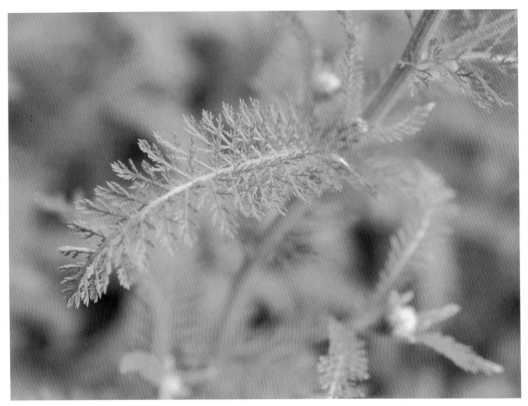

The feathery leaves of yarrow clearly distinguish it, even when the plant is not in flower.

and prickly pear in the Hill Country and continuing northward into the prairies and oak woodlands of Oklahoma. Begin noticing the plant in flower from late spring in Texas to mid-summer in high-elevation conifer forests. Cut back flowering stalks in larger stands, or clip basal leaves when flowering stalks aren't available. The rhizomes are best dug in early autumn but can be dug whenever the plant is identifiable.

Medicinal uses

Legion. Yarrow was perhaps the most widely used and variously applied herb of indigenous North Americans. The tea was given for headache, cold and flu, cough, sinus and chest congestion, and other respiratory complaints.

This aromatic bitter enables digestive secretions, improves appetite, and relieves pain and inflammation. It helps resolve a variety of bowel complaints, including diarrhea and constipation. Yarrow may be considered the superior remedy for any sort of bleeding, both internally and externally. Similarly, it's been applied for vaginal hemorrhaging (combine with rhatany) as well as delayed menses (combine with estafiate), in addition to being used during labor and postpartum to expel afterbirth and as an aid in healing the uterus. It's specific for uterine fibroids with bright red blood.

A hot infusion of the leaf and flower is decidedly diaphoretic, serving to break a fever whether due to cold or tension, and it provides cooling relief when drunk in a hot climate. Drinking a steaming cup of yarrow tea on a hot day is an intense experience but well worth the cooling aftereffects.

As a stimulating diuretic, yarrow is prized for its influences on the genitourinary system. It relieves gout (by helping clear uric acid) and inflammation in the urinary tract.

Topically, the fresh plant poultice, tea, or tincture can be applied to bleeding, infected wounds, swellings, burns, sores, bruises, or hematomas.

The roots serve a special role as a very effective toothache remedy. Simply chew on the fresh roots, or take a squirt of the fresh root tincture, and hold it on the affected area; this often brings swift relief. The root shares much of the leaf and flower's medicinal qualities, yet it is less bitter and more nutritious.

Future harvests

Gather only from large stands, and even then sparingly. Consider digging up root sections in the autumn to replant in new areas.

HERBAL PREPARATIONS

Herb Tea
Standard Infusion
Drink 2–4 ounces, up to 4 times per day.

Herb/Root Tincture
1 part fresh herb (or root), by weight
2 parts menstruum (95% alcohol),
   by volume
or
1 part dry herb, by weight
5 parts menstruum (50% alcohol,
   50% spring water), by volume
Take 10–40 drops, up to 4 times per day; apply the root tincture directly to teeth and gums.

yerba mansa

Anemopsis californica
bavisa
PARTS USED whole plant

*Look no further. No less an herbalist than Michael Moore called
yerba mansa "the most useful plant you will find."*

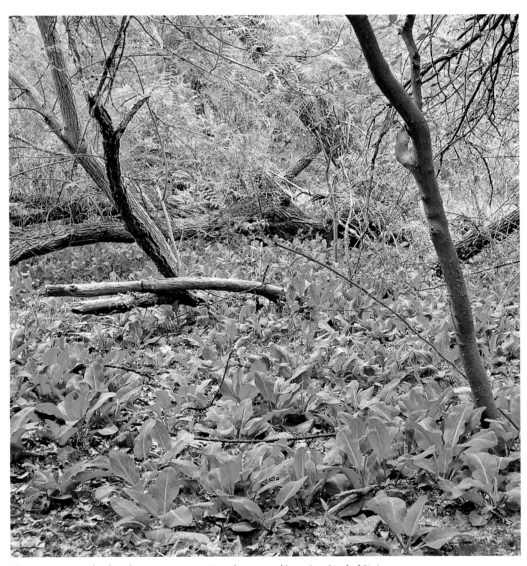

The spring growth of yerba mansa, carpeting the ground in a riparian habitat.

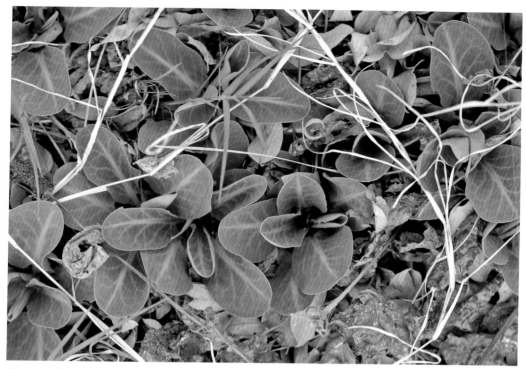
Clusters of basal leaves emerging in spring.

How to identify

This renowned herb colonizes marshy areas with its clusters of bright green, elliptical basal leaves with milky white venation throughout. Runners (sometimes over 10 feet long) may be sent out from the center of the basal rosette, seeking to root down from the nodes as they crawl along the earth. The long, rounded leaf stems, pinkish to dark red and often hairy, have a U-shaped groove where the leaf blade meets the stem. The solitary, terminal inflorescences are composed of bright white tepals (often pinkish on the outside) surrounding a conical spike of about 100 densely packed flowers, each with a tiny, rounded white bract at its base. The seedhead, along with the entire plant, turns brick-red in late autumn and emits the pungent aromatics of the plant when crushed.

Where, when, and how to wildcraft

Yerba mansa occurs predominantly in the western two-thirds of our region and is particularly fond of waterways, springs, and seeps. In areas of abundance, gather the whole plant in mid- to late spring, or the leaves throughout the summer. In areas of great density, digging up sections of root will reinvigorate the patch.

Medicinal uses

Michael Moore had it right. Beginning with the digestive tract, yerba mansa can be used for mouth sores, inflamed gums, abscesses, gingivitis, sore throat, esophageal and stomach ulcers, stomachache, diarrhea, dysentery, intestinal parasites, and hemorrhoids. The tea of the leaf, or whole plant, is a wonderful remedy for all the aforementioned. The tea relaxes the kidneys, is diuretic, and disinfects

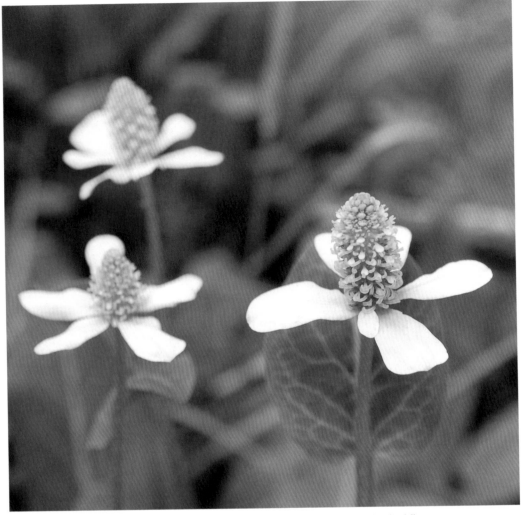

The conical inflorescences of yerba mansa are composed of around 100 individual flowers.

the urinary tract; it can be helpful to relieve edema or prostate pain.

Yerba mansa has a particular affinity for the sinuses. Chronic congestion, sinus infections, colds, allergies, viral or fungal infections—all are well addressed by this herb. It is mildly decongestant (combine with yerba santa and oshá) and drying to dampness within the lungs. One cannot go wrong with yerba mansa as an immune tonic during cold and flu season, during the acute stages

of inflammation, or during the cleanup phase after the infection has quieted down.

It is a mucous membrane tonic, helping to tonify the tissue when torpor sets in, while simultaneously relieving congestion and helping the body to move waste products through the lymph, enhancing the recovery process. As a fluid mover and a mild blood mover, yerba mansa is a valuable addition to formulas addressing a wide range of chronic infections.

Topically, the poultice, tea, or oil infusion can be applied to a variety of conditions: ulcers, boils, abscesses, wounds, fungal infections, or skin irritations, as well as arthritic or rheumatic joints. Also, take internally for arthritis.

Future harvests

As for so many of our Southwest plants, the future of yerba mansa depends largely on the longevity of our groundwater. Particularly in its drier desert habitats, yerba mansa often relies upon nearby deciduous trees to pull moisture from deeper down, bringing it up to the surface and out into the air. Safeguard our waterways, safeguard our trees.

HERBAL PREPARATIONS

Leaf Tea
Standard Infusion
Drink 4–8 ounces, as needed; apply topically, as needed.

Whole Plant Tincture
1 part fresh plant, by weight
2 parts menstruum (95% alcohol),
  by volume
or
1 part dry plant, by weight
5 parts menstruum (50% alcohol,
  50% spring water), by volume
Take 30–60 drops, up to 5 times per day; apply topically as a liniment to injuries and sore joints and muscles.

Oil Infusion
1 part dry leaf, by weight
5 parts extra virgin olive oil, by volume
Prepare as alcohol intermediate oil infusion (see page 38).

yerba santa

Eriodictyon angustifolium
mountain balm
PARTS USED leaf, stem, flower

*A warming remedy to open the lungs and clear phlegm, yerba santa restores
vitality during acute and chronic respiratory and genitourinary tract infections.*

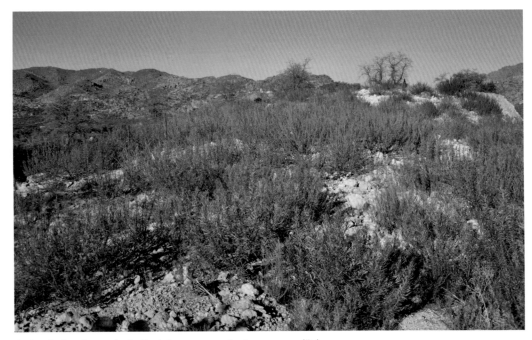

A stand of yerba santa, in the late summer of a "new normal" dry year.

How to identify

This woody, colony-forming shrub is normally
3–6 feet in height. Leaves are lance-shaped,
pointed, and toothed; they are sticky, shiny
green above, woolly white below. The bark of
the mature stem is light gray, and the young
stems are reddish brown to yellowish green.
Clusters of 5-lobed, somewhat crinkled white
flowers unfurl on slightly scorpioid stalks at
the branch tips. This plant may remain evergreen when not exposed to severe drought or
deep freezes.

Where, when, and how to wildcraft

Within our region, yerba santa occurs in
mid-elevation oak and piñon-juniper woodlands, chaparral, along trails, roadsides,
and other disturbed areas in well-drained
soils. This range corresponds to the area
running along the Mogollon Rim from the
eastern edge of Arizona heading northwest
to southern Nevada, southwestern Utah,
and the northern Mojave Desert in southern
California. Gather the young leaf and stem,
whenever present, by pruning branch tips.

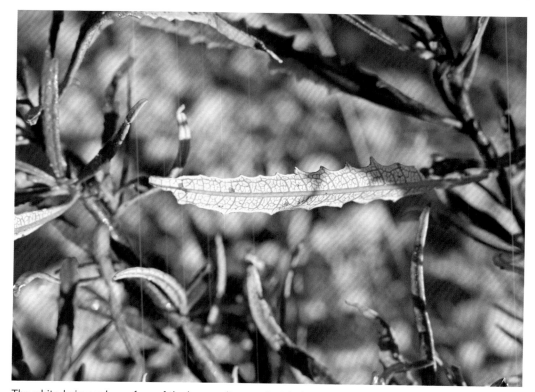

The white-hairy undersurface of the leaves aligns well with the first part of the genus name (*erion*, "woolly"); it is interspersed with a webbed network of raised yellow-green veins and midrib.

Flowering stems can also be gathered from abundant stands in the late spring. Dry for tea, or tincture the plant fresh.

Medicinal uses

Yerba santa is a warming, drying remedy with a sweet, pungent flavor. Having a particular affinity for the lungs, it is well suited to address cold, damp respiratory conditions, such as coughs, colds, flu, pneumonia, and smoker's cough. It will also aid in cases of hay fever, sinus congestion, sinusitis, bronchitis, asthma, and sore throat.

The leaf preparations (tea, tincture, poultice) are antimicrobial and can be used on skin sores and wounds, as well as eczema, poison ivy, insect bites and stings, sprains, and bruises. The tincture will curb UTIs and vaginitis and be helpful for hemorrhoids, leukorrhea, gas, bloating, and rheumatic joint pain.

The leaf is often used to improve the flavor of herbal formulas. Other useful preparations of yerba santa include oxymel, syrup, steam inhalation, smoke, smudge, or chew. As a low-dose remedy or flower essence, yerba santa enables us to hold true to our integrity despite adversity.

Future harvests

Yerba santa propagates freely via underground rhizomes. Gather modestly from established stands, and they should continue to produce for many years. Consider transplanting young suckers into your home landscape or to other suitable habitats.

Yerba Santa Oxymel

Combine the following dry herbs, by weight, and prepare as a vinegar decoction (see page 38); take 1 tablespoon in hot water, 2-6 times per day.

- 6 parts yerba santa leaf
- 3 parts spikenard root
- 3 parts pine inner bark
- 2 parts wild oregano leaf
- 1 part ginger
- ½ part anise seed or clove

Leaf Tea
Standard Infusion
Drink 2-4 ounces, up to 4 times per day.

Leaf Tincture
1 part fresh leaf, by weight
2 parts menstruum (95% alcohol),
  by volume
or
1 part dry leaf, by weight
5 parts menstruum (65% alcohol,
  35% spring water), by volume
Take 20-30 drops, up to 5 times per day.

⚠ Caution

Excessive use of yerba santa may induce nausea and vomiting. Follow the dosage guidelines to avoid potential problems.

yucca

Yucca species
palmilla, amole, Spanish dagger
PARTS USED leaf, root

A traditional remedy for arthritis, gout, and muscle aches, yucca can also be taken as a therapy for giardia and other protozoan infections.

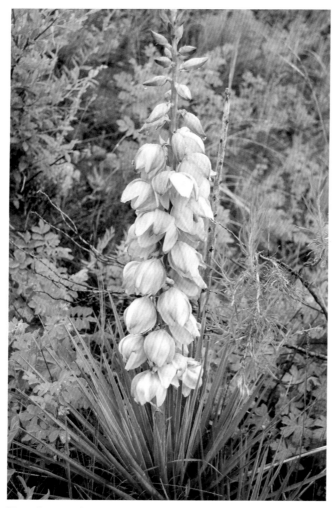

Yucca baccata, banana yucca, flowering mid-spring in the Sonoran desert.

How to identify

Yucca is most easily and clearly identified by its leaves, which always end in a sharp point. The leaves of *Agave* species, which are closely related, also end in a sharp point but most have toothed margins, whereas *Yucca* leaves do not. Yucca leaves appear as a U when cut in cross section and are generally stiff and straight (*Y. rupicola* produces twisted leaves). The margins of *Y. angustissima* and *Y. baccata* show frayed and curly white fibers. Leaf length (and width) varies by species, with some approaching 5 feet in length whereas others are only 8 inches long (and proportionately narrow). Flowers occur annually on long stalks emerging from the center of the leaf rosette (some species flower within the height of the leaves); the large-petaled blossoms are creamy white to pink, succulent to the touch, and usually hang down. The roots have white flesh and are covered in a thick brown bark.

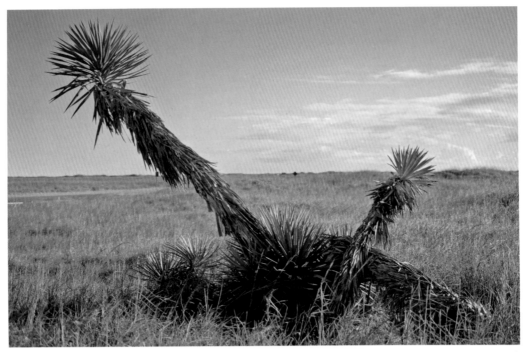

Yucca grows in a wide variety of Southwest habitats. Pictured here is *Yucca treculeana* on the Padre Island National Seashore.

Where, when, and how to wildcraft

Yucca is absent only from our lowest, driest deserts and high-elevation conifer forests. Leaves can be gathered any time of year, but roots are best gathered in late autumn or early spring before flowering. Gather the root from young plants or within large stands only. The long, creeping stems of some species can be included in root harvests.

Medicinal uses

The value of yucca to reduce musculoskeletal pain has been known by indigenous North Americans, and more recently within the folk medicine tradition, for centuries. It has been used for arthritis, gout, and general muscle aches and pains. Yucca should be considered an important therapy for those with chronic joint pain and concurrent inflammation of the digestive tract; infectious bacteria have been found in the joints of those with chronic gut inflammation, and research indicates that yucca's saponins can inhibit the growth of protozoa, distant relatives of bacteria, in the digestive tract. The root tincture or capsules are the best options for addressing this symptom picture. Be sure to include the root bark when tincturing or powdering for capsules, as the bark contains resveratrol, an important anti-inflammatory compound. The root tea is laxative at low doses but may relieve inflammation of the genitourinary tract.

The root was also used as a traditional remedy for snakebite, both topically and internally. A poultice or wash was traditionally used for sores and skin infections.

Saponins are also present in the leaf. The leaf, in addition to being used as an ingredient in emetic tea blends among indigenous peoples of the Southwest, inhibits the growth of *Giardia* as effectively as the antibiotic metronidazole. Ingest the powdered leaf, or a tea or tincture of the dry leaf.

Yucca is also used to lower cholesterol, LDL in particular; again, this action is attributed in large part to the presence of saponins. Consider the root capsules for this purpose.

The root is made into a shampoo and hair rinse by decoction. It is used ceremonially, but it is also known to stimulate growth, increase luster, and thicken the hair.

Future harvests

Gather seeds and sow them in spring, where appropriate.

 Caution

Yucca should not be ingested by those with iron-deficient anemia: the saponins it contains inhibit iron absorption. Consuming yucca may provoke nausea or promote intestinal distress; lower the dosage or discontinue therapy to resolve symptoms.

HERBAL PREPARATIONS

Root/Leaf Tea
Standard Decoction
Drink 2–4 ounces, up to 3 times per day.

Root/Leaf Tincture
1 part dry root or leaf, by weight (or combine the two in equal parts)
5 parts menstruum (50% alcohol, 50% spring water), by volume
Take 20–60 drops, up to 3 times per day.

Root/Leaf Capsules
Take 2–3 "00" capsules, morning and evening.

METRIC CONVERSIONS

INCHES	CENTIMETERS	FEET	METERS
¼	0.6	1	0.3
⅓	0.8	2	0.6
½	1.3	3	0.9
¾	1.9	4	1.2
1	2.5	5	1.5
2	5.1	6	1.8
3	7.6	7	2.1
4	10	8	2.4
5	13	9	2.7
6	15	10	3
7	18		
8	20		
9	23		
10	25		

TEMPERATURES

degrees Celsius = 0.55 × (degrees Fahrenheit − 32)

degrees Fahrenheit = (1.8 × degrees Celsius) + 32

TO CONVERT LENGTH:	MULTIPLY BY:
Yards to meters	0.9
Inches to centimeters	2.54
Inches to millimeters	25.4
Feet to centimeters	30.5

REFERENCES

Bigfoot, Peter. 2010. *Natural Remedies for Bites and Stings*. Reevis Mountain School of Self-Reliance.

Buhner, Stephen Harrod. 2002. *The Lost Language of Plants*. Chelsea Green.

―――. 2004. *The Secret Teachings of Plants*. Bear & Co.

―――. 2012. *Herbal Antibiotics*. 2d ed. Storey.

―――. 2014. *Plant Intelligence and the Imaginal Realm*. Bear & Co.

Cheatham, Scooter, et al. 1995–. *The Useful Wild Plants of Texas, the Southeastern and Southwestern United States, the Southern Plains, and Northern Mexico*. 4 vols. Useful Wild Plants, Inc.

Coffman, Sam. 2014. *The Herbal Medic*. Herbal Medics.

Curtin, L. S. M. 1997. *Healing Herbs of the Upper Rio Grande*. Rev. ed., Michael Moore, ed. Western Edge.

Easley, Thomas, and Steven Horne. 2016. *The Modern Herbal Dispensatory*. North Atlantic Books.

Epple, Anne Orth. 1997. *A Field Guide to the Plants of Arizona*. Falcon Guides.

Felger, Richard, and Mary Beck Moser. 1985. *People of the Desert and Sea*. University of Arizona Press.

Felter, Harvey Wickes. 1922. *The Eclectic Materia Medica, Pharmacology and Therapeutics*. John K. Scudder.

Foster, Steven, and Yue Chongxi. 1992. *Herbal Emissaries*. Healing Arts Press.

Frawley, David, and Vasant Lad. 1986. *The Yoga of Herbs*. Lotus Press.

Holmes, Peter. 2006. *The Energetics of Western Herbs*. 4th ed. Snow Lotus.

Kane, Charles W. 2011. *Medicinal Plants of the American Southwest*. Lincoln Town.

Kay, Margarita Artschwager. 1996. *Healing with Plants in the American and Mexican West*. University of Arizona Press.

Minnis, Paul, ed. 2010. *People and Plants in Ancient Western North America*. 2d ed. University of Arizona Press.

Moore, Michael. 1989. *Medicinal Plants of the Desert and Canyon West*. Museum of New Mexico Press.

―――. 1995. *Los Remedios*. Red Crane Books.

―――. 2003. *Medicinal Plants of the Mountain West*. Rev. ed. Museum of New Mexico Press.

Powell, A. Michael. 1987. *Trees and Shrubs of Trans-Pecos Texas*. Big Bend Natural History Association.

Slattery, John, and Maria Luiza Martinez. 2011. *Medicinal Plants of the Seri*. Unpublished.

Slattery, John. 2016. *Southwest Foraging*. Timber Press.

Tierra, Michael. 1992. *Planetary Herbology*. Lotus Press.

Verrier, James T. 2018. "Annotated Flora of the Santa Catalina Mountains, Pima and Pinal Counties, Southeastern Arizona." *Desert Plants*, vol. 33, no. 2. The University of Arizona for the Boyce Thompson Arboretum.

Wood, Matthew. 1997. *The Book of Herbal Wisdom*. North Atlantic Books.

Yetman, David, and Thomas R. Van Devender. 2002. *Mayo Ethnobotany*. University of California Press.

ONLINE REFERENCES

BMC Complementary and Alternative Medicine. Equisetum arvense (common horsetail) modulates the function of inflammatory immunocompetent cells. August 4, 2014. 14:283. https://www.ncbi.nlm.nih.gov/pubmed/25088216. Retrieved July 7, 2018.

Iranian Red Crescent Medical Journal. 2015, Mar. 31; 17(3). https://www.ncbi.nlm.nih.gov/pubmed/26019907. Retrieved July 7, 2018.

Journal of the International Association of Providers of AIDS Care. 2017 Jan/Feb; 16(1):11–13. https://www.ncbi.nlm.nih.gov/pubmed/27903949. Retrieved July 7, 2018.

Kindscher, Kelly. Echinacea Research. http://kindscher.faculty.ku.edu/research/medicinal-plants/echinacea. Retrieved July 25, 2018.

King's American Dispensatory, 1898, written by Harvey Wickes Felter, M.D., and John Uri Lloyd, Phr.M., Ph.D. henriettes-herb.com/eclectic/kings/index.html. Retrieved July 19, 2018.

Kress, Henriette. henriettes-herb.com. Retrieved April–September, 2018

Lady Bird Johnson Wildflower Center. wildflower.org/plants/. Retrieved January–September, 2018.

Native American Ethnobotany Database. naeb.brit.org. Retrieved January–September, 2018.

Natural Product Research. 2014 Vol. 28 No. 21. A new phenyl glycoside from the aerial parts of Equisetum hyemale. https://www.ncbi.nlm.nih.gov/pubmed/25117054. Retrieved July 7, 2018.

Phytotherapy Research. 2014, Apr; 28(4). In vitro inhibition of human CYP1A2, CYP2D6, and CYP3A4 by six herbs commonly used in pregnancy. https://www.ncbi.nlm.nih.gov/pubmed/23843424. Retrieved July 7, 2018.

SEINet. swbiodiversity.org/seinet/index.php. Retrieved January–November, 2018.

Texas Parks and Wildlife. Wildscapes: Plant Guidance by Ecoregion. tpwd.texas.gov/huntwild/wild/wildlife_diversity/wildscapes/ecoregions. Retrieved January–July, 2018.

The American Materia Medica, Therapeutics and Pharmacognosy, 1919, written by Finley Ellingwood, M.D.

The Pinecone Apothecary. Is Horsetail Dangerous? May 27, 2013. https://thepineconeapothecary.blogspot.com/2013/05/is-horsetail-dangerous.html. Retrieved July 7, 2018.

The Plant List. theplantlist.org. Retrieved January–November, 2018.

Tropicos.tropicos.org/Home.aspx. Retrieved January–July, 2018.

USDA Plants Database. plants.sc.egov.usda.gov. Retrieved January–November, 2018.

Vascular Plants of the Gila Wilderness. wnmu.edu/academic/nspages/gilaflora/scientific.html. Retrieved January–November, 2018.

Voyage Botanica. https://www.voyagebotanica.net/blogs/yerba-mansa-anemopsis-californica/the-lovely-graceful-powerful-anti-fungal-desert-willow-chilopsis-linearis-2. Retrieved on September 19, 2018.

Wikipedia. Chihuahuan desert. https://en.wikipedia.org/wiki/Chihuahuan_Desert. Retrieved July 8, 2018.

INDEX

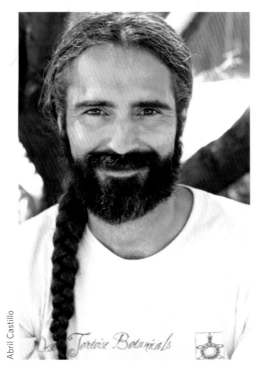

John Slattery is a bioregional herbalist, educator, and forager who is passionate about helping people develop deep and meaningful relationships with wild plants. His work has been influenced by indigenous healers throughout the Americas, herbalist Michael Moore, and, most importantly, the wild plants and places of the Sonoran desert. John is the founder of Desert Tortoise Botanicals (desertortoisebotanicals.com), a bioregional herbal products company in Tucson, Arizona; Desert Forager (desertforager.com), which specializes in prickly pear products; and the Sonoran Herbalist Apprenticeship Program, believing as he does that all education is ultimately experiential. His first book, *Southwest Foraging*, was released in 2016 by Timber Press. You can find out more about his work at johnjslattery.com.